CARDIAC DOPPLER DIAGNOSIS, VOLUME II

Previously published:

Cardiac Doppler Diagnosis Volume I, edited by M.P. Spencer. 1984.
ISBN 0-89838-591-1.

CARDIAC DOPPLER DIAGNOSIS, VOLUME II

edited by

MERRILL P. SPENCER, MD

Institute of Applied Physiology and Medicine
Seattle, WA 98122
USA

1986 **MARTINUS NIJHOFF PUBLISHERS**
a member of the KLUWER ACADEMIC PUBLISHERS GROUP
DORDRECHT / BOSTON / LANCASTER

Distributors

for the United States and Canada: Kluwer Academic Publishers, 190 Old Derby Street, Hingham, MA 02043, USA
for the UK and Ireland: Kluwer Academic Publishers, MTP Press Limited, Falcon House, Queen Square, Lancaster LA1 1RN, UK
for all other countries: Kluwer Academic Publishers Group, Distribution Center, P.O. Box 322, 3300 AH Dordrecht, The Netherlands

ISBN-13: 978-94-010-8383-6   e-ISBN-13: 978-94-009-4241-7
DOI: 10.1007/978-94-009-4241-7

Preface

My personal interest in cardiac Doppler arose from long experience in diagnosing carotid artery disease using Doppler continuous wave ultrasound with frequencey spectral analysis. The work of Dr. Liv Hatle of Trondheim, who was then using analogue tracings for cardiac Doppler, inspired me to try CW Doppler combined with spectral analysis and high-pass filtering techniques. The results with this system, without benefit of standard echocardiography were so productive that a special instrument was produced by Carolina Medical Electronics for worldwide marketing. Our experience led to the development of an international symposium and training program. These symposia gave birth to the International Cardiac Doppler Society and Volume I of this book series. This second volume on Cardiac Doppler Diagnosis is an outgrowth of the success of Volume I and the excellent work of many clinical scientists.

Doppler instrumentation continues to improve with integration of both continuous wave and pulsed wave Doppler with echocardiography. Color directional Doppler imaging techniques led by our Japanese colleagues is finding acceptance as a rapid screening method to find special regions of interest where more quantitative continuous wave with its quantitative capabilities of Doppler can be brought to bear.

I wish to thank the many fine authors of these two volumes for their excellent efforts and, again, Marian Wienker for her prodigious assistance. Acknowledgement is also given to my United States National Institutes of Health Grant #R01 HL19341 for my research in clinical applications of spectral analysis of CW Doppler signals which led to my chapters in both Volumes I and II of Cardiac Doppler Diagnosis.

MERRILL P. SPENCER, M.D., Editor

Contents

VIII

List of contributors

DANIELS, O., M.D., Pediatric Cardiology, St. Radboud Ziekenhuis Catholic University, NL 6500 Nijmegen, The Netherlands

DIEBOLD, B., M.D., Institut National de la Santé et de la Recherche Medicale – Unite INSERM 256, Hospital Broussais, 96 rue Didot, 75674 Paris, France

GARDIN, J.M., M.D., Cardiology Sections, Department of Medicine, University of California, Irvine Medical Center, Orange, CA, U.S.A.

IKWUEKE, M.R.C.P(UK), Senior Lecturer, Faculty of Medical Sciences, Department of Medicine, University of Jos, Private Mail Bag 2084, Jos, Nigeria

IWASE, M., M.D., 1st Department of Internal Medicine and Department of Thoracic Surgery, Nagoya University School of Medicine, 65 Tsurumai Showa-ku, Nagoya, Japan

KITABATAKE, A., M.D., Ph.D., The First Department of Medicine, Osaka University Medical School, 1-1-50 Fukushima, Fukushima-ku, Osaka 553, Japan

LIGHT, L.H., M.D., Bioengineering Division, Clinical Research Center, Watford Road, Harrow, Middlesex HA1 3UJ, England

NIMURA, Y., M.D., M.Sc., Director General, National Cardiovascular Center Research Institute, 5-125 Fujishiro-dai, Suita, Osaka 565, Japan

NOWICKI, A., Ph.D., Polska Akademia Nauk, Instytut Podstawowych Problemow Techniki, Swietokrzyska 21, 00-049 Warszawa, Poland

OMOTO, R., M.D., Professor of Surgery, Vice-Director, Saitama Medical School, Department of Surgery, 38 Morohongo, Moroyama, Iruma-Gun, Saitama, 350-04, Japan

REID, J.M., Ph.D., Biomedical Engineering and Science Institute, Drexel University, Philadelphia, PA

RITTER, S.B., M.D., F.A.A.P., F.A.C.C., Physician in Charge, Non-Invasive Cardiology, Michael Hazan Children's Heart Center, Department of Pediatrics and Pediatric Cardiology, The Brookdale Hospital Medical Center, Assistant Professor of Pediatric Cardiology, State University of New York-Downstate Medical Center, Brooklyn, NY, U.S.A.

SALMASI, A.M., M.D., Ph.D., Waller Cardiac Department, St. Mary's
Hospital, Praed Street, London W2, England

SHIMADA, H., M.D., The Kitasato Institute, 5-9-1 Shirokane, Minato-ku,
Tokyo 108, Japan

SKJAERPE, T., Ph.D., Regionsykehuset, Department of Medicine,
University of Trondheim, Postdqiro 5 873880, Trondheim 7000, Norway

SPENCER, M.P., M.D., Director, Institute of Applied Physiology and
Medicine, 701 16th Avenue, Seattle, WA 98122, U.S.A.

TAKAGI, S., M.D., 1st Department of Internal Medicine, Nagoya University
School of Medicine, 65 Tsurumai, Showa-ku, Nagoya, Japan

WEN, J.W., M.D., Department of Medicine, Division of Cardiology,
University of Virginia Medical Center, Charlottesville, VA, U.S.A.

WRANNE, B., Associate Professor of Clinical Physiology, Linkoping
University, Department of Clinical Physiology, Regionsjukhuset, S-581 85
Linkoping, Sweden

1. A history of echocardiography

JOHN M. REID

INTRODUCTION

This will be a rather personal narrative, based on recollected history backed by publications where possible. More details and illustrations are in a number of publications by the early workers [1, 2]. The chronological tables show the parallel time course of development in Europe, Japan and the United States.

During the initial, pre 1957, development of diagnostic ultrasound the heart seemed a very difficult target. The recording speed required was a formidable technical obstacle, and the question of access through lung was unanswered. Cardiac disease was, in fact, a difficult subject for all of medicine. The catheterization procedures that were available were of more interest to the physiologist than to the clinician since any surgical approach to the heart had formerly been impossible. It was a real surprize when the pioneering group in echocardiography published their first work outside of Scandanavia [3]. I was then working with Dr. John Wild, and finishing a masters' degree at the University of Minnesota, where the early experiments with circulation bypass through machines and with cross-circulation were about to make cardiac diagnosis of real clinical importance by allowing surgical therapy. Subsequent ultrasound developments thus took place amidst an upsurge in all types of medical imaging advances directed at cardiac disease.

The first observations of heart echoes were reported by Greenwood in 1949 at a Gordon Research Conference [4]. He used a gallstone locator produced by General Precision Laboratories after the early work of Ludwig and Struthers [5]. This was the first commercially available ultrasonic diagnostic equipment, although none were ever sold! He observed rapidly moving echoes when the transducer was placed over the anterior chest wall, presumably due to the heart.

SWEDEN AND EUROPE

The real history of pulse-echo cardiography began in the town of Lund, which was important enough to be visited by King Canute when he was king of England, Sweden, and Denmark. See Table 1 for the subsequent chronology. Doctor Inge Edler of the Hospital of the University of Lund expressed a desire to a young physicist, Hellmuth Hertz, to possibly use radar to investigate the motions of the heart. Dr. Hertz had knowledge of the first ultrasonic 'reflectoscope' that had been delivered to the shipyard in the nearby port city of Malmo and, after trying it out on his own heart, was able to persuade the Siemens Company to lend an insgtrument to the hospital for a year. This was a remarkable research effort since neither worker knew anything about the previous work in medical ultrasound [1].

Because the echoes from the heart moved back and forth very rapidly and could not be measured on the 'A' scope, a recorder was developed to record

Table 1. Time chart of beginnings of echocardiography.

	Europe	Japan	United States
1953.	Hertz & Edler, start		
1954.	Hertz & Edler, publish [6]		
1956.	Hertz & Edler, Acustica [3]		
1957.		Satomura, Doppler [8], Kikuchi et al., observation of echoes [9]	Reid & Joyner, start
1961.	Edler, valve ident [7]		
1963.	Ohlofssohn, scanner built [10]		Joyner & Reid, ceramics, verification [19], power measurement [17]
1965.		Oka et al., Esoph scans, heart stopped [11]	Feigenbaum, effusion [22]
1966.	Bleifeld & Effert tricuspid v. [21]	Tanaka, gated scans [12]	
1967.	Asberg, slow scans [13]	Nimura, tricuspid v.	Joyner & Reid, tricuspid v. [20], Flaherty, real-time scans [14]
1968.	Somer, phased array [15]		
1969.			Gramiak, contrast [25]

the position of the echoes from an intensity modulated cathode ray tube. This camera was apparently home built under the direction of Dr. Hertz. They thus invented the 'M' or motion, mode of echo display. The film moved at right angles to the intensity-modulated amplitude vs. distance display. Dr. Edler discovered that a very distinctive echo motion trace was obtained in cases of mitral stenosis and not at all in the case of mitral regurgitation [6].

Because of the limited sensitivity of the instrument, which used a quartz transducer designed for coupling into steel, no useful echoes were obtainable from most normal individuals. The clinical discovery, however, was of great utility, since the heart-lung machines were still experimental and patients with mitral stenosis could be subject to the much safer closed-chest commissurotomy.

A side effect of this effort was the aid given to Dr. Leksell of the Department of Neurosurgery in Lund, who was looking for a method to detect cerebral hemorrhage. Standard flaw detectors did not have enough sensitivity but he was successful with the Siemens instrument in Lund. This effort led to the discovery of the shift of the midline echo from the brain, a clinical determination which was, for many years, the mainstay of clinical centers in diagnostic ultrasound.

The first published report of the heart work was 1954 [6]. The publication which made this work known outside of Scandinavia was in the journal 'Acoustica' [3]. This paper reported the Siemens Company had developed a barium titanate transducer especially for Edler and Hertz which allowed them to record mitral valve motion curves from normal individuals and to detect the echoes from other heart structures and valves. They quickly identified cases of pericardial effusion, thrombosis, and myxoma of the left atrium.

This progress was made despite a fundamental problem in the misidentification of the anatomical structure which was responsible for what is now called the mitral valve echo. From physiological considerations it had been termed the echo from the 'anterior wall of the left atrium'. This was not cleared up until 1961 [7].

JAPAN AND SCANNING

The start of work in Japan must have preceded the publication, in 1957, of the first efforts of the two pioneering groups. Satomura, who worked with Nimura, published a report in English of the observation of Doppler-shifted reflections from the heart, indicating that not only wall motion but probably valve motions were observable [8].

Kikuchi et al. from Sendai reported only an observation of a rapidly moving cardiac echo [9], but this started a very significant effort in cardiac scanning that resulted, in 1966, in the first reported cross-sectional scan images of a beating human heart.

Scanning was begun first by the Swedish group who published their large ultrasonic mirror system in 1963 with a scan of a dead heart [10]. The Japanese group at Sendai started by building an esophageal scanner and imaged a living dog heart in 1965, but had to stop the heart briefly to make a scan [11]. (Joyner and Reid, Philadelphia, made some ECG gated scans on humans with a manual scanner that year but the poor quality and my imminent departure for Seattle caused us to shelve the effort.) Tanaka et al. [17], used ECG gating to accomplish their human imaging in 1966, just in time [12]!

The Swedish scanner was applied by Asberg et al. whose report appeared the following year [13]. At 6–7 frames per second it was faster than the other real-time machines that had been developed, such as the 'B' scanner built by Reid in Minneapolis. It was, however, neither the first or the fastest heart scanner up to that time, but it produced the best images. The first real time cardiac scanner was reported in 1967 by Flaherty et al. and it was even offered for sale by Magnaflux Corp [14]. This 16 frame per second scanner was built into a fluroscopy unit since the X-ray was believed essential for localization of the scan plane. The transducer was made very small and perhaps as a consequence had limited depth, being used primarily for detecting anterior effusion.

Scanning was clearly the way to go although good image quality would be elusive for many years. A hint of the future was given in Europe by Somer, whose 1968 paper proposed a full phased array, which seemed like a nearly unattainable goal with the technology available before [14]. The semiconductor revolution, however, was to change the world before long.

PERSONAL EFFORTS, AND THE UNITED STATES

The preceeding stories we know from the published histories. Reid's personal involvement began back in 1956 when he found a position which would allow him to pursue studies toward the Ph.D. degree at the University of Pennsylvania, while building an echocardiograph system at the University.

The first problem was to decide what to use for a transducer. This can best be seen in light of the development of medical ultrasound at that time. The Howry and Holmes group, in Colorado, had developed their own transducers using lithium sulphate, a high coupling coefficient but water-soluble

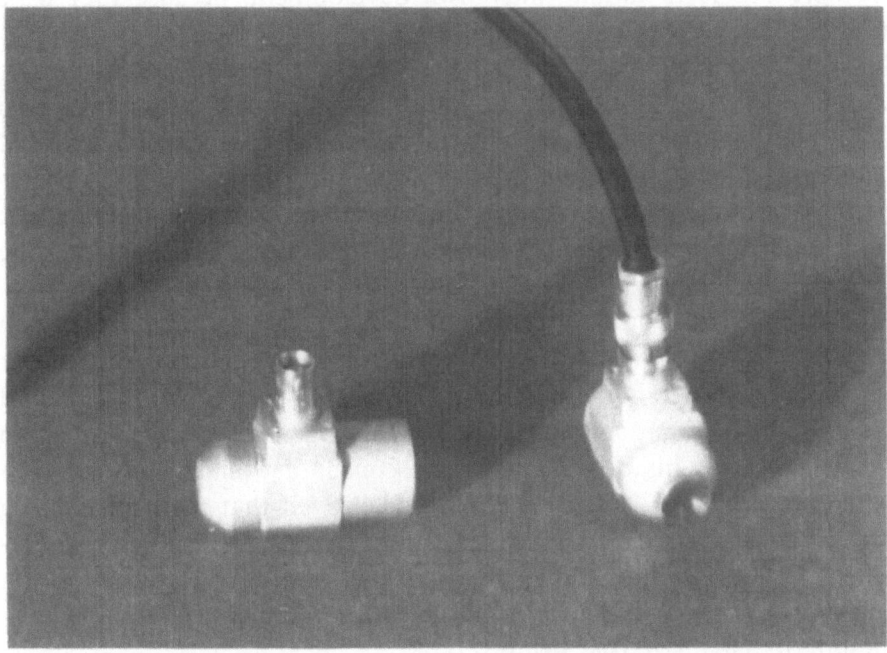

Figure 1. The first U.S. ceramic transducers for echocardiography. These used barium titanate ceramics with backing centrifuged in place in a lossy epoxy housing.

compound which could be grown in the needed single-crystal form only with considerable difficulty. The apparatus Reid constructed in Minneapolis used air-backed quartz crystals obtaining the necessary bandwidth through the use of a high (15 MHz) operating frequency. Although Siemens had produced a ceramic transducer, these were not known in the United States. On a trip to the Sperry Reflectoscope Company Reid was shown a report being completed for the Navy 'proving' that ceramic transducers could not be used for short pulses!

A lithium sulphate transducer was manufactured by the Curtiss-Wright Corporation, but it had high level echoes presumably from the walls of the housing, as well as uncomfortably sharp corners on the front. They declined to disclose or modify any of the technology they used; Reid commenced an investigation into methods of using ceramics and coupling them to the electronic apparatus. This work involved analysis of the equivalent circuit and the development of a design method to maximize transducer bandwidth, minimize radial mode voltages and maximize power transfer to the receiver. The transducers are shown in Figure 1. These methods were disseminated through scientific meetings, and a thesis published in microfilm which was widely distributed [16]. Industry apparently needed only the news that ceramics were usable to initiate their own development, because they have been available ever since.

The years from 1957 to 1963 were a rather low period for diagnostic ultrasound in the U.S. Only the midline echo technique was in widespread use. The National Institutes of Health approved a large grant for John Wild but later withdrew it when the sponsor dropped out, returning his equipment to Washington and putting it into a sub-basement storeroom. Dr. VonMicsky in New York had, perhaps, the only other active grant. The work in Philadelphia went maddeningly slowly for all of us.

The other technical difficulties of getting an operational echocardiograph in Philadelphia were overcome, and a wideband one and two megaHertz pulse echo system was built. A commercial moving film camera was found in the equipment storeroom and the apparatus was moved to the animal lab for initial testing. This difficult and time consuming phase was cut short with the news that Dr. Edler, in 1961, had proved that the echoes being recorded were actually generated by reflections from the mitral valves themselves [7]. All objections at this time as to the use of the equipment on humans were swept away and was installed in the catheterization laboratory, despite its large size (see Figure 2).

Although Reid was needed for the initial operation of the machine, the medical collaborators very quickly took over the actual patient examination. This was found to be somewhat of an anomaly in medical diagnosis. Dr. Joyner, took the records himself because this procedure was quite critical. Interpreting the mitral valve velocity, using the calibration marks placed on the film automatically, could be done with minimal training in a few minutes. This was an early indication of the importance of the clinical technologist.

In Pennsylvania further studies which were done on this early equipment included the first reported measurement of the power output of a diagnostic ultrasound system, measured through determining the radiation force on a suspended absorbing pad [17]. The radiation force measurement used a standard laboratory analytical balance which was modified by raising its center of gravity to compensate for the increased damping of the rubber target that was immersed in water. This was a rather delicate experiment conducted in the heat of the Philadelphia summer in a non-airconditioned storeroom. It was later felt it was necessary to cross-check our results by adapting Carstenson's self-reciprocity technique to calibrate the absolute sensitivity of our transducers as independent check [18].

The clinical results were good [19]. We identified the same echoes that had been seen by our European colleagues and added some examination features such as rocking the transducer to identify echoes from the tricuspid valve leaflets through their similarity to echoes from the mitral valve [20].

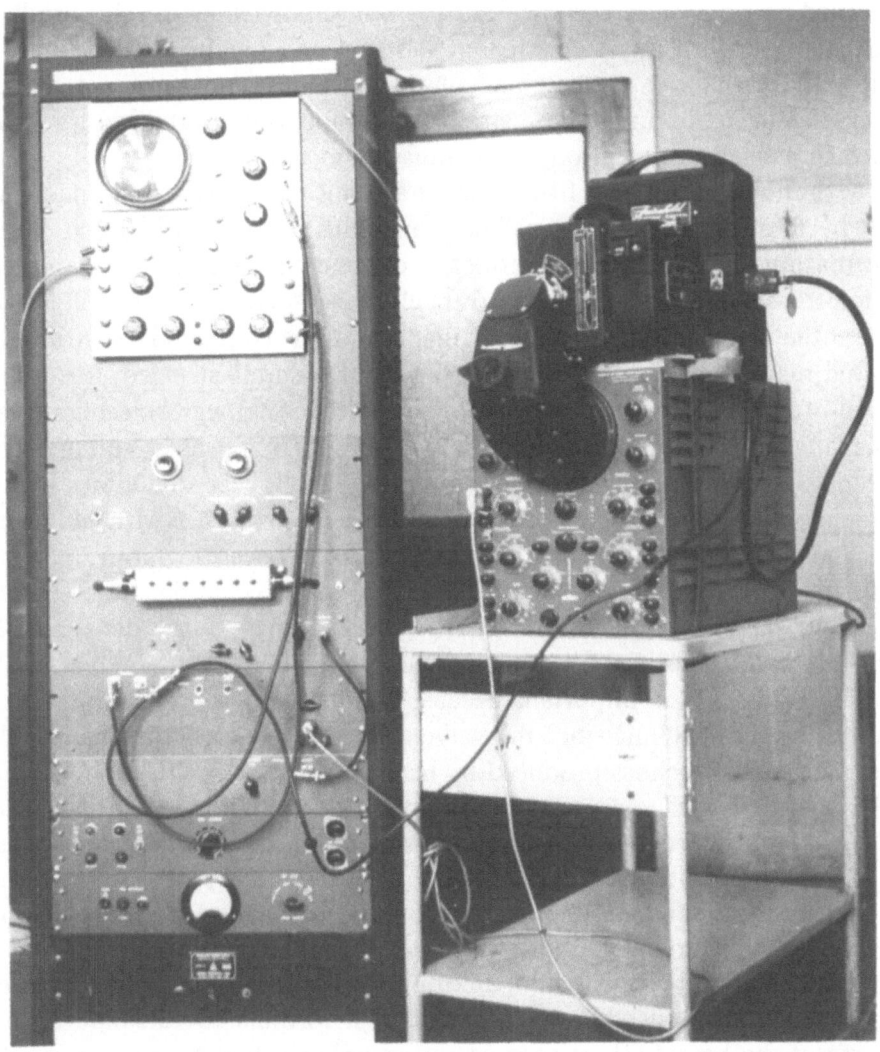

Figure 2. The research echocardiograph at the University of Pennsylvania, 1964. The M-mode moving film camera is on the right.

We did not know that Bleifeld and Effert had already reported such echoes (in German) [21], and that Nimura was to publish on them the same year! The final and best news, for the University of Washington was that Blue Cross had approved reimbursement for the echo examination.

Thus, the stage was set for the commercialization of these ideas into special purpose equipment. Up to that time all the other groups had been forced to use modified industrial flaw detection devices. In America commercialization proceeded through a parallel effort by the Sonomedic Corporation on one hand and Smith-Kline French Corporation on the other. The Sonomedic Corporation was the first to produce a machine in pilot production but, through a miscalculation of the gain and bandwidth required to deflect the cathode-ray tube, made modifications to my original design which resulted in an unusable instrument. Although this situation was corrected in a field modification, the company did not survive.

The Smith-Kline French firm adapted a small materials-testing machine, built by Branson, to the medical field and thus the Ekoline 20 was born. This machine is also an example of early commercial design using semiconductor transistors. The recording difficulty was solved by using Polaroid film, at the patient's expense. The availability of the commercial instrument allowed many clinicians to enter the field and progress speeded up.

One of the most vigorous early workers in this field was Feigenbaum at Indianapolis. He found the SKF machine was particularly suitable for detecting pericardial effusion, a determination that Joyner sometimes found extremely difficult to make [22]. Reid's heart is in contact with his chest wall and therefore, an excellent subject was for echocardiography. Testing these machines Reid brought about the realization that the signal processing in the two was quite different. A special effort was spent even after Reid left Philadelphia to assess the processing done by the Smith-Kline French Ekoline 20 [23]. This was important because Reid's original design was much easier to use in the clinic since the valve echoes were clearly distinguishable from all the other echoes produced by blocks of tissues, such as the septum and ventricular wall. As we finally discovered, the SKF machine used differentiation of the echoes to sharpen up the interfaces and by so doing lost the ability to separate the blocks of tissue from the blood spaces of the heart or at least to make this differentiation more difficult. One Japanese machine even had a switch and offered both direct and differentiated responses.

A contribution by Feigenbaum, an important factor in the rapid spread of echocardiography, was the development of a formula to calculate stroke volume of the heart [24]. It seemed rather unlikely that a simple formula based upon a single linear dimension which could not even be guaranteed to be perpendicular to the axis of the ventricle could be used to calculate volumes. The work was based, at least in part, in calculations of stroke volume using two dimensional data from contrast studies of the heart. Subsequently, with the survival of many individuals with scarred, nonmoving myocardium through the later development of bypass grafts, the population of sick individuals having strangely moving myocardial walls has increased. The calculations have thus passed from favor and have been supplanted in large part by dynamic assessment with real-time scanners.

To reach general medical acceptance, however, something more was needed to give clinicians full confidence in the technique. This was provided by the work of Gramiak. In 1969 Gramiak published the results of his studies using the echoes from rapidly injected fluids to identify the anatomical site of the different echoes received from the heart [25]. At one stroke he established not only the use of contrast material for echocardiography but was able to give a persuasive anatomical interpretation to all of the echoes seen in the standard views and in certain others which he described. Subsequently echocardiography was more widely accepted, and developed rapidly as a standard method of examining the heart. Contrast media consisting of gas bubbles produced by rapid injection of fluids (saline, blood, or X-ray contrast media) became routinely used, particularly to demonstrate flow jets and shunts inside the heart.

2-D SCANNERS

At this point, 1969, we leave the medical history and follow the technical history. The chronology of scanner development is given in Table 2. What was needed was a scanner capable of producing real-time cross-sectional pictures of quality comparable to those being obtained in other areas of medical ultrasound. Manually driven mechanical scanners were in wide use in ultrasound and motor driven models adaptable to heart imaging were coming [26]. There was clearly a clinical use for ultrasound sector scanners fast enough to image the heart even before these were available. This was

Table 2. Scanner development time chart.

	Europe	Japan	United States
1970.			Thurstone, phased array [27]
1972.			King, gated scans [28]
1973.	Bom, Multiscan [31] Somer, phased array [30]		Griffiths & Henry, mech. sector scanner [32]
1974.	Organon Technica, intro.		Von Ramm & Thurstone, phased array [35] Grummar, intro, phased array Barber et al., Duplex [34] Unirad, Cardio IX'er, gated
1975.			Hofferel, Picker, SKI exhibit mech. sector scanners, AHA mtg.

difficult because of the rapid speed of the heart. For example, Reid had made some efforts to develop a time-to-voltage convertor circuit for following the mitral valve while in Pennsylvania. It became apparent that the automatic tracking circuits used in World War II radar to follow airplanes were completely inadequate. The rate of change of range of a moving mitral valve, in wavelengths, is approached in the radar case only by a reentering ICBM!

By 1968 the efforts of Somer to produce a true phased array fast imager were well known through his progress was slowed by ever present funding problems [15]. A parallel effort with similar difficulties was undertaken by Thurstone and co-workers at Duke University [27]. Industry opted for a different approach. Scan lines collected, at a given time in the cardiac cycle, could be assembled from samples taken at different times in the following heartbeats to produce an image of the heart. Even irregular rates could be handled, but extra or anomalous beats could not. King, in New York, used this type of system [28]. By introducing the long axis scan he also freed future users from the imaginary restriction of having always to scan in planes parallel to the ribs. Gramiak and Waag also used the sampling approach [29].

The Unirad Corp. built this type of system, called the Cardio-IX'er, into the early analog grey scale scan-converter equipped instruments. It assembled nine images on the converter tube and replayed them back in rapid sequence to produce a pseudo 'motion picture' of the heart. These units did not sell too well since the majority of echo-cardiographers were satisfied with the 'M' mode display.

Electronic scanning was still proceeding. At the Rotterdam World Meeting in 1973 Somer reported an operating phased array system [30], and Bom introduced a linear scanner which stepped the sound beam along the length of an array, as proposed originally by Buschmann [31]. This latter system was introduced commercially into the U.S. the following year. It caused great excitement even though it was plagued by poor resolution and cross-plane directivity. Some heart structures were seen during a part of the cardiac cycle in planes where they were not supposed to be. The resulting confusion caused problems for the unwary clinician.

A small, simple, oscillating sector scanner was built by Griffiths and used by Henry which captured the attention of the field [32]. They showed that wall motion was well visualized, and that short-axis views could image the mitral orifice for direct observation of the valve area [26]. Industry saw the mechanical sector scanner as an economical way to get high-quality images. In rapid order Hofferel, Smith-Kline French, and Picker introduced these units (1975–1976) and seemingly every cardiologist, even the 'M' mode holdouts, converted to scanning!

Besides the myriad of oscillating sector scanners, there was a constant velocity sector scanner reported in 1969 by Tomey and myself[33]. This started life as a high resolution, real-time, compound scan system for peripheral blood vessels. It went through several changes in configuration, but most of the basic design was adopted by Barber as the basis for the duplex scanner commercialized with and without Doppler by Advanced Technology Laboratories[34]. This is currently a popular mechanical heart scanner.

Efforts were continued to bring the phased array to fruition. The most extensive effort in this country was that of Thurstone and his co-workers at Duke University. This culminated in the report in 1974 of a full scale phased array system which was shortly to be commercialized by Grumann[35]. The system was so obviously adaptable to high quality real-time cardiac images that other manufacturers eagerly brought out new versions. A lower cost version using microprocessor controlled switched delay lines was soon announced by Varian and after about the same time lag a version using three rows of transducers to improve the cross plane directivity problem was introduced at an even lower price by Toshiba.

The current state is one of competition between phased arrays and mechanical scanners. The mechanical scanners have good cross plane directivity and suffer less from stray signals because they have no switching signals and can concentrate on a single input stage of increased dynamic range. The phased arrays are improving quite rapidly. The adoption of large apertures with many elements, manufactured using modern semiconductor saws to yield small element spacings, combined with full scale dynamic focusing (an idea which was proposed by Sven Larson for some of the earlier scanner work done back in Minneapolis) and apodisation has yielded some truly outstanding results in linear phased-arrays for the abdomen. These ideas could possibly be applied to heart instruments for scans parallel to the ribs where sufficient aperture is available. The mechanical scanners may well disappear. Only the future will show which type will win out.

The engineers and clinicians who developed this field have shown the advantages of cooperation just as industry has shown the benefits of competition, in improving the human condition!

REFERENCES

1. Hertz CH: The interaction of physicians, physicists and industry in the development of echocradiography. Ultrasound in Medicine and Biology 1(1):3–11, 1983.
2. Edler I: Ultrasound cardiography. In: Fundamentals of medical ultrasonography. Gilbert Baurm (ed.), 1975.
3. Hertz CH, Elder I: Die registrierung von hertzwandbewegungen mit hilfe des ultraschall-impulsverfahrens. Acustica 6:361, 1956.

4. Kelly (-Fry) E (ed.): Ultrasonic energy, University of Illinois, Press, Urbana, p 300, 1965.
5. Ludwig GD, Struthers FW: Consideratins underlying the use of ultrasound to detect gall-stones and foreign bodies in tissue. Project No. NM 004 001, Report No. 4, U.S. Naval Medical Research Instit, Bethseda, MD.
6. Elder I, Hertz CH: The use of ultrasonic reflectoscope for the continuous recording of movements of heart walls, Kungl. Fysiogr sallsk, i Lund forhandl 24:5, 1954.
7. Edler I et al.: Ultrasoundcardiography. Part II. Mital and aortic valve movements recorded by an ultra-sonic echo-method. An experimental study. Acta Med Scand, Suppl 370:67–82, 1961.
8. Satomura S: Ultrasonic doppler method for the inspection of cardiac functins. J Acoust Soc Am 29(11):1181–1185, 1957.
9. Kikuchi Y et al.: Early cancer diagnosis through ultrasonics. J Acoust Soc Am 29(7):824, 1957.
10. Ohlofssohn S: An ultrasonic optical mirror system. Acoustica 13(5):361, 1963.
11. Oka S et al.: Ultrasono-tomography for the heart, great vessels and other mediastinal organs, Digest of the 6th Int'l Conf on Med Electronics and Biological Engineering, 294–295, 1965.
12. Tanaka M et al.: Ultrasonotomography of the heart and great vessels in living human subject, Medical Ultrasonics 4:47, 1966.
13. Asberg A, Hertz CH: Ultrasonic pictures of the human heart. Digest of the 7th Int'l Conf on Med and Biological Engineering, p 322, Stockholm, 1967.
14. Flaherty JJ et al.: Simultaneous fluoroscopic and rapid scan ultrasonic imaging. 7th Int'l Conf on Med and Biol Engineering, p 321, Stockholm, 1967.
15. Somer JC: Electronic sector-scanning for ultrasonic diagnosis. Digest of the 7th Int'l Conf on Medical and Biological Engineering, p 314, Stockholm, 1967.
16. Reid JM: Ultrasonic diagnostic methods in cardiology, Ph.D. Thesis, University of Pennsylvania, by University Microfilms, Ann Arbor, Michigan, Order No. 55–4683, 1965.
17. Reid JM, Joyner CR, Jr: The use of ultrasound to record the motion of heart structure. Ultrasonic energy-biological investigations and medical applicatins, Kelly E (ed.), 278–293, University of Illinois Press, Urbana, 1963.
18. Reid JM: Self-Reciprocity calibration of echo ranging transducers. J Acoust Soc of Am 55:862–868, April, 1974.
19. Joyner CR, Jr, Reid JM, Bond JP: Reflected ultrasound in the assessment of mitral valve disease, Circulation 27:503–511, 1963.
20. Joyner CR, Jr, Hey EB, Jr, Johnson J, Reid JM: Reflected ultrasound in the diagnosis of tricuspid stenosis, Am J of Cardiology 19:66–73, 1967.
21. Bleifeld W, Effert S: Uber das ultraschallkardiogramm der tricuspidalklappe, Ztschr Kreislaufforsch 55:154, 1966.
22. Feigenbaum H, Waldhausen JA, Hyde LP: Ultrasound diagnosis of pericardial effusion. JAMA 191:711, 1965.
23. Reid JM: An evaluation of intensity-modulated recording for ultrasonic diagnosis, J Acoust Soc Am 44:1319–1323, 1968.
24. Feigenbaum H, Zaky A, Nasser WK: Use of ultrasound to measure left ventricular stroke volume. Circulation 35:1092, 1967.
25. Gramiak R, Shak PM, Kramer DH: Ultrasound cardiography. Contrast studies in anatomy and function. Radiology 92:929, 1969.
26. Griffith JM, Henry WL: Electromechanical ultrasonic scanning for dynamic cardiac imaging. In: Cardiac Ultrasound, Gramiak R, Waag R (eds.), pp 228–238, 1975.
27. Thurstone FL, Melton HE, Jr: Transducers for pulse-echo ultrasound imaging. Proc 15th Ann Mtg, Amer Inst Ultr in Med., 1970.
28. King DL: Cardiac ultrasonography: a stop-action technique for imaging intra-cardiac ana

tomy. Radiology 103:387, 1972.

29. Gramiak R, Waag RC, Simon W: Cine ultrasound cardiography. Ultrasound in medicine & biology 1(1):59, 1973.

30. Somer JC: Electronic sector scanning in cerebral diagnosis: principle and technical development. Excerpta Medica No 277:7, 1973.

31. Bom N: A multi element system and its application to cardiology. Excerpta medica No 277:1–2, 1973.

32. Griffiths JM, Henry WL: A real time system for two-dimensional echocardiography. Proc of the 26th Annual Conf on Eng in Med and Biol, Minneapolis 15:422, 1973.

33. Tomey GG, Reid JM: Rotational compound scan, 8th Int'l. Conf on Medicine and Biological Engineering, Chicago, 1969.

34. Barber FE, Baker DW, Nation AW, Strandness DE, Reid JM: Ultrasonic duplex echo-doppler scanner. IEEE transactions on biomedical engineering BME-21: 109–113, March, 1974.

35. Von Ramm OT, Thurstone FL: Thaumascan: Design considerations and performance characteristics. Proc 19th Annual Conf of the American Inst of Ultrasound in Medicine, p 48.

2. Physics for ultrasonic diagnosis

MERRILL P. SPENCER and JOHN M. REID

INTRODUCTION

Ultrasound is a mechanical vibration which is basically no different than audible sound waves. The limits of human hearing ability are between 20 and 20,000 Hertz (cycles per second) but the upper limit decreases with age. Middle-C on the piano is a note caused by vibrations of the piano string 262 times per second (262 Hz). This frequency of vibration is usually called the fundamental carrier *frequency* on which some higher frequencies (harmonies) may be superimposed. Each octave, on the piano, represents a doubling of the fundamental frequency as we go up the scale and higher frequencies have a higher pitch. Sound waves having frequencies higher than the human hearing are called ultrasound. Frequencies which are 100 times higher than those of the human hearing range 2–10 million Hertz or megahertz (MHz) are the most commonly used frequencies in medical diagnosis. The concepts summarized in this chapter are discussed in more detail in many available textbooks [1–11].

BASIC PROPERTIES OF SOUND WAVES

Ultrasonic waves have a short wave length and travel with properties which we usually associate with light rays rather than with sound. That is, ultrasonic waves can be formed into narrow beams instead of spreading out in all directions. The wave length is a particular dimension of the wave which helps to define many of its properties. Figure 1 shows a vibrating surface at the left in contact with a compressible material represented by the rows of dots. These dots can be thought of as molecules in the tissues of the body. As the source vibrates, it moves back and forth from left to right, pushing against and pulling apart the molecules. Each push moves the com-

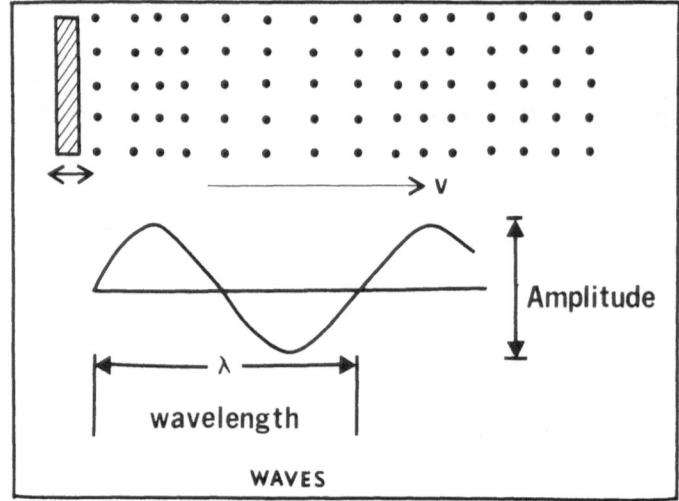

Figure 1. Definition of wave length. The wave length is the physical distance between corresponding points of a repetitive waveform. At the upper left a transducer face is shown alternately compressing and spreading out the molecules of the transmitting medium. The wave is propagated from left to right with velocity v.

SOUND WAVES

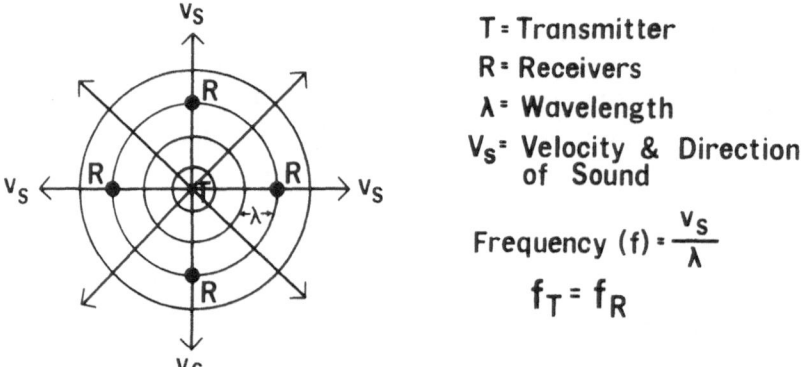

T = Transmitter
R = Receivers
λ = Wavelength
V_S = Velocity & Direction of Sound

Frequency $(f) = \dfrac{V_S}{\lambda}$

$f_T = f_R$

Figure 2. The relationship between a sound wave frequency, its velocity and wave length. When the transmitter source and the receivers are stationary with respect to one another the frequency detected at the receiver is the same as that at the transmitter.

pressed region to the right. This series of compressions is a *wave* and the distance between the compressed regions is the *wave length*. Figure 2 introduces a concept of an omnidirectional transmitter and multiple receivers or detectors. If an ultrasonic transmitter is radiating waves throughout the space around it and is stationary with respect to receiving detectors, the frequency detected at receiving points is exactly the same as that of the transmitter. The waves are moving at a relatively constant velocity in all directions. The wave length leaving the transmitter is equal to the wave length at any one of the receivers. We therefore have the mathematical relationship shown in Figure 2 between sound frequency, velocity, and the wave length. When ultrasound is formed into beams we find that the minimum width of the beam possible to attain is about one wavelength. Thus, a wave length is an important parameter in setting the resolution of any diagnostic system using soundwaves. To form such beams it is necessary to use such sources of sound which are large with respect to the wave length. The probes, which are applied to the skin, are therefore usually one centimeter or greater in diameter.

INTERACTION OF SOUND WAVES AND TISSUES

The primary characteristics that affect the propagation of ultrasound within the body are the speed of sound in tissue, the magnitude of the ultrasonic attenuation coefficient, and the density of the tissue. For most ultrasonic imaging and measurement systems the speed of sound within body tissues is assumed to be a constant. This is only approximately true, with variations of 5% from the mean value being common Goss et al. [12]. Of particular interest for calculations related to the Doppler effect, is the speed of sound in blood at a normal body temperature of 37 °C. The normal speed of sound in blood is reported to be from 1580 to 1585 m/sec with the speed of sound being slightly higher for males than females due to differences in percent hematocrit Kikuchi et al. [13] and Bakke et al. [4]. These figures are for 44 percent hematocrit for men and 41 percent for women. For patients with a low hematocrit, the velocity of sound will be less by approximately 1 m/sec for each percent hematocrit.

The density of tissue within the body is also one of the prime determinants of ultrasonic propagation within the body. The acoustic impedance, z is defined by the equation

$$z = \rho c \tag{1}$$

where ρ is the density and c is the speed of sound in tissue. Reflection of part of the ultrasonic wave occurs whenever the ultrasonic wave reaches a boundary where there is a change in acoustic impedance as defined above. Thus, either variations in the density of tissue or variations in the speed of sound within tissue, or both, can be responsible for the reflections which are the basis for ultrasonic B-Scan or sector scan images.

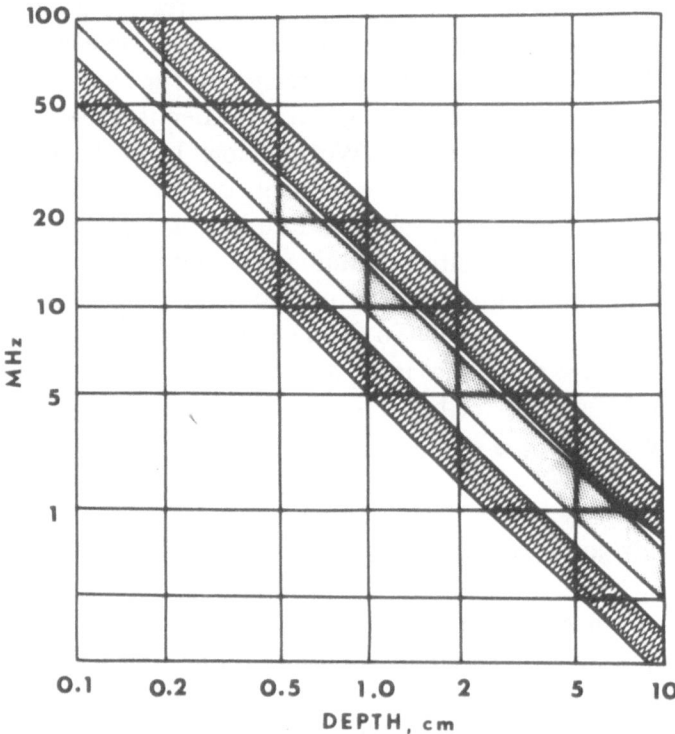

Figure 3. Chart of ultrasound frequency giving the maximum echo strength from small scatterers (red cells) theoretically determined for various depths of three intervening tissues.

As ultrasonic waves travel through the soft tissues of the body, they are absorbed, reflected or scattered. In most soft tissues, sound is absorbed to a degree which is proportional to the frequency. When travelling into the body by 1 cm and back again, the power in the sound wave is reduced by one-half for every megahertz of frequency. For example, at a frequency of 5 MHz sound waves travelling 1 cm into and out of the tissue will be reduced in power to 1/32 of their original energy. Lower frequencies are, therefore, used for deeper penetration into the body (Figure 3). Absorption figures in the body are about average for muscle; they are less for fat and considerably less for blood (about 1/10 of that for muscle). Absorption is caused primarily by conversion of sound energy into heat.

Ultrasound waves can be bent or refracted when passing into tissues transmitting sound with greater or lesser velocity. The velocity in fat, for example, is approximately 10% lower than that of other tissues. The bending effect can be calculated from Snell's Law of Optics.

Scattering is a major process by which ultrasound radiation is deflected.

THE DOPPLER EFFECT

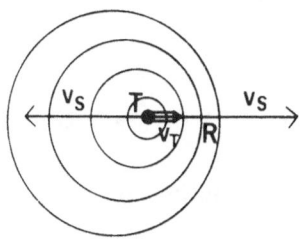

T = Moving Transmitter
R = Stationary Receiver
V_T = Velocity of Transmitter
V_S = Velocity of Sound
f_T = Frequency of T
f_R = Frequency at R

$$\frac{V_T}{V_S} = \frac{f_R - f_T}{f_T}$$

Figure 4. Principle of the Doppler effect produced when a transmitter (T) is moving toward a stationary received (R). When the Doppler shift ($f_R - f_T$) is measured and the frequency of the transmitter as well as the velocity of sound in the medium are known the velocity of the transmitter can be calculated.

The scattering of ultrasound is a much more pronounced and useful effect. The reflections which are sent back towards the examining ultrasonic probe from tissues in the body are used by a variety of medical ultrasonic diagnostic instruments.

THE DOPPLER EFFECT

Scattering particularly results from erythrocytes or groups of erythrocytes in the blood because their diameter is small compared to the wave length of the ultrasound. The wavelength of a 5 MHz ultrasound is 308 micra while the diameter of a red cell is between 7–8 micra. The scattered ultrasound is re-radiated in all directions. The scattering red cells vibrate at the same frequency as the incident wave. They may, therefore, be considered a multitude of small transmitters which are moving with the blood velocity. Since the velocity of sound in blood is constant (1560 m/s), the moving wave length in front of the transmitter as the ultrasound is radiated, is shortened and behind the direction of movement, the wave length is lengthened. A remote receiver will detect a frequency different from the frequency of the transmitter which difference is called the *Doppler effect,* Figure 4. The ratio between the velocity of the transmitter and the velocity of sound is equal to the ratio of the difference frequency and ultrasonic frequency of the transmitter. The Doppler effect is a common everyday observation, when the sound of a moving vehicle such as an automobile or train appears to emit frequencies greater when coming towards the observer than when moving away from the observer. The angle between the line of motion and the

THE REMOTE TRANSMITTER
Doppler Effect vs Scattering Direction

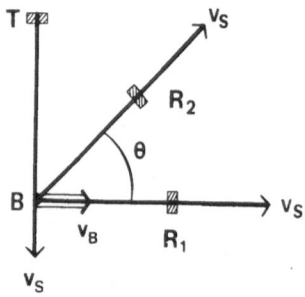

T = Transmitter ; R_1 & R_2 = Receivers

B = Moving Scatterer

V_S = Velocity & Direction of Sound

V_B = Velocity & Direction of B

θ = Angle Between V_B & BR

$$\Delta f = \frac{f_T \cdot V_B}{V_S} \cos \theta$$

Figure 5. A remote transmitter is used to produce scattering from a moving particle. The resultant Doppler frequency is dependent upon the angle between the direction of the moving particle and the direction between the particle and the receiver.

Ultrasound Probe Frequency (MHz)	\(\frac{KHz}{m/s}\) \(\frac{m/s}{KHz}\)					
	Angle of Sound Beam (Deg)					
	0	10	20	30	45	6 0
2	2.56 / 0.39	2.53 / 0.40	2.41 / 0.42	2.22 / 0.45	1.81 / 0.55	1.28 / 0.78
2.25	2.88 / 0.35	2.84 / 0.35	2.71 / 0.37	2.5 / 0.40	2.04 / 0.49	1.44 / 0.69
2.50	3.21 / 0 .31	3.16 / 0.32	3.01 / 0.33	2.78 / 0.36	2.27 / 0.44	1.6 / 0.62
3	3.85 / 0.26	3.79 / 0.26	3.61 / 0.28	3.33 / 0.30	2.72 / 0.37	1.92 / 0.52
3.5	4.49 / 0.22	4.42 / 0.23	4.22 / 0.24	3.89 / 0.26	3.17 / 0.32	2.24 / 0.45
5	6.41 / 0.16	6.31 / 0.16	6.02 / 0.17	5.55 / 0.18	4.53 / 0.22	3.21 / 0.31
6	7.69 / 0.13	7.58 / 0.13	7.23 / 0.14	6.66 / 0.15	5.44 / 0.18	3.85 / 0.26
7.5	9.62 / 0.10	9.47 / 0.11	9.04 / 0.11	8.33 / 0.12	6.8 / 0.15	4.81 / 0.21
10	12.82 / 0.08	12.63 / 0.08	12.05 / 0.08	11.10 / 0.09	9.07 / 0.11	6.41 / 0.16
COS	1	0.98	0.94	0.87	.71	.5

$$f_D = \frac{v \cdot f_u \; .2 \cos \emptyset}{c}$$

f_D = Doppler-shifted frequency (Hz)
v = Velocity of blood (m/s)
u = Ultrasonic frequency (Hz)

$\emptyset$ = angle between soundbeam and flow direction
c = velocity of sound in blood (1560 m/s)

THE DOPPLER TRANSDUCER

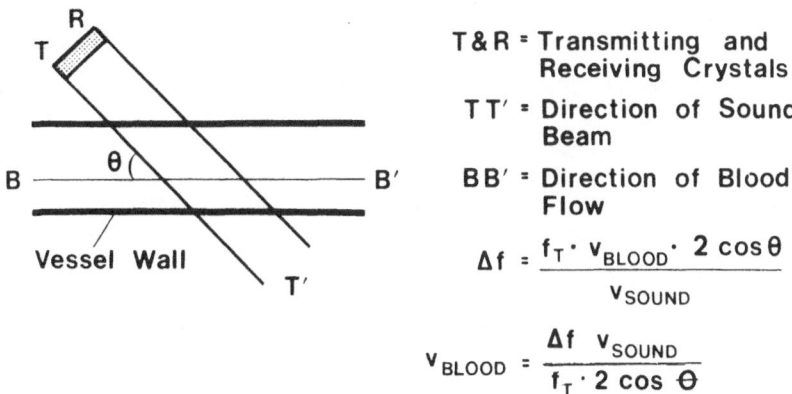

T & R = Transmitting and Receiving Crystals

T T' = Direction of Sound Beam

B B' = Direction of Blood Flow

$$\Delta f = \frac{f_T \cdot v_{BLOOD} \cdot 2 \cos \theta}{v_{SOUND}}$$

$$v_{BLOOD} = \frac{\Delta f \; v_{SOUND}}{f_T \cdot 2 \cos \theta}$$

Figure 6. The Doppler equation when both transmitter and receiver are at the same position in space remote from the moving scatterers. The effect of the angle between the direction of the scatterer and the direction of the sound is doubled i.e. $2 \cos \theta$.

observer has an effect on the Doppler shift, Figure 5. The difference frequency (f) varies in direct proportion to the cosine of the angle between the direction of the moving particle and the direction of the receiver.

In a practical medical Doppler probe, the transmitter and receiver are incorporated side-by-side. This means that the angle between the transmitter beam and the receiver direction to and from moving blood cells is the same and, therefore, doubling the Doppler effect for any angle, Figure 6. To make the calculations in the Doppler equation, the frequency units should be in Hz and the velocity units in m/sec. Table 1 provides a convenient reference for several frequently used ultrasonic probe frequencies for various probe angles. It should be particularly noted that the frequencies evoked by the Doppler shift are directly proportional to the ultrasonic frequency; for example, a pitch provided by a 10 MHz flow meter is twice that produced by a 5 MHz flowmeter. The fortunate result of using ultrasound for blood velocity detection is that the Doppler shift frequency falls within the range of human hearing. Simply listening to the Doppler frequencies and using the discriminating abilities of the human ear and brain is a useful technique when interpreting many dynamic features of the blood flow in the arteries, veins, and heart. If the velocity is very high, as is often found in jets through constricting stenoses or valve regurgitations, the resulting pitch of the Doppler shift may be too high for some persons to hear. Spectral analyzers which provide a visual display of the frequencies and amplitudes continuously with time, are therefore convenient for observation while listening to

PARABOLIC PROFILE & DOPPLER SPECTRUM

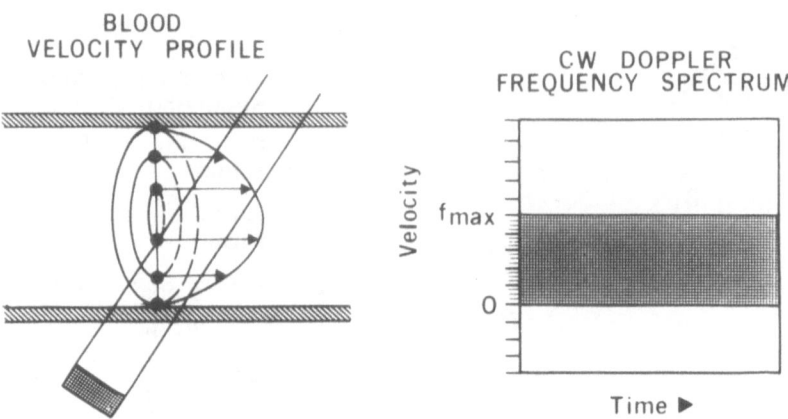

Figure 7. Relationship between the blood velocity profile and the Doppler frequency spectrum produced by a continuous wave ultrasound beam covering the entire cross section of a blood vessel. In the case of a parabolic laminar velocity profile of blood velocities, the resultant Doppler frequencies and energies are equally distributed across the frequency spectrum.

document the results of the examination and to teach the principles of Doppler ultrasound diagnosis.

FREQUENCY SPECTRAL ANALYSIS

Figure 7 illustrates the idea of representing the distribution of blood velocities flow streams by a corresponding distribution of frequencies on a display of a Doppler frequency spectrum. This type of translation of velocity to frequency is most often provided by the FFT spectral analyzer. This display is derived from the concept of the Fourier series. It has been shown, mathematically, that any complex frequency such as any sound heard by the ear, can be described by a set of fundamental sinusoidal waveforms each with a specified amplitude and frequency of some multiple of the fundamental or lowest frequency of the sound wave (Figure 8). The Fast-Fourier transform provides a very practical updating of the frequencies as they occur (generally every 10 m/sec). Each 10 m/sec sample interval is first adjusted so that the beginning and ending of samples do not produce artificial frequencies (Figure 9). Each sample can then be treated as a separate Fourier series and displayed every 10 m/sec to provide an apparently continuous frequency analysis. This whole process may be thought of as passing the original sound wave in the form of an electrical signal through a set of band-pass filters and displaying the range the filters represent in terms of

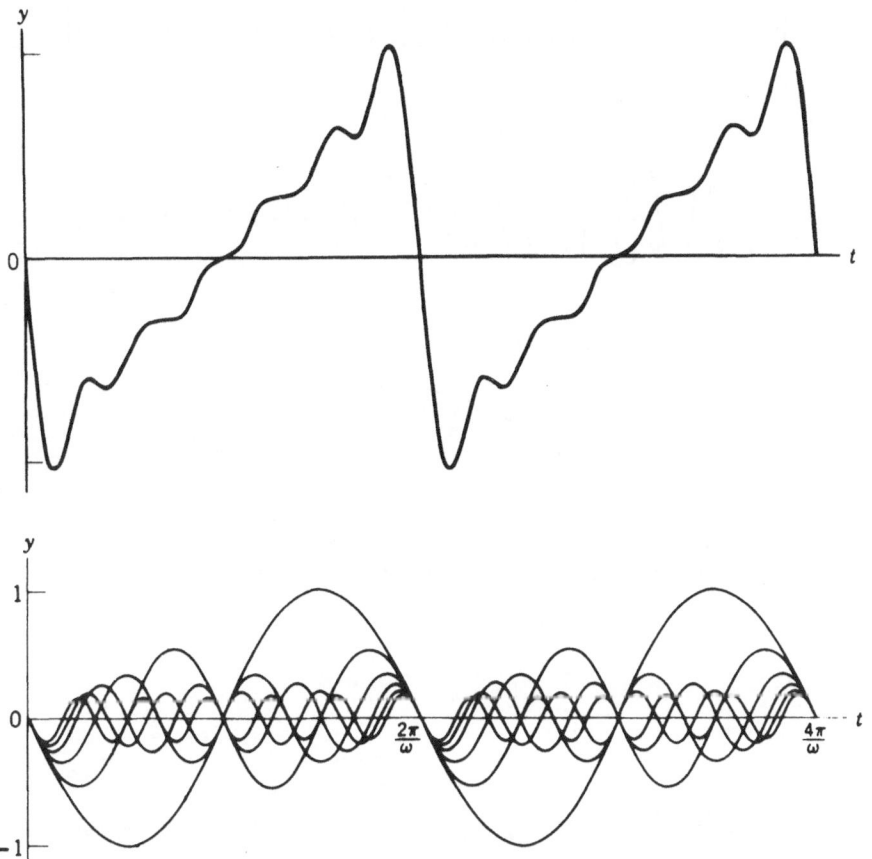

Figure 8. The basis for frequency spectral analysis in the Fourier series. Any arbitrary waveform such as in the upper section of the figure can be represented by a series of sinusoidal waveforms of varying frequency and amplitude shown in the lower section of the figure.

frequency on a vertical scale, while the amplitude of each frequency is represented as the density or brightness of each line representing the individual frequency sampled. This continuously running display can then be spread out on a time base as shown.

Since the continuous wave Doppler sound beam can pass through a broad region of blood velocities in the heart or a blood vessel without focussing in depth it provides a representation of many hemodynamic phenomena occurring within the beam. When, therefore, the CW transducer is placed against the chest wall and directed at the heart, a rather confusing set of repetitive sounds are heard and displayed on the frequency spectrum display. Without filtering the spectrum is dominated by enormous low frequency energies which override the more subtle high frequencies present. These unwanted low frequency energies are conveniently removed by means

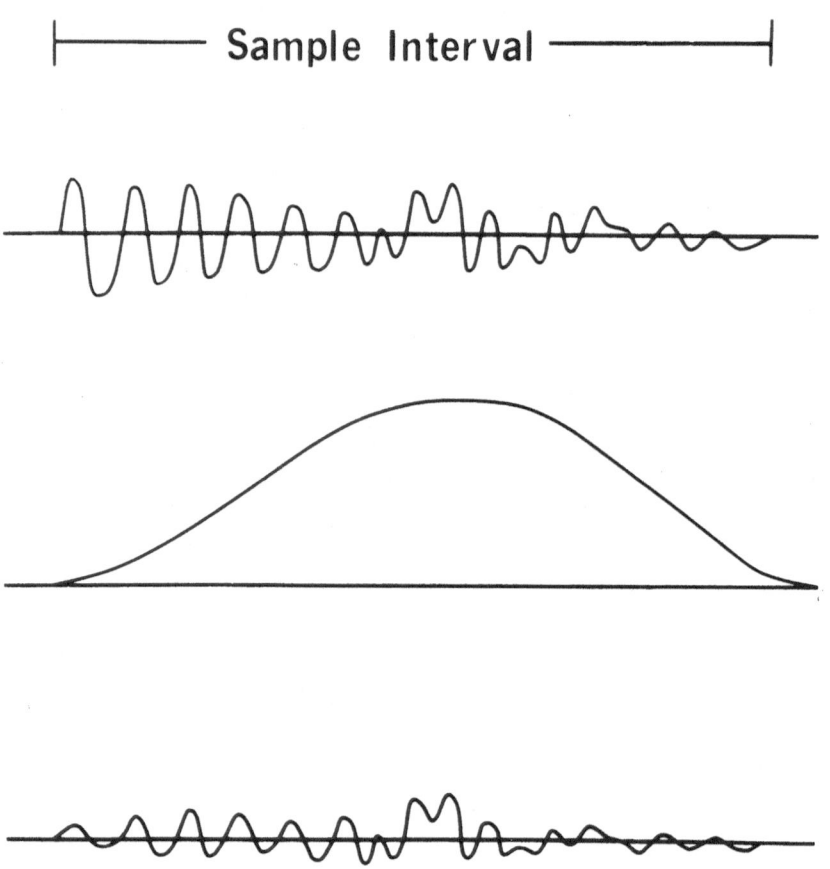

Figure 9. Diagram of how Fourier analysis can be applied to a short pulse of sound wave shown in the upper section. The middle section illustrates the amplication function applied over the sample interval. The lower section illustrates how the amplication function eliminates the discontinuities at the beginning and ending of the sample interval.

of a high-pass filter which eliminates most of the frequency energies below 1 kHz. Figure 10A and 10B. These high energies are produced by reflections from the moving cardiac walls and valve structures while we are actually more interested in the more subtle frequencies representing the blood flow streams within the cardiac chambers. Another application of filter processing of the spectrum is that of using a high-pass filter or a 'high boost' to accentuate the high frequency, low amplitude components of the spectrum.

THE ULTRASOUND TRANSDUCER

The 'heart' of a transducer is a material which will change its dimensions when an electric field is applied to it or which will generate an electrical

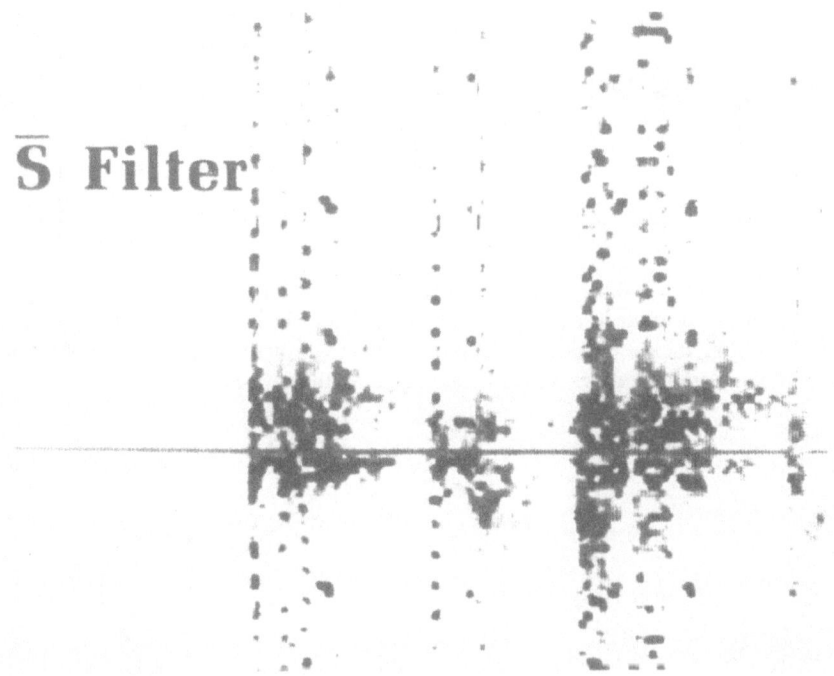

S̄ Filter

Figure 10A. Continuous wave Doppler generated frequencies from a probe held over the normal mitral valve.

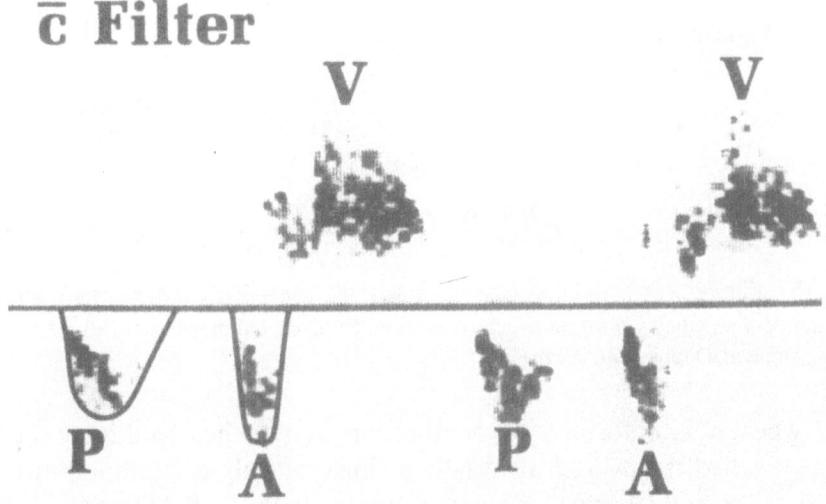

c̄ Filter

Figure 10B. Application of a high-pass filter eliminates the high energy low frequencies present in '10A' and with further amplification the more meaningful velocity signals emerge. 'P' represents the passive inflow velocities upon opening of the mitral valve. '10A' represents the Doppler frequencies generated by atrial contraction. Both P & A represent velocities moving towards the transducer. 'V' equals the velocities moving away from the transducer in the ventricular outflow track.

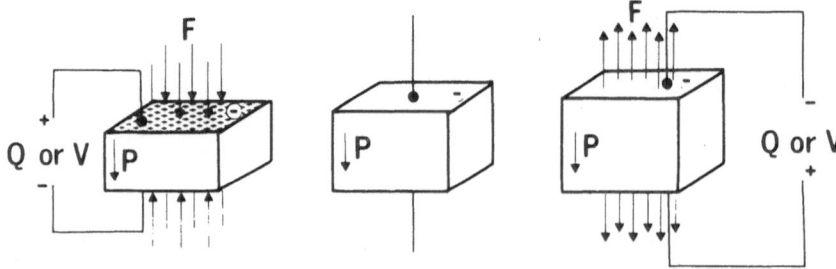

Figure 11. In the center is illustrated a biased ceramic material with electrodes on opposing faces. On the left application of a voltage results in a change in thickness. On the right application of a reversing voltage polarity produces an opposite change in thickness. Application of pressure on the material produces an electrical charge on the surfaces.

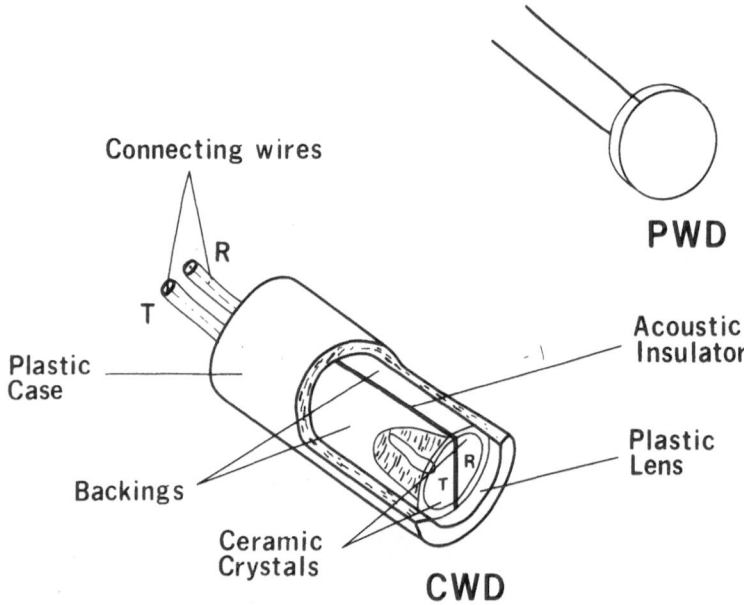

Figure 12. Cut-away view of ultrasound transducer. Two elements are shown for CWD operation but both may be used for pulse echo operation. PWD crystal may be substituted for a more efficient pulsed Doppler operation.

field when it is deformed by a vibration as sketched in Figure 11. This element called the *crystal,* is usually a single or poly-crystalline material in which the crystal structure is aligned suitably with the field produced by the electrodes and to the surfaces of the material. Practically all medical transducers use a poly-crystalline ceramic which has the property of being electrostrictive; that is, it will change its shape in response to an electrical field. These ceramics are a poly-crystalline, lead zirconate titanate. The components of the transducer (Figure 12), including the ceramic are placed in a

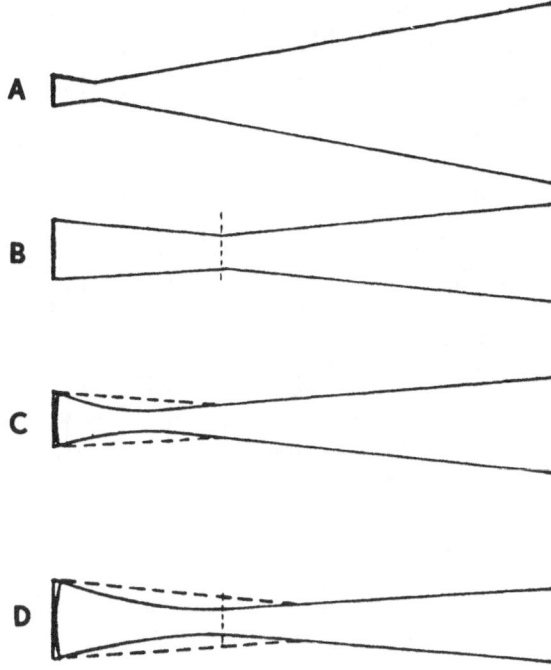

Figure 13. Outline of approximate field shape for focussed and unfocussed transducers. A: small unfocussed transducer, B: larger unfocussed transducer, C: transducer with focussing. The sound field can be narrowed only in the near field region. D: large transducer with focussing producing a smaller field at a greater range.

protective case with suitable lead wires connecting it and the crystals to the electronic apparatus. Generally, a backing material is used for isolation to provide greater strength and to wider the bandwidth of the transducer. Various means of focussing may be built into the continuous wave transducer.

The most sensitive frequency, for operation of a ultrasound transducer is the fundamental resonant frequency inherent in the ceramic crystal element. The frequency at which the electronics operate the transducer, is usually adjusted to coincide with the resonant frequency of the transducer.

FOCUSSING

The natural focussing of an ultrasonic transducer may be illustrated in Figure 13A and B. Three major points are illustrated:

1) The near field, close to the face of the transducer is approximately the shape of the crystal itself but narrows down towards a focal zone. The far field, at greater ranges, diverges as shown in Figure 8.

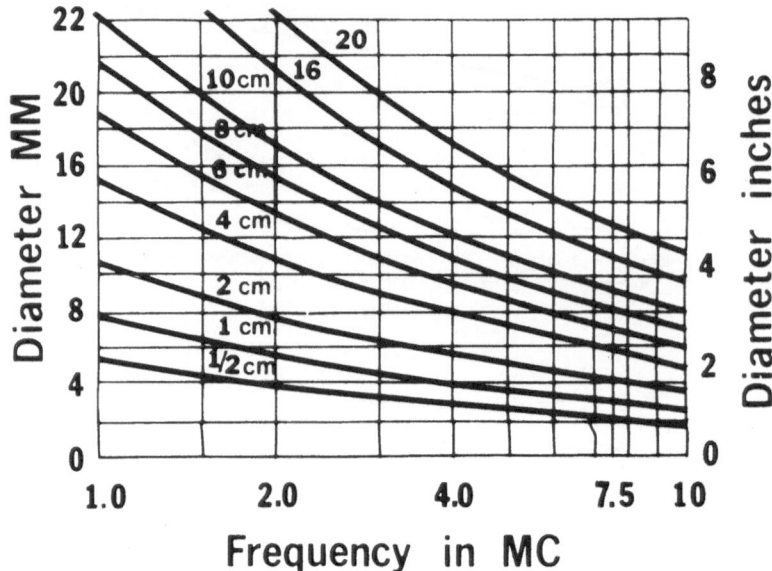

Figure 14. Chart of near-field extent as a function of transducer diameter and ultrasound frequency. Curves are numbered according to the near-field length.

2) The minimum field occurs at the focal zone where the near field changes to the far field and is approximately equal to the radius of the transducer. This narrowest focal point of the beam is found by dividing the square of the radius by the wave length (Figure 14).

3) In the near field, the width of the beam is directly proportional to the size of the transducer, while in the far field the width is inversely proportional to the size of the diameter of the transducer. The longer the diameter focuses more sharply than the narrow diameter. In addition, the focal zone represents a region of sensitivity where the transmitted beam and the projected reveiving 'beam' maximally overlap.

Figure 12 also illustrates how additional focus to the sound beam can be provided by means of the lens placed over the transducer or using a spherical-shaped crystal element. The lens, as provided, is generally in a concave shape because the velocity of sound in the lens material is higher than that of the coupling jel and body tissues. It is interesting to note that with light using glass lenses in air, a spherical lens is necessary for focussing because speed of light in the optical lenses is lower than the velocity in air.

The photographs of the actual focused acoustic fields are shown in Figure 15 were taken with a Schlieren optical system, which makes the sound waves visible. For very strong focussing, the field is concentrated with a short focal zone, while for deeply focused transducers the focal zone is longer.

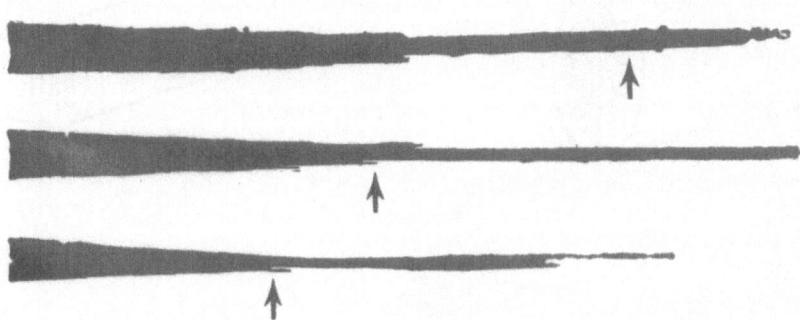

Figure 15. Schliren photograph of an actual sound field shapes for three different lenses applied to the same diameter transducer. Arrows mark focal length.

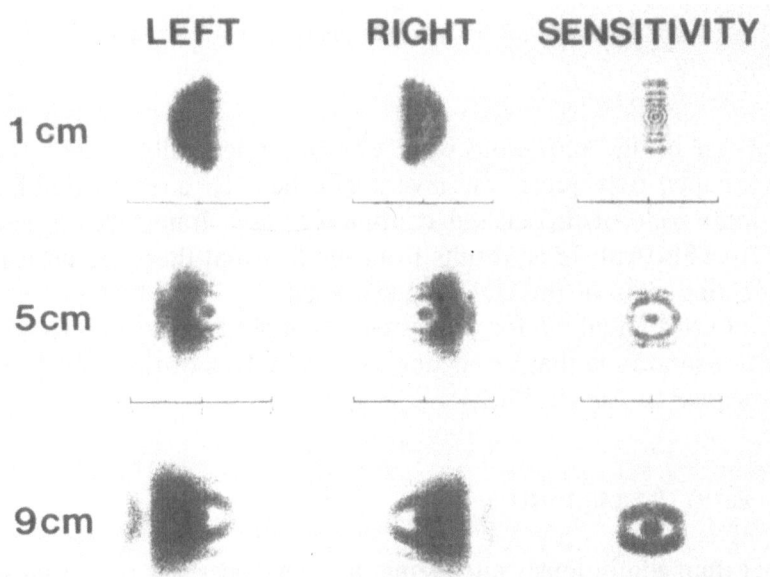

Figure 16. Ultrasonic beam field profiles of a continuous wave Doppler transducer. Individual fields of the left and right 'D' shaped crystals are shown individually at 1, 5, and 9 cm. The right hand column represents the combined sensitivity produced by the overlap of transmit and receive fields.

CW DOPPLER TRANSDUCERS

The face of the transducer containing the elements of a *continuous wave transducer* are shown in Figure 12.

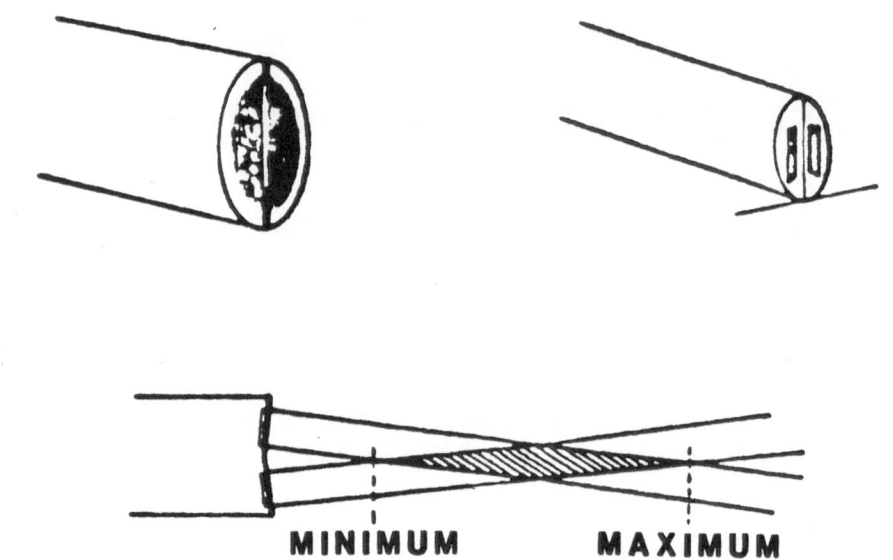

Figure 17. Method for focussing CW transducer by tilting the transmit and receive crystals to the desired focal zone.

In the case of the continuous wave transducer generally made by splitting the disc-shaped transducer, we have a so-called 'D' shaped sound field.

The focal zone of a focussed continuous wave transducer is shown in Figure 16. This oval shape results from the fact that there are basically two principle diameters of the 'D' shaped crystal.

An additional method for focussing available to continuous wave 'D' shaped transducers is that of angling the two halves of the transducers in a fashion shown in Figure 17.

PULSED ECHO ULTRASOUND

Rather than continuously energizing the transducer, a series of pulses may be applied by repeatedly switching the electrical energy to the transducer off and on in a pulse train. Generally, the duration of the pulse is considerably shorter than the interval between pulses, Figure 18. The pulse repetition rate (PRF) represents the rate at which the pulses are applied, generally, around 1–2 kHz. The internal content of the pulse is an ultrasonic frequency itself of only a few oscillations. During the interval between pulses, when the transmitter is turned off, the crystal serves as a receiver and the receiving amplifiers are 'listening'. If the pulse is travelling through the tissues at a rate of approximately 1500 m/sec, an echo from considerable depth may be received before the next pulse is sent. By listening at any interval at a specific

Ultrasonic Pulse Train

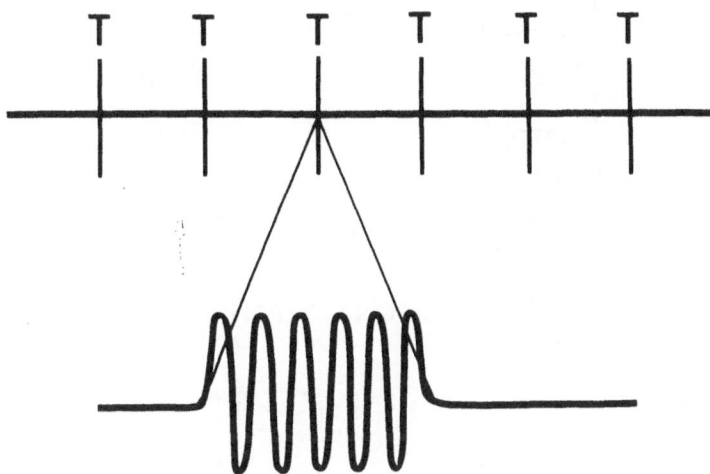

Figure 18. Diagram of an ultrasonic pulse train from typical transmitter. Below is an expansion of an individual pulse showing the sinusoidal ultrasonic waveform content.

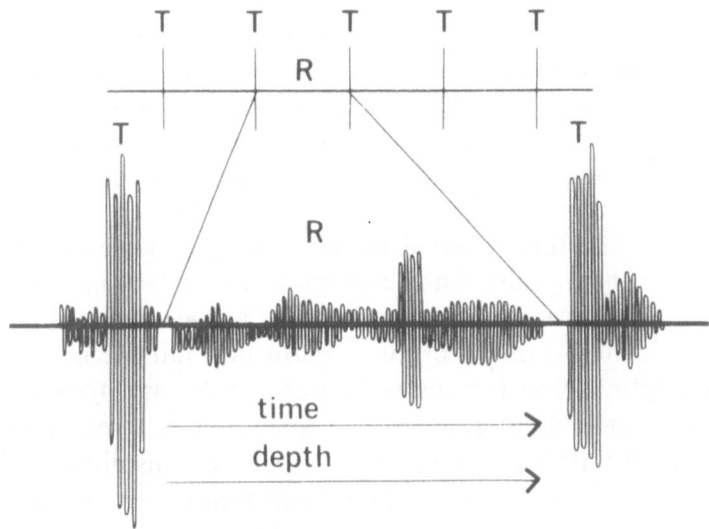

A· Mode Ultrasound

Figure 19. Upper section: transmitted pulse train. Lower section: amplified received signal of ultrasonic echos between repeated pulses. The amplitude of the received signal is modulated according to the reflectivity of tissue interfaces. Time between pulses is calibrated in depth of tissue.

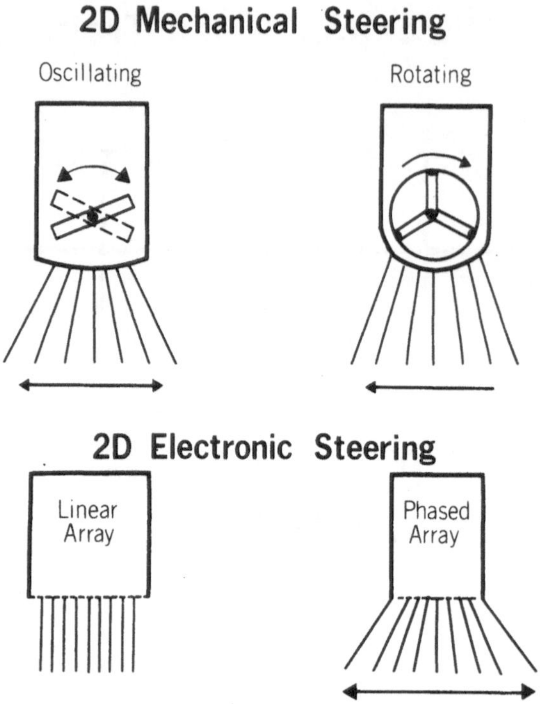

2D Mechanical Steering

Oscillating   Rotating

2D Electronic Steering

Linear
Array

Phased
Array

Figure 20. Methods of producing two-dimensional imaging.

interval of time after each pulse, the reflections from a specific section of tissue can be examined. There is a limit to the depth in the tissues from which echoes can be detected before another pulse is transmitted. For deeper structures longer intervals between pulses must be used. This principle of echo ranging was developed for sonar and radar using sound and radio waves. In echocardiography the echo display is termed the 'A' mode display, Figure 19. The time interval on the display is proportional to the distance between the transducer and each successive reflecting structure producing amplitudes. Because sound waves travel at such a high speed in soft tissues (approximately 1 mile/sec), they return in a rather short time. The time which elapses between transmission of a pulse and reception of an echo, from a structure 1 cm away, is 13.3 millionths of a second (microseconds). This short time interval also means that the transmitting pulse cannot last very long or it would occupy several centimeters in space. Pulse lengths of the order of microseconds occupy distances in space in the order of millimeters.

Since one 'A' mode display is repeated for each pulse there are e.g. 2000 displays per second. This enormous data rate can be used to produce a two-dimensional image by use of 2-D transducers. Various means of sweeping the sound beam back and forth while the beam is spread over a 2-D

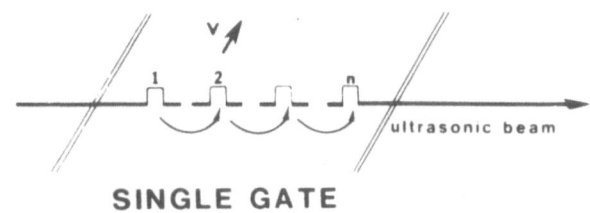

SINGLE GATE

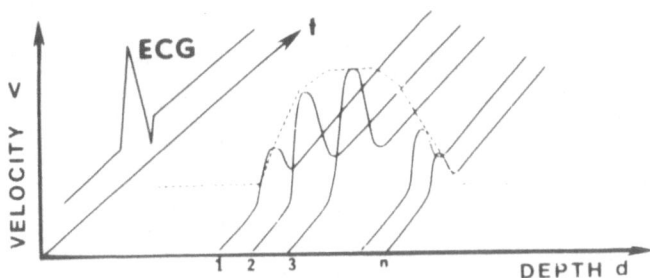

Figure 21. Method of using a movable single gait pulsed Doppler to interrogate velocity profiles.

space the amplitudes of the A-mode are used on a graded gray scale to produce an image of structures both static and moving. Figure 20 Two-dimensional echocardiography is an example of this use. The resolution of the image is dependent on the shortness of the pulse but is generally higher along the line of the sound beam because focussing in depth is better by means of short pulses than is allowed by the attainable width of the sound beam.

PULSED DOPPLER

Pulsed wave Doppler (PWD) utilizes a special amplifier which listens for short gated intervals of time. The listening gate can be moved throughout the interval between pulses to provide by 'range gating' a method of focussing in depth for the Doppler shifted signal. Figure 21. The Doppler shift occurs only during each pulse because the ultrasound frequency is present only within the pulse. The depth of focus is determined by the duration of the original pulse and the duration of the range gate in the amplifier. While a short pulse and a short range gate provides the smallest sample volume, a larger sample volume may be often helpful in finding the signal of interest. The effect of the pulse wave Doppler on the frequency spectrum is shown in

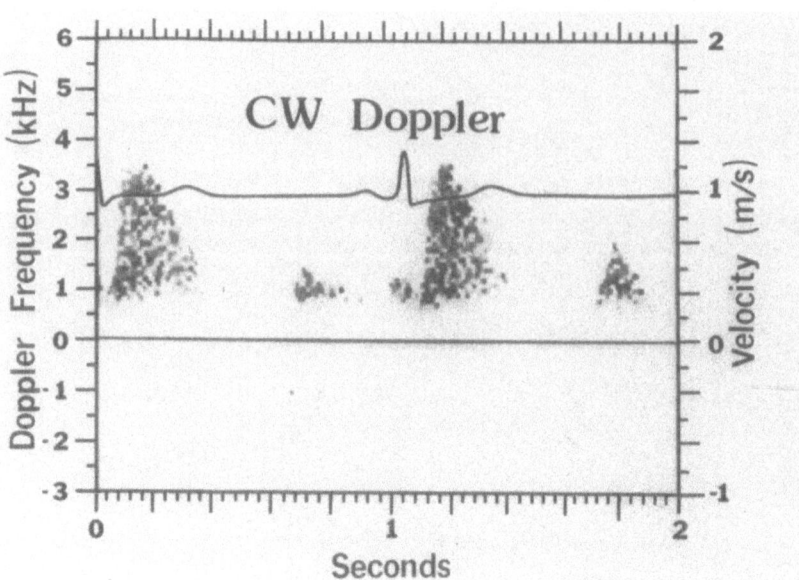

Figure 22A. Continuous wave Doppler spectrum of normal aortic ejection velocities through the aortic valve. Hihg pass filtering eliminates the low frequency interferences.

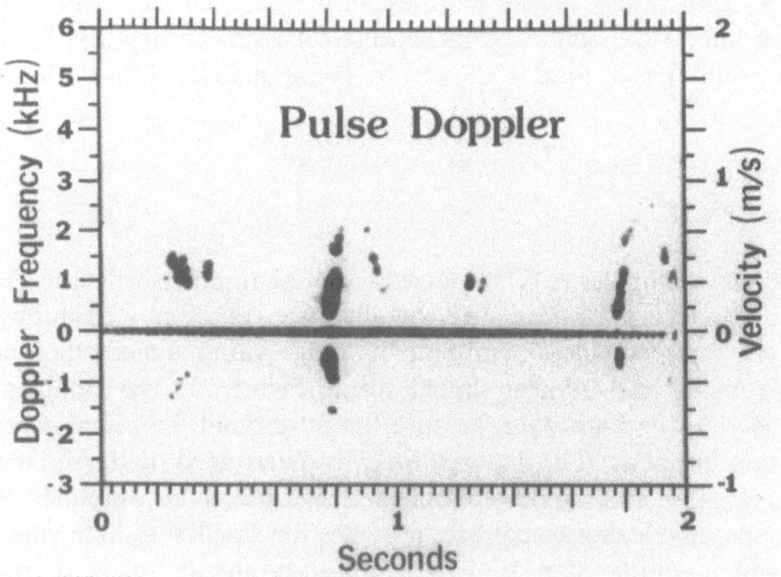

Figure 22B. Pulsed Doppler spectrum of the same aortic ejection velocities.

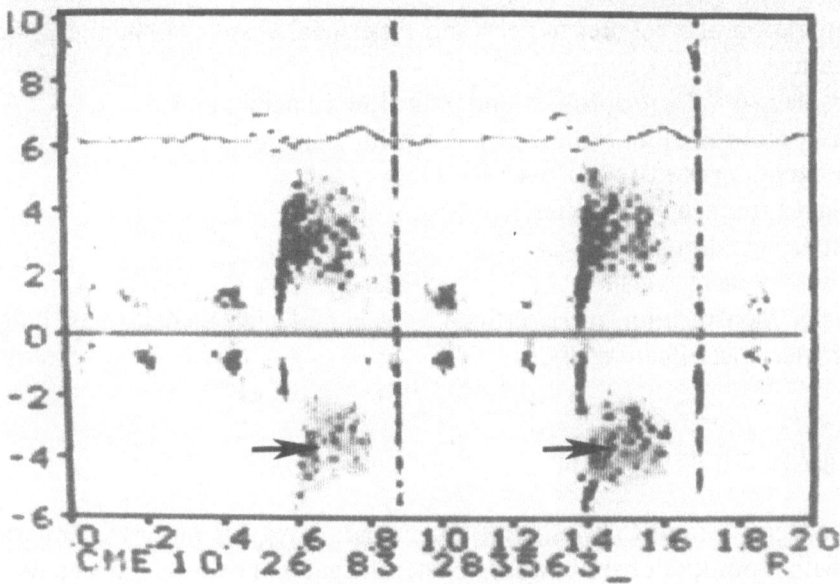

Figure 23. Effect of aliasing on the pulsed Doppler frequency spectrum in the presence of high velocities produced by aortic valve stenosis. Upward directed velocity spectrum is amputated at 6 kKz and is displaced below the zero line.

Figure 22. Here, when only a small portion of the blood flow streams are sampled, only the narrow band of frequencies representing the range of velocities within the sample volume, are represented.

ALIASING

While PWD is very good at focussing in depth it suffers difficulty in resolving blood velocities which are greater than one half the PRF. This produces frequencies in a false range. A familiar example of this is seen when making a movie of a turning wheel with spokes. The wheel appears to move slowly and backwards when the movie frame repetition rate is less than the 'spoke rate'. Figure 23 illustrates the limitations of pulsed Doppler in following the maximum velocities which occur in stenosis of the aortic valve. Aliasing occurs in any sampling process when the PRF is not high enough to follow the velocities of blood within the sample volumes. Thus, when the Doppler shift frequency exceeds one half the PRF the sampling process fails to represent the velocities in their proper frequency range, hence, the term aliasing.

The advantages of PWD over CWD:
1) Separation of velocities in deep and superficial vessels or channels of the heart,
2) Display of velocity profiles and 2-D flow imaging, and
3) Easier combination with 2-D pulse echo imaging.
  The advantages of CWD over PWD:
1) Higher frequency response,
2) Better signal/noise,
3) Lower power levels,
4) Easier identification of superficial vessels and high velocity jets, and
5) Greater cost effectiveness.

MULTIGATE PULSED DOPPLER

In concept, a multigate pulsed Doppler uses a regular pulse transmission train with a number of simultaneous listening gates. The received signals are range gated at various time delays into a number of parallel channels for parallel processing.

DOPPLER IMAGING

Either CWD or PWD can be used to make a map representation of the location of blood flow similar to an X-ray contract angiogram. Doppler imaging helps in the search for diagnostic signals by scanning for regions of special interest. When, for example, an abnormal jet is found the high velocities produce characteristic colors on the Doppler image. Quantitative evaluation may then be made by freezing the image and dwelling on the regions with quantitative modalities. Particularly useful is the ability of Doppler imaging to produce a cross section of flow channels in 2-D. Figure 24. Color coding of direction of blood flow is particularly helpful. Figure 25 illustrates a color Doppler instrument with separate screens for sector scans

Figure 24. Method of producing 2D color Doppler imaging. The blue represents blood velocities simultated for the pulmonary artery which are moving away from the transducer while red represents velocities in the aortic root and left main coronary artery moving away from the transducer. A, B and C represent single line A mode Doppler signals.

Figure 25. Aloka color Doppler imager, IREX ᵀᴹ880, which mixes both blood velocity imaging and 2D echocardiography. Courtesy IREX cardiology group at Johnson and Johnson Ultrasound, Inc.

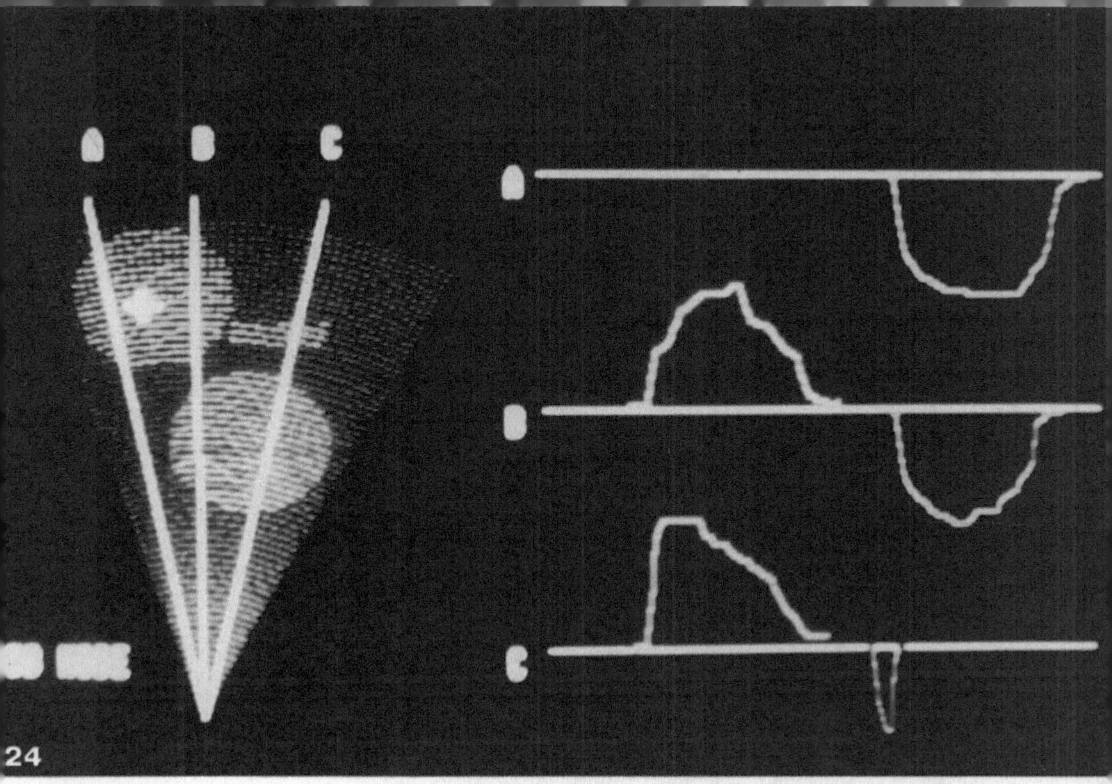

24

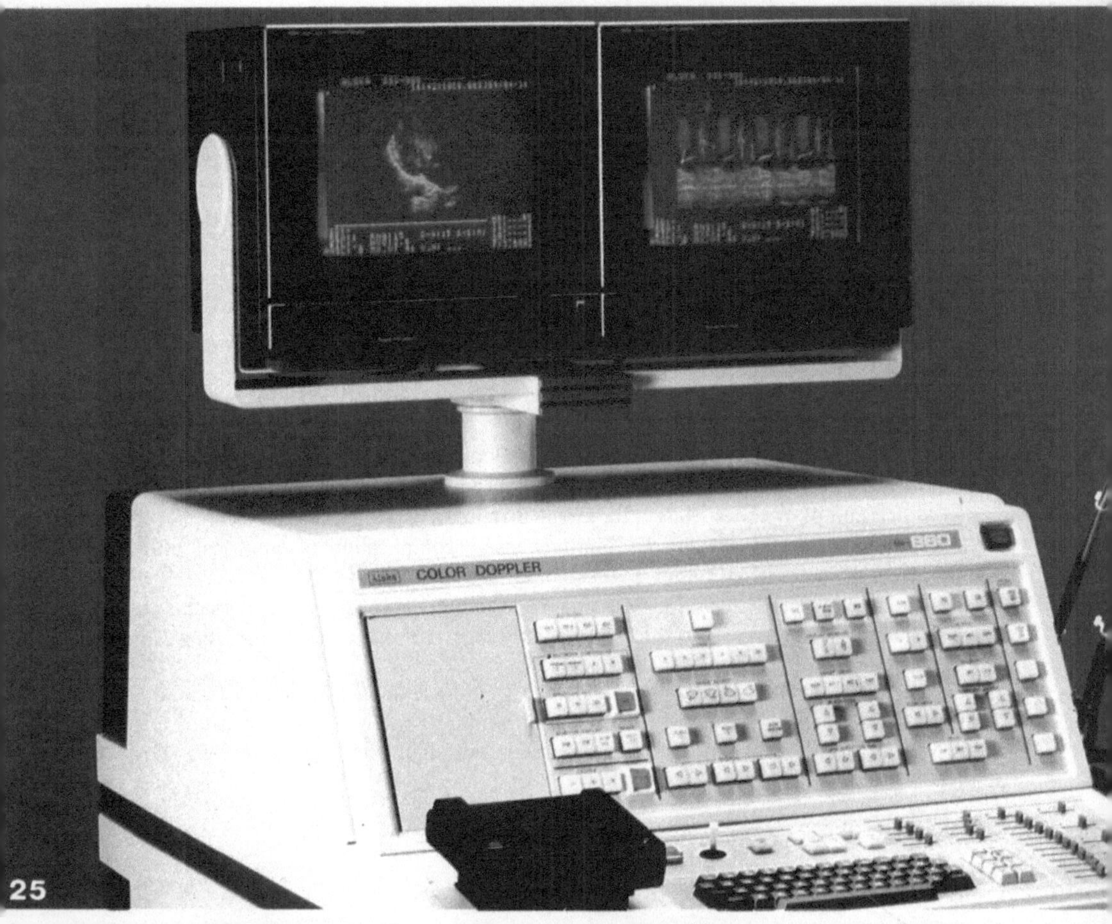

25

38

and M-mode Doppler. Chapters 9 and 10 of this book provide examples of how Doppler imaging has been applied to the cardiac Doppler diagnosis. A color or grey scale can be applied to the image to code whose intensity is proportional to the Doppler frequency. Since Doppler signals are directional, the use of two different colors is necessary to represent this feature. The equipment for 2-D color Doppler imaging is illustrated in Figure 25.

REFERENCES

1. Wells PNT: The possibility of harmful biological effects in ultrasonic diagnosis. In: Cardiovascular applications of ultrasound. Robert S Reneman (ed.). North-Holland Publishing Company, The Netherlands, 1:1-17, 1974.
2. Reid JM: Sound and ultrasound. In: Cerebrovascular evaluation with Doppler ultrasound. Merrill P Spencer and John M Reid (eds.), Martinus Nijhoff Publishers, The Netherlands. 2:23-40, 1983.
3. Wells PNT: Biomedical ultrasonics. London/New York: Academic Press, 1977.
4. Reneman RS (ed.): Cardiovascular applications of ultrasound. Amsterdam, London, New York: North Holland/American Elsevier Publishing, 1974.
5. Baum G: Fundamentals of medical ultrasonography. New York. GP Putnam's Sons. (See chapter 27, 'Principles of Doppler ultrasound'). 1975.
6. King DL: Diagnostic ultrasound. CV Mosby Company. (See chapter by Donald W Baker), 1974.
7. Reneman RS, Hoeks APG: Doppler ultrasound-principle, advantages and limitations. In: Doppler ultrasound in the diagnosis of cerebrovascular disease. Robert S Reneman and APG Hoeks (eds.). Published by Research Studies Press, a division of John Wiley & Sons, Ltd., Great Britain, 4:77-101.
8. Angelsen BAJ: Analog estimation of the maximum frequency of Doppler spectra in ultrasonic blood velocity measurements. Report 76-21-W. Div of Eng Cybernetics, NTH, Trondheim, Norway, 1976.
9. Mol JMF: The clinical use of Doppler hematographic investigation in cerebral circulation disturbances. In: Doppler ultrasound in the diagnosis of cerebrovascular disease. Robert S Reneman and APG Hoeks (eds.). Published by Research Studies Press, a division of John Wiley & Sons, Ltd., Great Britain, 6:129-156.
10. Klepper JR: The physics of Doppler ultrasound and its measurement instrumentation. In: Cardiac Doppler diagnosis. MP Spencer (ed.). Martinus Nijhoff Publishers, The Netherlands, 3:19-31, 1983.
11. Spencer MP: Frequency Spectrum Analysis in Doppler Diagnosis. In: 2nd Edition, Introduction of vascular ultrasonography. William J Zwiebel (ed.). Research Studies Press Limited, a division of Wiley & Sons, Ltd, Great Britain, in press.
12. Goss SA, Johnston RL, DUnn F: Comprehensive complication of empirical ultrasonic parameters of mammalian tissue. J Accoust Soc Am 64(2):423-457.
13. Kikuchi Y, Okuyama D, Kasai C, Yoshida Y: Measurement of sound velocity and absorption of human blood in 1-10 MHz frequency range. Rec. Elec. Commun, Eng Convers Tokohu Univ 41:152-159, 1972.
14. Bakke T, Gytre T, Haagensen A, Giezendanner L: Ultrasonic measurement of sound velocity in whole blood. A comparison between an ultrasonic method and convention packed-cell-volume test for hematocrit determination. Scand J Clin Lab Invest 35:473-478, 1975.

3. Time interval histogram – An alternative in the detection of the maximum velocity in the heart

A. NOWICKI, P. KARLOWICZ, M. PIECHOCKI, W. SECOMSKI and M. PLESKOT

INTRODUCTION

Up to late seventies the essentially only method of Doppler frequency measurement was the counting of zero crossings (ZCC) of Doppler signal. The response of the ZCC to the signal is in direct proportion to the second moment of the spectrum of the measured signal.

For real spectra the dependence between the second moment (f_{ZCC}) and mean Doppler frequency (f_{av}) is quite complex and difficult to evaluate directly. It is only in the case of spectrum with a uniform distribution in the band analysed that this dependence is known being $f_{av} = 0.87 f_{ZCC}$. The same limitation concerns the estimation of the maximum frequency.

Different signal processings were proposed to extract the maximum frequency from the Doppler spectrum. The most complex is obviously Fourier analysis permitting evaluation of the spectrum; its broadening, mean and maximum frequency etc. However, Fourier analysis requires expensive equipment and as Light [1] has shown in most cases a purpose-built system of band pass filters over the Doppler frequency range permits quantitative measure of blood flow, particularly in the aorta.

A competitive device designed by Angelsen [2] functioning as a filter tracing the maximum frequency of the Doppler spectrum has been widely used in investigations of intracardiac flow (Hatle, Angelsen [3]).

PRINCIPLE OF THE MAXIMUM FREQUENCY MEASUREMENT BY MEANS OF TIME INTERVAL HISTOGRAPH

Forster and Baker [4] described the principle of the measurement of the instantaneous Doppler frequency, using time interval histograms of Doppler signals (TIH).

They investigated the possibility of using histograms in evaluating flow turbulences, assuming a Gaussian distribution of the Doppler spectrum. From mathematical analysis and model investigations, they showed that the variance of the spectrum of the Doppler signal is a good measure of the intensity of flow turbulence and can be determined directly from a histogram.

The apparent simplicity of interpretation of histograms and their comparison to the power spectrum have recently caused a critical analysis of the method (Angelsen [5], Burckhardt [6]).

A histogram of zero crossings, in contrast to the power spectrum, does not contain all information on the signal. In view of the random character of the Doppler signal, the time intervals between its successive zero crossings are random. A theoretical description of the histogram is only possible in terms of probability. Therefore, the histogram description used lies in the probability distribution of the time intervals between successive zero crossings. This distribution describes the mean occurrence rate of particular instantaneous quasi-frequencies. It is determined by the character of the signal.

The theoretical considerations of Angelsen and the computer simulation by Burchardt have shown that the probability distribution in question does not represent the shape of the spectrum, but only permits its second moment and the 'broadening of the spectrum' to be evaluated.

The present investigation used the approximate theoretical relationship between the power spectrum of the Doppler signal and the probability distribution of the instantaneous frequencies of this signal.

$$p(f_c) = \frac{\sigma_s^2}{2\,[(f_c-\bar{f})^2+\sigma_s^2]^{3/2}} \tag{1}$$

where σ_s^2 is the variance of the power spectrum of the signal, $\bar{f}$ the mean frequency of the power spectrum of the signal, f_c the instantaneous frequency of the signal.

This relationship was given by Angelsen, on the assumption that $\sigma_s/\bar{f}<0.1$, i.e. for relatively narrow spectra. In view of its simplicity, this relationship was used to show the probability distributions of the instantaneous frequencies for several signals with rectangular power spectra (Figure 1). These signals were subsequently used in experimental investigations of the present detector of the maximum frequency in the spectrum. In fact, they have their analogues in real flows. In the systole the flow profile in the arteries becomes flattened and therefore higher frequencies dominate in the spectrum. For stenoses the flow profile becomes elongated, which is manifested by a broadening of the Doppler spectrum. An increase in the ampli-

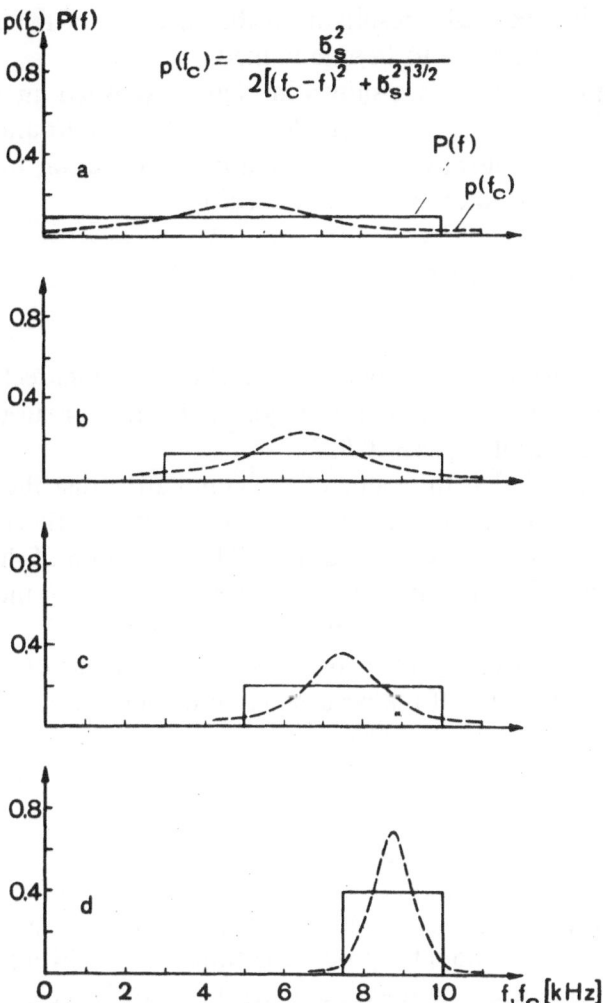

Figure 1. Spectra P (f) and probability distribution of Doppler instantaneous frequencies p (f$_c$) for the bandwidth (a) 0-10 kHz, (b) 3-10 kHz, (c) 5-10 kHz, (d) 7.5-10 kHz.

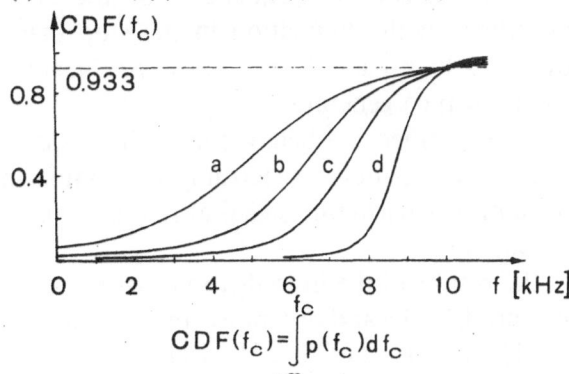

Figure 2. Cumulative distribution function calculated for the probability distributions p (f$_c$) from Figure 1.

tude of successive rectangles results from the necessity of the constant total power of particular signals to be maintained.

The probability distributions shown in Figure 1 (dashed line) do not indicate the existence of the characteristic feature of the maximum frequency in the spectrum. When, however, the cumulative distribution function of the distributions mentioned above is calculated, i.e.

$$\text{CDF}(f_c) = \int_{-\infty}^{f_c} p(f_c)\, df_c \tag{2}$$

it will appear that for all the power spectra shown in Figure 1 the value of the cumulative distribution function (Figure 2) for the maximum frequency is constant, being $\text{CDF}(f_{max}) = 0.933$.

It can be repeated that the value of the cumulative distribution function of a given frequency f_c determines the probability of the occurrence of instantaneous frequencies not exceeding f_c. The definition of the method for the measurement of the maximum frequencies resulsts from the fact that the value of the cumulative distribution function is constant for the maximum frequencies of the spectra shown. It is necessary to measure the frequency for which the probability of the occurrence of higher frequencies is close to 0.1.

EXPERIMENTAL INVESTIGATIONS

The main purpose of the present investigation was to show that the system designed by the authors for processing time interval histograms permitted the measurement of the maximum frequency of Doppler signals.

White noise was analyzed in the acoustic band 65 Hz–10 kHz, by changing the upper and lower cut off frequencies of the spectrum. Special, RFT HP 601 type filters, with attenuation in the stop band of 80 db/oct., were used as low- and high-pass filters. Noise was generated by a Sine-Random B and K 1024 type generator.

The investigations examined the behaviour of the system for tracing the maximum frequency of the noise spectrum, by comparing it with the response of the system to a harmonic signal at frequency equal to the upper frequency of the spectrum.

Figure 3 shows the results of the investigations for frequencies of 3.5 kHz, 5.5 kHz, 7.5 kHz and 10 kHz and for noise in the bands 65 Hz–3.5 kHz, 65 Hz–5.5 kHz, 65 Hz–7.5 kHz and 120 Hz–10 kHz.

These photographs show the grey scale of the histogram with increased brightness for the center frequencies of the band in question (greater bright-

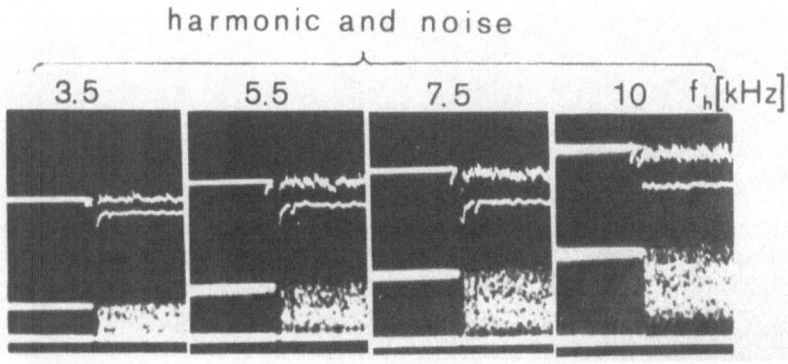

Figure 3. Maximum frequency output (upper line) and ZCC (middle line) for different spectral noise inputs and a harmonic signal. Noise was investigated in the bandwiths 65-3.5 kHz, 65-5.5 kHz, 65-7.5 kHz and 120-10 kHz.

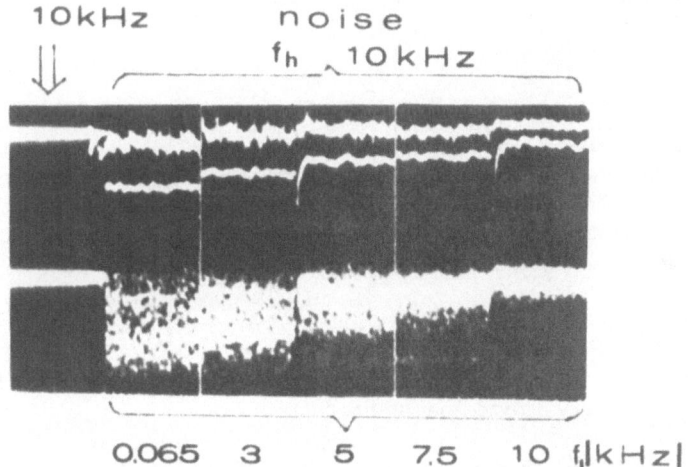

Figure 4. Maximum (upper line) and ZCC (middle line) frequency output for noise with an constant upper cut off frequency of 10 kHz. The lower cut off frequency was varied between 65 kHz and 10 kHz.

ness corresponds to a larger number of points, i.e. a larger number of zero crossings of the Doppler signal).

The system tracing the maximum frequency of the spectrum behaves as assumed. Figure 3 shows that its response to the noise signal is the same as the response of the system to a simple harmonic signal at a frequency equal to the maximum noise frequency.

Figure 4 shows the results for noise with an upper cut off frequency of 10 kHz and different lower cut off frequencies: 65 Hz, 3 kHz, 5 kHz,

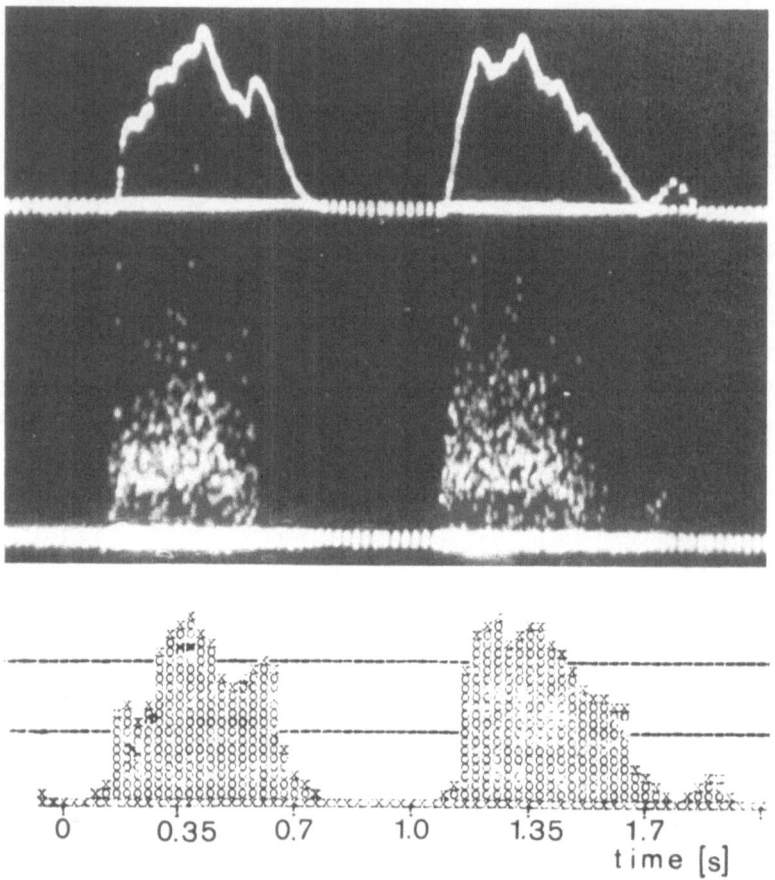

Figure 5A. TIH of the aortic flow (lower trace) and maximum frequency (upper trace), Figure 5B: Maximum frequency derived from off-line FFT.

7.5 kHz and 10 kHz. For comparison, the behaviour of the system for one frequency of 10 kHz is also shown. In this case the system measures correctly the maximum frequency, irrespective of the spectrum width, whereas the frequency of zero crossings (ZCC) increases as the upper cut off frequency increases.

Figures 5A and 5B show a comparison of measurements of the maximum frequency in the descending aorta by the TIH method and those by spectral analysis. Fourier transforms were calculated at time intervals of 20 ms. The value below which 95 per cent of the power of the signal investigated fell was taken as the maximum frequency.

The frequency analysis of the regurgitant flow in Figure 6 has shown frequency components up to 15 KHz but their level was 36 dB below the power of middle range components and only 5 db over the noise level.

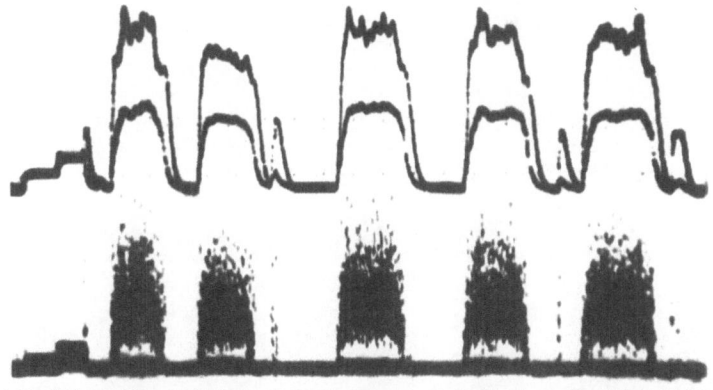

Figure 6. Monitor display of the TIH and maximum frequency recording of the mitral regurgitation. Calibration pulses correspond to 1 and 2 kHz Doppler shift. The peak frequency in the systole is 11 kHz.

CONCLUSIONS

The possibility of tracing the maximum Doppler frequency by means of TIH offers an inexpensive and wide range of application of Doppler flowmeters in investigation of the hemodynamics of blood circulation system.

Although the Fourier analysis gives more information on the received flow signal, properly processed time interval histogram can reveal the maximum flow velocity in most clinical studies. In the case of low power high velocity signals, e.g. small and middle grade valvular insufficiency, additional L.F. filtering plus differentiation up to 20 kHz should be done.

REFERENCES

1. Light LH: Transcutaneous aortovelography a new window on the circulation, Br Heart J 38:433-442, 1976.
2. Angelsen BAJ: Analog estimation of the maximum frequency of Doppler spectra in ultrasonic blood velocity measurements, Dep Eng Cybern Norwegian Inst Technol, Trondheim, Norway, Rep 76-21, 1976.
3. Hatle L, Angelsen BAJ: Doppler Ultrasound in Cardiology, Lea and Febiger, Philadelphia, 1982.
4. Forster FK, Baker DW: Quantitative flow measurement utilizing a time interval histogram of Doppler shifted ultrasound, Ultrasound in Medicine, Vol 4, White D (ed.), Plenum Press: 349-353, 1976.
5. Angelsen BAJ: Spectral estimation of a narrowband caussian process from the distribution of the distances between adjacent zeros, IEEE Trans Biom Enging: 27(2), 1980.
6. Burchardt CB: Comparison between spectrum and time interval histogram of ultrasound Doppler signal. Ultrasound Med Biol 7:79-82, 1981.

4. Velocity profiles in the aortic arch and Doppler determination of cardiac output: The normal and the pathological

B. DIEBOLD and P. PERONNEAU in collaboration with

R. ESSIAMBRE and A. DELOUCHE

INTRODUCTION

Our present knowledge of blood flow dynamics in the healthy or diseased aorta, on both sides of normal and abnormal aortic valves, provides an elaborate although incomplete appreciation of their complexity and direct implications in cardiovascular pathophysiology. Flow pulsatility, the aortic valve, the particular configuration of the thoracic aorta with its branching and its intrinsic elastic properties all contribute in shaping velocity profiles. Shearing forces are also significantly involved in the dynamic modifications of aortic blood flow. These give rise to secondary flows and turbulences which are directly affected by disease processes particularly those giving rise to jet formation such as valvular aortic stenosis or regurgitation. The influence of these phenomena on the quality of cardiac output determination is considerable.

The thoracic aorta is asymmetrically curved in three dimensions, has a progressively tapering circular cross-section and its main plane of curvature allows it to arch over the left pulmonary vessels. This geometry is further complicated by the emergence of three major arterial trunks in its transverse portion.

The wall of the aorta has longitudinal stiffness far greater than in the transversal plane. The aortic wall is viscoelastic but its viscosity is low. Therefore, the elasticity generates volume variations essentially through radius modifications.

Due to this compliance, part of the blood ejected from the left ventricle in systole is trapped in the aorta and the great vessels. The diastolic recoil of this structure restores blood to the periphery.

Pressure waves propagating in the vascular system are partially transmitted and partially reflected at all points in the system where the cross-sectional area or the elasticity change, namely at major branching points and all along the tapering aorta. Therefore at each point, the pressure curve is the sum of distally travelling and proximally reflected waves. In practice, as emphasized in studies of aortic impedance, the spectrum of velocity curves, in the absence of valvular disease, is far from the sum of a continuous component with a pure sinusoidal wave. Therefore, quantitative analysis can only be drawn from either *in vivo* measurements or *in vitro* studies in which fluid viscosity and flow pulsatility approach physiological conditions.

NORMAL AORTA

Basic elements

In the aorta, as in other conduits, fluid elements are forced to roll and stretch along the boundaries, within a region called the boundary layer. As a fluid flows into a tube, the viscosity of the fluid is such that this shearing effect is progressively transmitted to fluid elements away from the wall, thus increasing gradually the width of the boundary layer. Those events lead to modifications of velocity profiles. In case of a steady flow in a straight rigid tube, the developed flow depends on the longitudinal velocity (v), the radius of the tube (R), and the kinetic viscosity (v) of the fluid as expressed in Reynolds' number (Re): $Re = 2\,Rv/v$.

In the aorta the distance traveled by the fluid before the flow acquires its developed profile is greater than the full length of the vessel.

In curves, the boundary layer contributes to secondary flows originally described by Dean. Simply stated fluid elements are moved by centrifugal forces from the inner to the outer part of the bend. These are then transferred along the wall by a rotational movement towards the inside of the bend (Figure 1a). The sum of these primary and secondary flows given rise to a double helicoidal motion. With steady flows the initial axial velocity profile is skewed along the curve and peak velocity moves towards the outside of the bend.

Pulsatility greatly modifies both primary and secondary flows. In 1971, Lyne suggested that an oscillatory flow may modify the twin vortex described by Dean into four helicoidal motions with inward centrifuging near the center of the tube (Figure 1b). Other theoretical studies have predicted the same four vortex motions and this has subsequently been experimentally verified in 'near' physiological models.

In the aorta, these phenomena are further complicated by flow development as blood enters the arch. Data concerning a comparable configuration was recently reported and included a detailed description of secondary

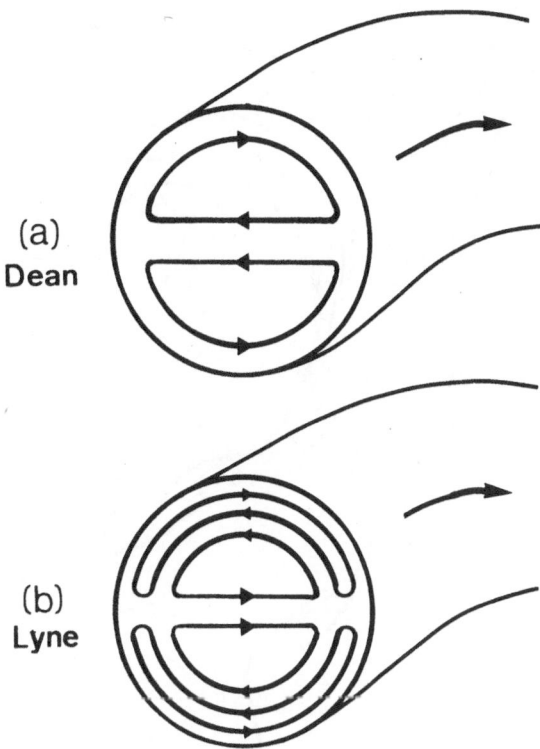

Figure 1. a) Dean type secondary flows, b) Lyne type secondary flows.

flows, Talbot [1]. They show clear Dean type secondary components during the beginning of ejection all along the bend. This is then modified into a Lyne type, during mid systole, in the second half of the bend. The development of secondary flow is clearly delayed with respect to axial velocity but it persists with high components during the decelerating phase.

Flow profiles in the aortic arch

The aortic orifice being in proximity to the mitral orifice in the same plane causes blood flow to undergo clear asymmetric contraction of its cross-section from the left ventricle to the aorta thus defining the aortic entry. This entrance phenomenon along with flow pulsatility should lead to a flat velocity profile at the level of the aortic orifice (Figure 2).

Downstream from the free edges of the aortic leaflets viscous forces induce systolic vortices which are trapped in the sinuses of Valsalva, Bellhouse [2]. In diastole, the geometry is modified by valve closure and two of the three sinuses are involved by flows feeding the coronary arteries. At the entrance of the ascending aorta, the velocity profile appears relatively blunt

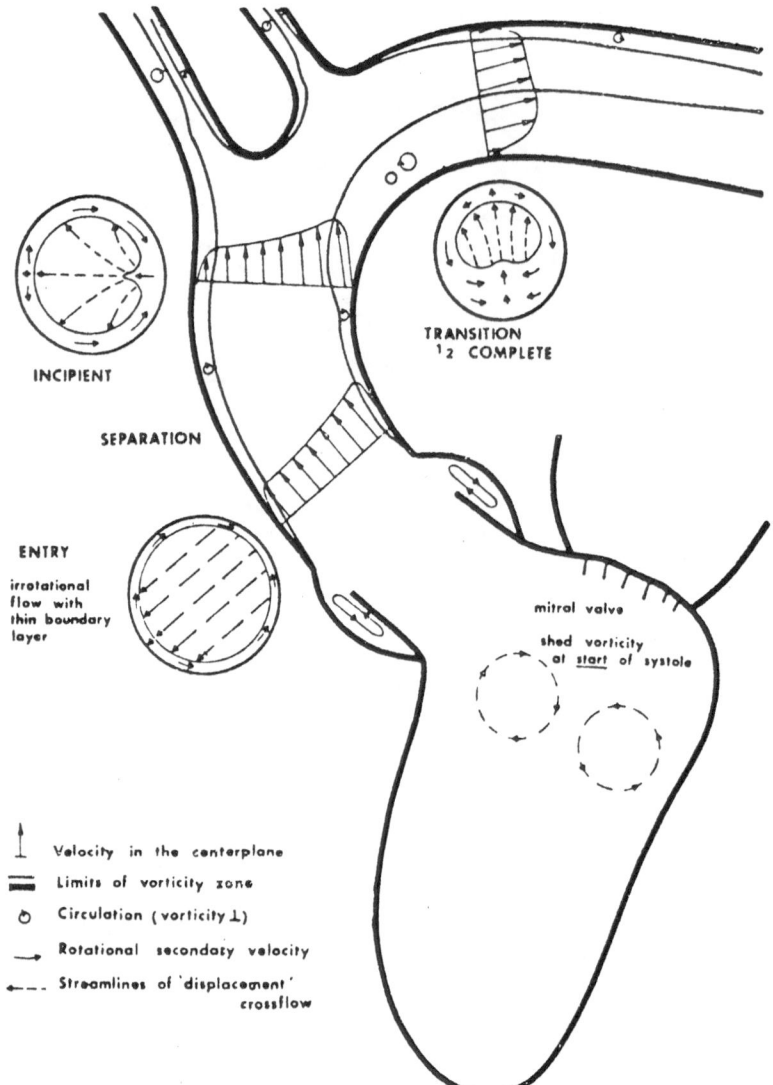

Figure 2. Final theoretical flow picture at mid-systole showing axial velocity in the centerplane, cross-sectional flow and the circulation in zones of vortices. The progression of inner and outer boundary layers is depicted (from Farthing, 1979).

across the diameter. Nevertheless significant misalignment between the axis of the left ventricle and the axis of the initial aortic segment may cause rapid skewing of the velocity profile in systole with maximal velocities developing close to the inside of the bend (Figure 3). Moreover, as blood is ejected into the ascending aorta it occasionally has a tendency to flow separation along the inner aspect of the bend thus inducing a brief flow reversal at end systole. Blood decelerates in the core region more slowly than in the

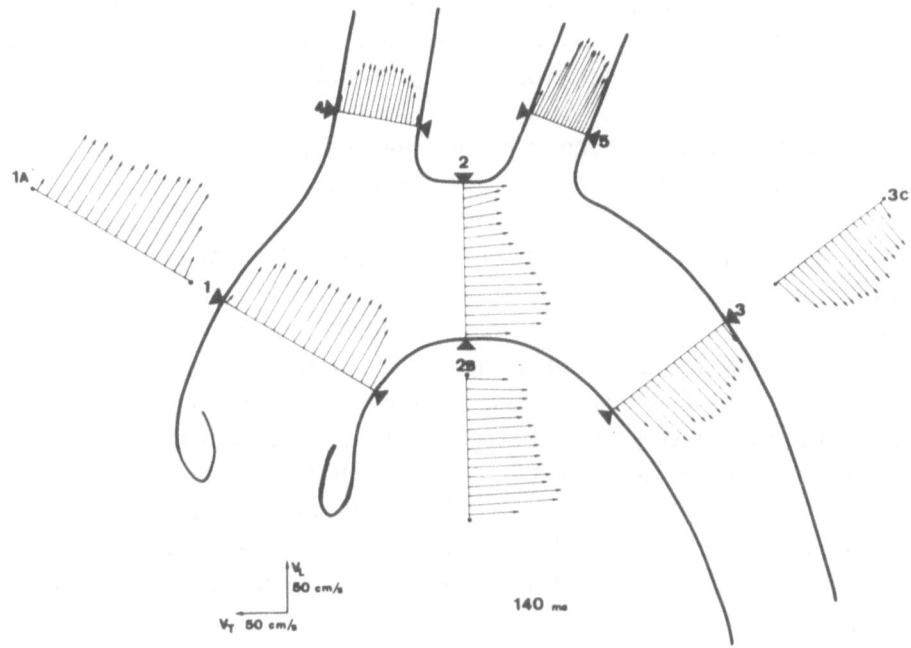

Figure 3. Modifications of velocity profiles along the canine thoracic aorta in early-systole. Profiles 1a, 2b and 3c are perpendicular to profiles 1, 2 and 3 respectively (from Farthing, 1979).

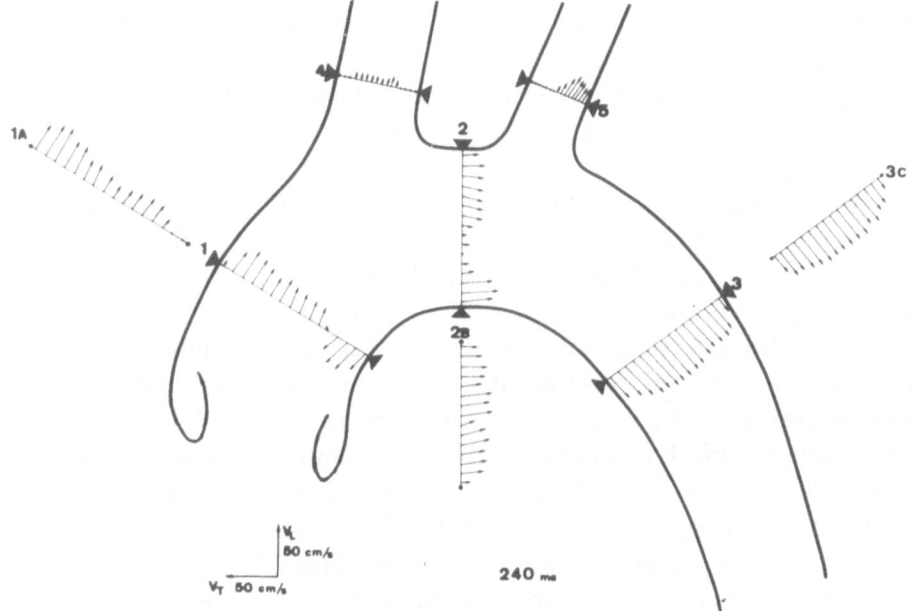

Figure 4. Velocity profiles along the canine thoracic aorta in early-diastole (from Farthing, 1979).

boundary layer giving rise to the development of an axial flow reversal along the inner aspect of the initial curvature, Farthing [3], Yearwood [4]. The consequences of which progressively disappear from mid to late diastole (Figure 4).

In the ascending part of the arch, the skewness of the axial velocity profile is more striking as blunt flow enters the main curvature, Jenni [19]. As mentioned previously, a pressure gradient is established within the boundary layer between the outer and the inner regions of the bend giving sufficient centripetal acceleration to contained elements to follow the curvature of the arch. The reduced axial flow velocity in the boundary layer confers less centrifugal force and thus fluid acceleration is oriented towards the inside of the bend. The boundary layer along the lateral walls develops strong cross-flows thus progressively increasing its thickness along the inside of the bend. Hence the axial velocity profile is progressively modified.

Fluid elements entering the inside of the bend are accelerated while those entering the outside are decelerated as skewing steepens. Therefore during systole, the instantaneous peak velocities are encountered close to the medial and posterior aortic walls, Farthing [3], Yearwood [4], Paulsen [5], Falsetti [6], Lucas [7]. Many groups have experimentally described in dogs this skewness in accordance with theoretical studies, Talbot [1]. Its importance varies from one subject to the other, Lucas [7], and is furthermore important in cases of increased cardiac output, Falsetti [6]. Moreover, the time course of secondary flows is very close to that of the deceleration instabilities or turbulences often described in the normal aorta (Falsetti [6], Yamaguchi [8].

In early and mid-diastole, a clear flow reversal appears along the inside of the bend while forward flow is still present along its outer part, Farthing [3], Yearwood [4] (Figure 5).

The data available concerning flow distribution in the transverse part of the aortic arch were obtained on dogs and therefore corresponds to a somewhat different anatomical situation, there being only two emerging trunks both showing significant anterograde flow in diastole as in the human left common carotid artery. Studies using branching arterial models do not allow application of their conclusions to aortic arch flow due to the particular configuration of the arch and rigid models, Chandran [9] are not suitable for studies in diastole due to the absence of both compliance and recoil feeding of the arch vessels. Nevertheless a few points need to be discussed. Tapering of the aorta prevents any dramatic decrease of mean flow velocity downstream which would otherwise result from branching. Conversely the fluid deviated from the main course into the arch vessels consists mostly of fluid elements moving within the boundary layer along the outer aortic curvature (Figure 2).

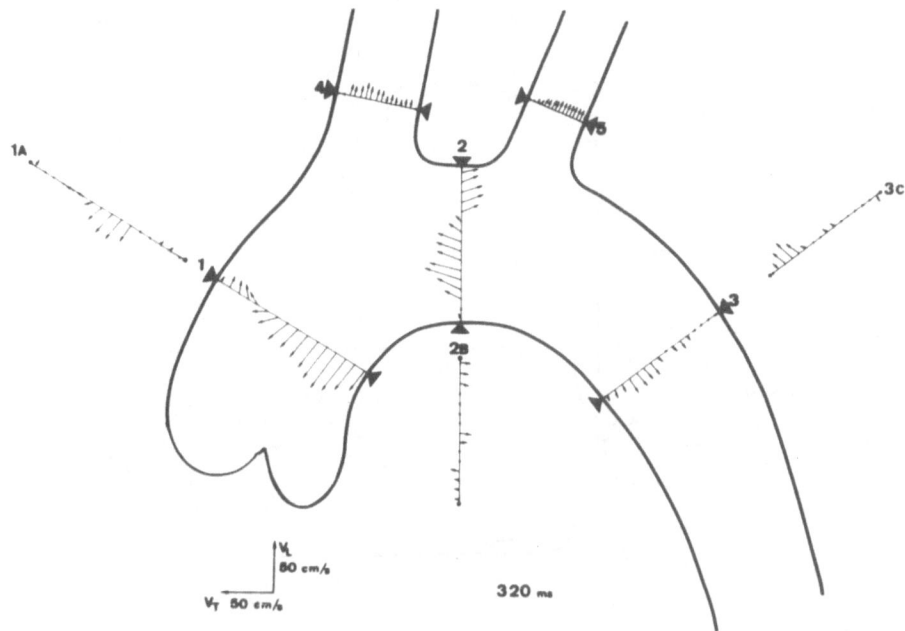

Figure 5. Velocity profiles along the canine thoracic aorta in late-diastole (from Farthing [3]).

When considering successive cross-sections, from the ascending to the transverse aorta, the increasing thickness of the boundary layer at the inner wall progressively moves the instantaneous peak velocity towards the centerline (Talbot [1], Farthing [3], Yearwood [4]). The profile thus modeled in the mid-portion of the arch is skewed towards the inner part of the curvature in early systole but displays during deceleration a clear 'hallow' with a peak maximal instantaneous axial velocity located centrally. In diastole, flow reversal persists along the inner aspect of the bend and a clear forward flow oriented towards the origin of the left common carotid artery is seen.

Entering the descending aorta the boundary layer along the outer aspect of the bend rapidly redevelops after being deviated into the arch vessels; thus, it is far thinner than its counterpart along the inside of the curvature. The secondary flows contained within this progressively thickening inner boundary layer favors flow separation from the aortic wall.

AORTIC STENOSIS

Blood crossing a narrowed aortic orifice successively passes through three different regions (Figure 6). Fluid elements are initially accelerated in the

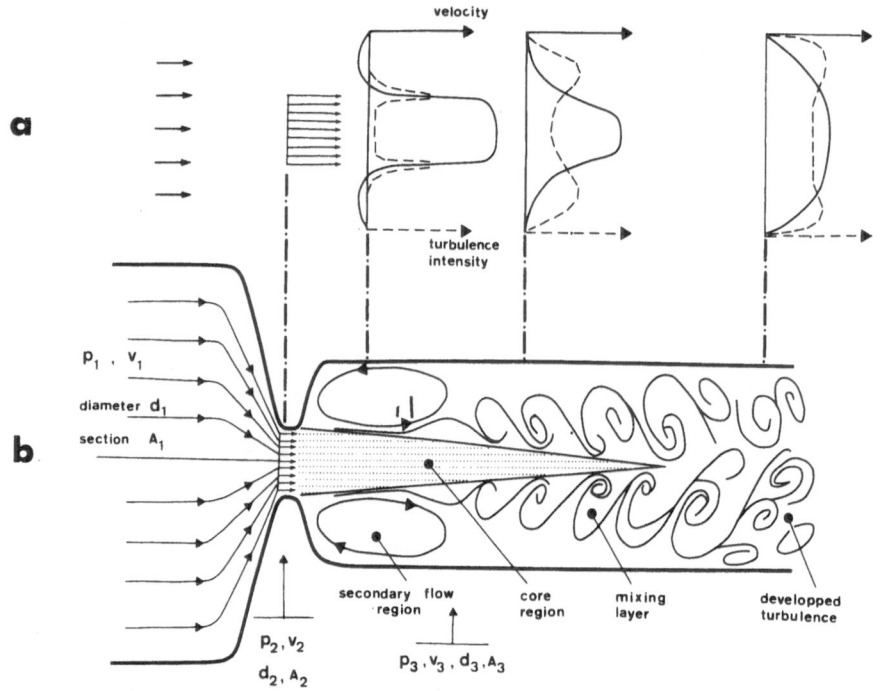

Figure 6. (a) Modification of both the velocity profile and turbulence intensity immediately beyond a stenosis until the region of developed flow. (b) Flow representation before, within and after a stenosis with the production of a jet.

area of convergence where a significant pressure drop occurs. These enter the downstream vessel forming a jet as an abrupt increase in diameter appears. Finally, this jet induces further downstream turbulences with a partial pressure recovery.

Flow velocities and pressure drop within the stenosis

The energy accumulated by the blood is the sum of pressure and kinetic energies. As streamlines converge, towards the orifice, fluid elements undergo a velocity increase corresponding to an energy transfer from pressure to kinetic energy. This energy conversion is also accompanied by an energy loss occurring around the orifice and depending upon the geometry of the stenosis. Its contribution has been introduced as the 'C' coefficient in Gorlin's initial formula. Fortunately the value of 'C' remains essentially constant around 0.9.

Flow unsteadiness induces both a time related flow acceleration and inertial phenomena which need consideration. The additional component is positive in early systole and negative during end-systole. The equation is as follows:

$$p_1 - p_2 = \frac{1}{2} \cdot \frac{\rho}{C^2} \cdot (v_2^2 - v_1^2) + \rho \int_1^2 \frac{dv}{dt} ds$$

where p_1 = upstream pressure,
$\quad\quad p_2$ = pressure at the orifice,
$\quad\quad v_1$ = upstream velocity,
$\quad\quad v_2$ = velocity at the orifice,
$\quad\quad\quad$ = volume mass of the fluid
and where dv/dt and ds respectively represent acceleration and the element of length of the converging segment.

Flow velocities within the jet

At the orifice, in spite of high velocities and an elevated Reynolds' number, flows are laminar, Clark [10]. Furthermore the upstream convergence of the streamlines, the shortness of the stenosis and to some extent, the pulsatility should induce a flat velocity profile during ejection.

Immediately downstream from the orifice, most of the available data concerning velocity profiles have been gathered from studies of free air jets. Nevertheless, they remain of interest since the qualitative description they provide agrees with the few measurements obtained on liquid jets and published so far, Clark [10] (Figure 7). However, all the reported studies have used stenoses or nozzles with a circular cross-section. The resulting geometry clearly differs from stenoses usually seen in patients, particularly in

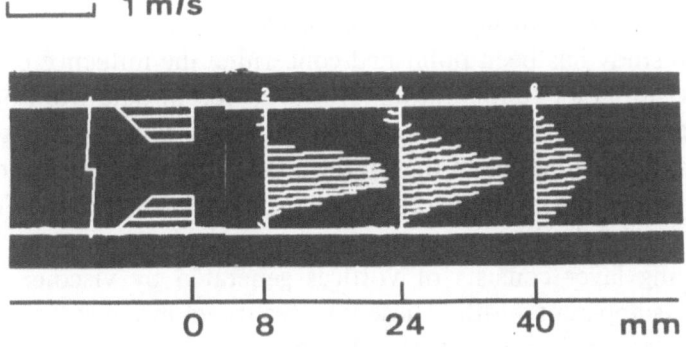

Figure 7. Modifications of peak systolic velocity profiles in a water-tank model of aortic stenosis. The orifice has a surface area of 0.4 cm² and the rigid receiving conduit has a diameter of 1.6 cm.

adults, and where the jet develops in a volume of blood bounded by the aorta. The following jet description is thus mainly qualitative.

Immediately away from the stenotic orifice an abrupt increase in cross-section appears. At the onset of ejection, the streamlines organized within the stenosis penetrate into a column of blood. This creates a boundary layer between a centrally located jet consisting of an accelerated laminar flow and a surrounding, initially almost immobile blood cylinder. This boundary layer is, in fact, a mixing layer, but differs from that previously described since the flow motion can be transfered from central to peripheral regions. Indeed peripheral fluid elements acquire a centripetal movement. Its orientation is perpendicular to the centerline before becoming more parallel as it approaches the boundary layer. During mid-systole the blood laminarly ejected with a high velocity, Clark [10], constitutes a central core enveloped by the mixing layer which is itself surrounded by a developing secondary flow. Therefore, three concentric volumes need to be described: a central laminar jet, a mixing layer and a secondary flow region.

When considering flows at increasing distance from the orifice, the velocity within the central laminar core is relatively uniform but the latter is progressively involved, along with peripheral blood, with turbulences arising in the progressively thickening mixing layer, Moore [11]. The central core thus occupies a definite distance corresponding to approximately four times the orifice diameter in a steady flow model.

Within the peripheral cylinder, the transversal components of the secondary flow induce the development of a clearly defined vortex walled by the edges of the stenosis and the oartic root. It has an annular shape. Its internal layer is thin with high forward velocity components. At the opposite, its external layer is thicker but contains backward components of smaller amplitude. The latter having a specific time course (Figure 8). The external secondary flow region is present from the orifice to the area where the mixing layer reaches the aortic wall. This corresponds to the 're-attachment point' which moves during the cardiac cycle.

So far no study has been published concerning the influence of the aortic wall on the initial jet configuration. However, recent data from our laboratory strongly suggest that, when a pansystolic jet is present, its apparent diameter is independent from that of the aorta although, with larger orifices, higher stroke volumes are necessary to generate a detectable jet (Figure 9).

The mixing layer consists of vortices generated by viscous forces and occupying its apparent width. These vortices travel in the same direction as the central jet while investing it. As they move, the vortices cohalesce through a pairing effect thus increasing in size but decreasing in number, Moore [11]. This accounts for the apparent widening of the mixing layer. It

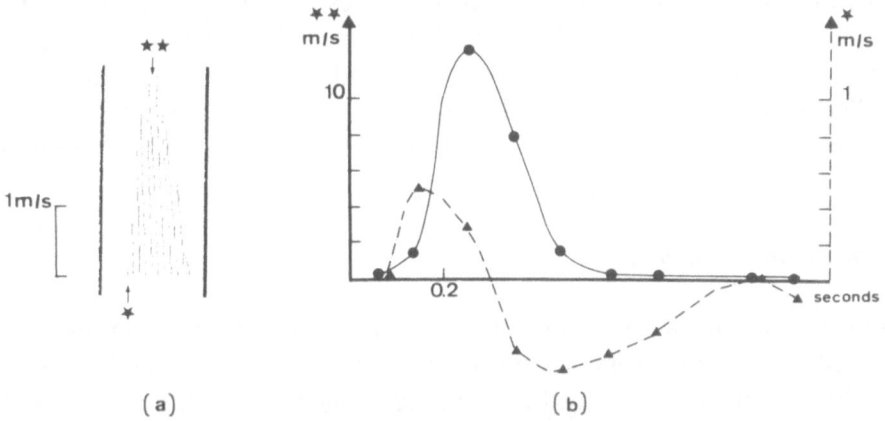

Figure 8. (a) Peak systolic velocities 8 mm away from a narrowed orifice. The secondary flow (*) and the centerline (**) are identified, (b) Time course of velocities in positions (*) and (**) respectively. The scale of curve (**) is ten times that of curve (*). The boundary layer appears initially involved with primary flow at the beginning of systole and later with secondary flow. The latter seems to be sustained beyond the end of ejection.

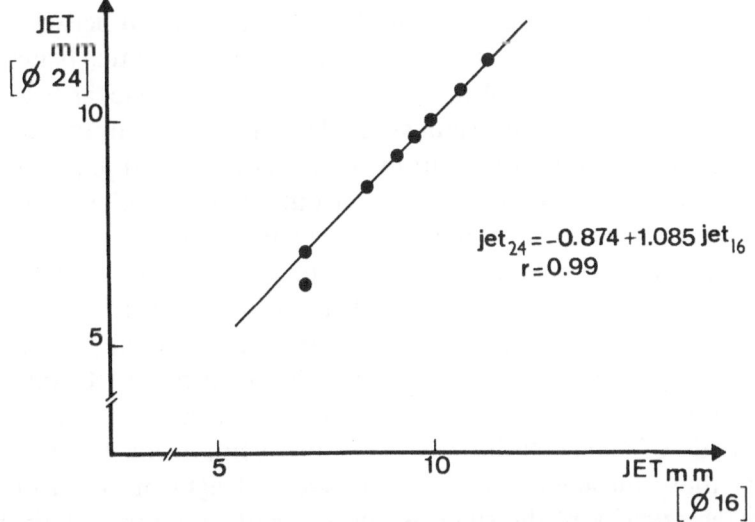

Figure 9. Apparent jet diameter (mm) measured with a multigate pulsed Doppler instrument in a water-tank model of aortic stenosis. A full range of narrowed orifices is included with two different 'aortic' diameters (16 and 24 mm). The only discrepant joint is within the theoretical accuracy of the method.

remains unclear whether this phenomenon is reproducible from one cycle to the other and whether it is axisymmetric or not since significant instabilities have been described in aerodynamic studies. The motion of mixing vortices modifies the apparent instantaneous length of the potential core. The influence of pulsatility is unknown.

Because of their very short life-span vortices can only be appreciated on flow visualization performed at high frame rate. Moreover large sized vortices progressively transfer their energy to middle sized vortices and so on to smaller ones. The smaller a vortex, the shorter will be its duration. Therefore these events appear as fluctuations of velocity curves thus defining turbulences.

Downstream turbulences

Downstream from the re-attachment point of the flow and from the tip of the central core, the cross-section of the aorta is totally invested by turbulent flows which are described for discrete elements of volume and time by a mean velocity $(v(t))$ and fluctuations $(u'(t))$ around this mean velocity. The amplitudes and frequencies of these turbulences have been studied in models of valvular and vascular stenosis, Clark [10]. Their amplitude is related to their energy content and their frequency to their size and duration. These studies correspond to models using straight rigid tubes and therefore do not introduce the damping effect due to aortic elasticity or the modifications related to the curve and to the misalignment between the axis of the jet and the initially curved ascending aorta. The latter being responsible for the impact lesion of the jet on the aortic wall. Nevertheless, qualitative elements seem well established. The site of maximum turbulence intensity is slightly downstream from the tip of the initial jet, varying with the severity of the stenosis and ith cardiac output. The profile of turbulences in this location depends on the geometry of the stenosis.

Further on, the profile of turbulences seems more flat but their intensity is related primarily to the aorta rather than to the stenosis. When studying those turbulences at increasing distance from the orifice, in pulsatile conditions, their appearance is increasingly delayed with respect to the onset of the forward systolic blood motion and therefore the beginning of the systolic flow is made of an increasing non disturbed component, Clark [13]. Furthermore those turbulences are present over a length of vessel depending both on the severity of the stenosis and on cardiac output, Clark [13].

AORTIC REGURGITATION

The aortic valve separates two mechanically distinct structures. On one side, the left ventricle, a muscular contractile cavity within which two different blood movements of opposite directions alternate: left ventricular filling during diastole and left ventricular emptying during systole, both normally isolated by the anterior leaflet of the mitral valve. On the other side, the aorta, which has already been described.

Within the left ventricle, a jet appears in diastole originating at the level of the valvular defect. Similarities between the initial diastolic jet of aortic regurgitation and the initial systolic jet of aortic stenosis are numerous and the qualitative description of the latter can be applied to the former. In particular, velocities within the central core seem to be in accordance with the simplified Bernoulli formula. When considering the jet further down, away from the orifice and within the left ventricle, significant differences occur since the anterior mitral leaflet is mobile and occupies only a given length. Therefore the jet of aortic regurgitation is less strongly bounded by the left ventricular outflow tract than the jet of aortic stenosis by the aorta. It thus behaves more like a free turbulent jet.

In a steady flow model, free turbulent jets are usually considered to present four flow patterns: (i) the initial jet, previously described, (ii) a transition zone, (iii) an established flow region (iv) a terminal region.

Immediately downstream from the tip of the central core, along successive cross-sections of the transition zone, Moore [11], the velocity profile acquires a Gaussian shape but the turbulence profile displays two velocity peaks separated by lower values along the jet axis (Figure 6). These peaks progressively disappear until the turbulence profile adopts also a Gaussian shape. Peak axial turbulence intensity will be measured in this region. Within the region of established flow, both mean velocity and turbulence profiles show a Gaussian distribution. They are all similar and can be approximated by the same curve of normal error. The predicted length of the established flow far exceeds the dimensions of the left ventricle.

Within the aorta, systolic velocity profiles are modified by the compensatory increase in stroke volume. This induces a more striking skewing along the inside of the arch and reinforces flow separation in regions where it tends to occur.

Diastolic velocity profile studies have not been reported. The only data available suggest that velocimetric measurements correlate with the severity of the aortic leak, either when calculating the ratio of diastolic reverse flow to systolic forward flow integrals, Nichols [14] or the ratio of end-diastolic to peak-systolic flow amplitudes on recordings performed at the origin of the descending aorta, Diebold [15].

OTHER LESIONS

Aneurysm of the ascending aorta creates an abrupt increase in the cross-section. It can induce a jet phenomenon similar to the one described in idiopathic dilation of the pulmonary artery.

Coarctation of the aorta is a vascular stenosis and as such produces a jet. The velocity within the initial jet obeys Bernoulli's formula but the C factor depend on the length of the stenosis. If the latter is short, C has about the same value as in valvular aortic stenosis. Furthermore, the compliance of the proximal aorta feeds a forward diastolic flow through the stenosis. This together with delayed flow waves travelling through the collateral circulation may induce a significant continuous component in the descending aorta.

In cases of patent ductus arteriosus the shunt usually occurs in both systole and diastole. In systole the ductus diverts fluid elements from the inner boundary layer into the pulmonary artery. In diastole, ductal flow comes both from the arch and the descending aorta. Upstream from the dent it induces a forward diastolic component. Downstream, it creates a diastolic flow reversal.

Aortic valve prostheses have been carefully studied, Chandran [9], Chandran [16], Yoganathan [17] in order to improve their design.

Flow modifications induced by bioprostheses are similar to those associated with mild stenosis, i.e. a jet phenomenon. Its importance depends on the surface area of the prosthesis.

Systolic velocity profiles immediately downstream from caged ball valves are axisymmetric. They display two peripheral peaks of almost equal amplitudes separated by a central negative velocity. The latter accounts for vortex formations due to the central obstacle created by the ball.

Tilting disc valves display two asymmetric channels. Systolic velocity profiles measured perpendicularly to the axis of disc rotation show two very asymmetric peaks, the higher velocity values corresponding to the larger orifice. The downstream influence of this asymmetry depends on the orientation of the prosthesis with respect to the arch. If the main channel is towards the inside of the bend, the initially asymmetric profile reinforces the skewing of the systolic profile. At the opposite, if the main channel is oriented towards the outside of the bend, it creates a flow separation along the inside part of the bend, inducing a large systolic vortex in the ascending aorta.

In systole, bileaflet valves display two symmetric lateral channels separated by a smaller central one. Systolic velocity profiles measured perpendicularly to the rotating axis of the prosthesis present two lateral peaks separated by a relatively smaller central one.

NON INVASIVE DETERMINATION OF AORTIC CARDIAC OUTPUT USING DOPPLER ULTRASOUND

The cardiac output is the product of stroke volume and heart rate. The stroke volume is the integral of the instantaneous volumic flow (Q(t)) over a cardiac cycle. The latter being the key information. Theoretically it is obtained using the following formula:

$$Q(t) = \int_x \int_y V(t, x, y)\, dx\, dy$$

where $V(t, x, y)$ is the local instantaneous velocity.

Unfortunately real time 2D Doppler measurements are far from being accurate enough for this type of computation.

At the opposite, multage Doppler velocimeters have technical features allowing them to measure accurately velocities along a fixed ultrasonic beam. They have a specific number of gates extracting twice as many Doppler signals, the latter being usually processed through a zero-crossing counter. Provided a known angle with respecto to flow direction, they give a quantitative assessment of velocity profiles.

Available date, Farthing[3], Paulsen[5] reasonably support the assumption that in the ascending aorta velocity profiles measured across a diameter are comparable with those existing across others. It is, therefore, possible to consider the aorta as the sum of concentric rings themselves being divided into half-rings and to assume that the instantaneous velocity $(V_i(t))$ is the same over the area of each half-ring. If r_i is the distance separating the middle of the ring from the centerline, the area of each half-ring equals $\pi \cdot r_i \cdot g$, where g is the length of each sample volume. The volumic flow within each half-ring is $V_i(t) \cdot \pi \cdot r_i \cdot g$.

The instantaneous total volumic flow is obtained by computing the sum of all the rings:

$$Q(t) = \sum_i V_i(t)\, \pi\, r_i \cdot g$$

This approach has been validated invasively in dogs, Rumberger[18]. The reported results provide accurate velocity measurements and good correlations for volumic flows despite limitations in the assessment of aortic wall position. This kind of measurement has the main advantage of being applicable in the ascending aorta when considering skewing of systolic profiles. Recent data suggest that it can be performed noninvasively in humans, Jenni[19]. It may be applied both to normal or regurgitant flows in the absence of turbulence. In fact, the presence of the latter precludes any accurate measurement of the mean velocity at each gate. Therefore this approach cannot be used downstream from the initial jet in cases of aortic stenosis. Furthermore, the application of the multigate pulsed Doppler velocimeters to study the initial jet would necessitate an accurate determination of its diameter. So far this has not yet been possible.

Multigate Doppler velocimeters are available for research purposes in a few centers only. However, single gate pulsed Doppler velocimeters are widely available. Their use for cardiac output determination has required a few simplifying hypotheses: (i) processing of the Doppler signal takes into account the profile related spectral broadening, Fisher [20], (ii) the velocity profile is uniform within the sample volume, Fisher [20], Goldberg [21], Lewis [22], (iii) an angle correction can be successfully performed using 2D echo imaging although the angle in the orthogonal plane must be neglected, Goldberg [21].

All the above mentioned evaluations have used a spectral and a visual determination of velocities of interest. Other studies have used zero-crossing counters, Loeppky [23], Ihlen [24]. Despite the non linearities when Doppler frequencies are close to the Nyquist limit, Steingart [25], the latter processing seems to lead to correlations as good as the former.

All agree that the most difficult and unreliable measurement is that of aortic diameter. Theoretically this should be measured at the same level as the velocity. In practice, the two measurements are obtained from different regions on the assumption that the velocity does not differ significantly between the two sites. For example, the diameter is measured at the aortic anulus and the velocity either upstream, Lewis [27] or downstream, Ihlen [24] from it, therefore introducing further sources of error. Furthermore, the accuracy of ultrasonic measurements seems to be too low, Godlberg [21]. Those problems may account for the apparent negligible influence of velocity profiles, although their importance has been mentionned in experimental studies focused on cardiac output measurements, Lucas [7].

In aortic regurgitation, systolic velocities are modified by an increased stroke volume and the results are similar to those reported in states of high cardiac output as induced, for example, by dobutamine.

Downstream from the initial jet, aortic stenosis precludes any reliable mean velocity measurement. Within the jet, cardiac output computation would require a measurement of the cross-section of the orifice.

The ultimate simplification of the method was obtained using continuous wave Doppler, Huntsmann [26], Chandraratna [27]. Since this method does not allow any depth discrimination two further hypotheses have been introduced: (i) it is possible to extract accurately frequencies corresponding to the highest velocities encountered along the beam, (ii) the highest velocities correspond to aortic components in line with the ultrasonic beam, provided a careful aiming of the transducer.

These principles should lead to measurements in the ascending part of the aorta and to the extraction of the top of the skewed profile introducing therefore an overestimation. The reason why the latter has not been reported may be the use of the trailing to leading edge method for aortic diameter measurement.

From the above mentioned clinical studies it is important to stress out that reasonable correlations have only been achieved with an artificially increased range of cardiac outputs. When only considering values corresponding to likely clinical situations, the method lacks accuracy.

CONCLUSION

The above reflections on aortic blood flow dynamics in normal and diseased states, will contribute to a better understanding of the underlying processes. This should improve, as a result, the design of methods developed for investigating patients using Doppler echocardiography.

ACKNOWLEDGEMENT

The authors wish to express their appreciation to Miss Paola PARADISI for preparing this manuscript.

REFERENCES

1. Talbot L, Gong KO: Pulsatile entrance flow in a curve. J Fluid Mech 127:1-25, 1983.
2. Bellhouse BJ: Fluid mechanics of heart valves. Cardiovascular Dynamics, 111-139, by Bergel Dott (ed.). Academic Press New York, 1972.
3. Farthing S, Peronneau P: Flow in the thoracic aorta. Cardiovascular Research 13:607-620, 1979.
4. Yearwood TL, Chandran KB: Physiological pulsatile flow experiments in a model of the human arch. J Biomechanics 15:683-704, 1982.
5. Paulsen PK, Hasenkam JM: Three dimensional visualization of velocity profiles in the ascending aorta in dogs measured with a hot film anemometer. J Biomechanics 16:201-210, 1983.
6. Falsetti HL, Carrol RJ, Swope RD, Chen CJ: Turbulent flow in the ascending aorta of dogs. Cardiovascular Research 17:427-436, 1983.
7. Lucas CL, Keagy BA, Hsia HS, Johnson TA, Henry GW, Wilcox BR: The velocity profile in the canine ascending aorta and its effects on the accuracy of pulsed Doppler determination of mean blood flow. Cardiovascular Research 18:282-293, 1984.
8. Yamaguchi T, Kikkawa S, Parker KH: Application of Taylor's hypothesis to an unsteady convecture field for the spectral analysis to turbulence in the aorta. J Biomechanics 17:889-895, 1984.
9. Chandran KB, Cabell GN, Khalighi B, Chen CJ: Pulsatile flow past aortic valve bioprostheses in a model of human aorta. J Biomechanics 17:609-619, 1984.
10. Clark C: The fluid mechanics of aortic stenosis. II. Unsteady flow experiments. J Biomechanics 9:567-573, 1976.

11. Moore CJ: The role of shear layer instability waves in jet exhaust noise. J Fluid Mechanics 80:321–367, 1977.
12. Clark C: Turbulent velocity measurements in a model of aortic stenosis. J Biomechanics 9:677–687, 1976.
13. Clark C: The propagation of turbulence produced by a stenosis. J Biomechanics 13:591–604, 1980.
14. Nichols WW, Pepine CJ, Conti CR, Christie LG, Feldman RL: Quantitation of aortic insufficiency using a catheter-tip velocity transducer. Circulation 64:375–380, 1981.
15. Diebold B, Peronneau P, Blanchard D: Non invasive quantification of aortic regurgitation by Doppler echocardiography. Brit Heart J 49:167–173, 1983.
16. Chandran KB, Cabell GN, Khalighi B, Chen CJ: Laser anemometry measurements of pulsatile flow past aortic valve prostheses. J Biomechanics 16:865–873, 1983.
17. Yoganathan AP, Chaux A, Gray RJ, Woo Y-R, DeRobertis M, Williams FP, Matloff MJ: Bileaflet, tilting disc and porcine valve substitutes: *in vitro* hydrodynamic characteristics. JACC 3:313–320, 1984.
18. Rumberger GA, Fastenow CF, Laughlin DL, Marcus ML: Validation of a third-generation Doppler system for studies of detailed aortic flow. Am J Physiol 247 (Heart Circ Phys 16) H 847–856, 1984.
19. Jenni R, Vieli A, Ruffmann K, Krayenbuehl HP, Anliker M: A comparison between single gate and multigate ultrasonic Doppler measurements for the assessment of the velocity pattern in the human ascending aorta. European Heart J 5:948–953, 1984.
20. Fisher DC, Sahn DJ, Friedman MJ, Larson D, Valdes Cruz LM, Horowitz S, Goldberg SJ, Allen HD: The effects of variations on pulsed Doppler sampling site on calculation of cardiac output: An experimental study in open-chest dogs. Circulation 67:370–376, 1983.
21. Goldberg SJ, Sahn DJ, Hallen HD, Valdes-Cruz, Hoenecke H, Carnahan Y: Evaluation of pulmonary and systemic blood flow by 2-dimensional Doppler echocardiography using fast Fourier transform spectral analysis. Am J Cardiol 50:1394–1399, 1982.
22. Lewis JF, Kuo LC, Nelson JG, Limacher MC, Quinones MA: Pulsed Doppler echocardiographic determination of stroke volume and cardiac output: clinical validation of two new methods using the apical window. Circulation 70:425–431, 1984.
23. Loeppky JA, Hoekanga DE, Greene ER, Luft UC: Comparison of non invasive pulsed Doppler and Fiek measurements of stroke volume in cardiac patients. Am Heart J 339–348, 1984.
24. Ihlen H, Amlie JR, Dale J, Forfang K, Nitter-Hauge S, Otterstad JE, Simonsen S, Myhre E: Determination of cardiac output by Doppler echocardiography. Br Heart J 51:54–60, 1984.
25. Steingart RM, Meller J, Barovick J, Patterson R, Herman MV, Teichholz LE: Pulsed Doppler echocardiographic measurement of beat to beat changes in stroke volume in Dogs. Circulation 62:542–548, 1986.
26. Huntsmann LL, Stewart DK, Barnes SR, Franklin SB, Colocousis JS, Hessel EA: Non invasive determination of cardiac output in man: clinical validation. Circulation 67:593–602, 1983.
27. Chandraratna PA, Nanna M, McKay C, Nimalasuriya A, Swinney R, Elkayan U, Rahimtoola SH: Determination of cardiac output by transcutaneous continuous wave ultrasonic Doppler computer. Am J Cardiol 53:234–237, 1984.

5. Influence of the geometry of the ascending aorta upon the velocity profile

T. SKJAERPE

INTRODUCTION

When the cardiac output (CO) is estimated noninvasively by echo and Doppler measurements in the ascending aorta, the velocity profile is generally assumed to be flat [1-4]. The recorded velocities will then represent the spatial mean velocity, and the stroke volume is obtained as the product of the integral of the velocity curve and the cross sectional area of the aorta at the same level.

Our first experience with this method did not fit the assumtion of a flat velocity profile. In some patients severe overestimation of CO, up to more than 200%, were made compared to thermodilution measurements. We therefore decided to have a closer look upon geometrical features of the ascending aorta that might influence the velocity profile.

PROCEDURE

Theoretical considerations

When the outlet from a flow channel with a large diameter is through a channel with a much smaller diameter (Figure 1), the velocity profile in the entrance region will be flat with a very thin boundary layer [5]. However, if the entrance region is curved, as the aorta, flow theory says that the profile is skewed with the highest velocities at the inner curvature during the first part of the bend, with a redistribution of the highest velocities to the outer curvature after a distance of 1-2 radii from the inlet [6].

Sometimes a vena contracta may form in the proximal part of the entrance region, where the effective flow area is smaller than the physical area (Figure 2A).

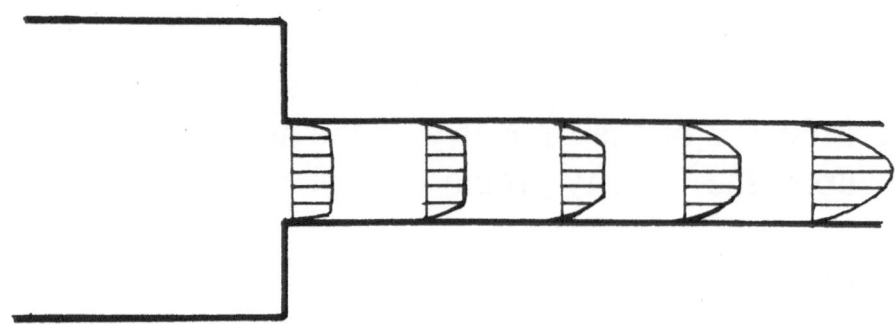

Figure 1. Flow pattern in a straight channel branching of from a much larger channel. In the entrance region the velocity profile is flat. Downstream, viscous friction gradually changes the shape of the profile into a parabola.

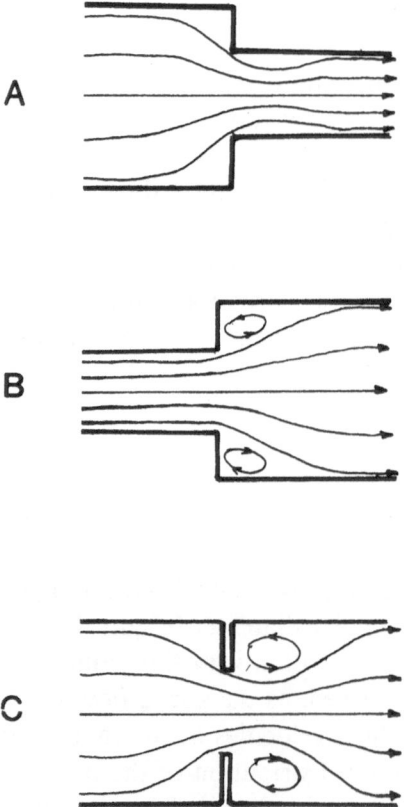

Figure 2. (A) In the entrance region a vena contracta may form, reducing the effective flow area. (B) The flow pattern when there is a sudden expansion of a flow channel. (C) The flow pattern in a channel which at one level is partly obstructed.

When there is a sudden expansion of a flow channel, a central, expanding core of flow is found where the velocity is higher than the cross sectional mean velocity (Figure 2B). Eddies are surrounding the core, giving rise to negative velocities close to the walls. Further downstream the expanding core will fill the channel, with a corresponding decrease in velocity.

If the models in Figure 2A and 2B are combined to form a channel which at one level is partly obstructed, the flow pattern will be as indicated in Figure 2C. Just proximal to the obstruction the velocity will increase, and the highest velocity is found at the obstruction or in the first part of the downstream flow, depending on if, or to what extent a vena contracta is formed. The important point to realize is that, when the highest velocities are measured, only the area of the obstruction can be used to calculate a sensible estimate of volume flow.

Patients

Fifty-five patients were selected from out- and inpatients referred for an echocardiographic study. The only criterion for inclusion was a normal aortic valve as judged by echocardiographic and Doppler examinations. There were 32 men and 23 women, aged 3 to 74 years (mean 35.8 years). Twelve patients had simple shunts, 8 had ischemic heart disease, 10 had mitral and pulmonary valve disease, and in 25 no cardiac disease were found (most of them had innocent murmurs).

Diameter measurements

The ascending aorta was visualized in the parasternal long axis view with two-dimensional echocardiography, and diameters were measured at four different levels (Figure 3). An ATL mark III (Advanced Technology Laboratories) with a 3 mHz mechanical sector tranducer, or an Irex III B (Irex Corporation) with a 2.5 mHz phased array transducer was used. The diameters were measured in systole using leading edge measurements.

Velocity measurements

To evaluate the importance of the curved course of the ascending aorta on the velocity profile, it was attempted to record flow velocities at the inner curvature, centerline velocities, and velocities at the outer curvature in patients where the diameter measurements indicated a fairly even calibred aorta (diameters at levels 1, 3 and 4 differing no more than 3 mm), and where the ascending aorta could be visualized from the suprasternal notch. The sample volume was placed at a level where the angle between the

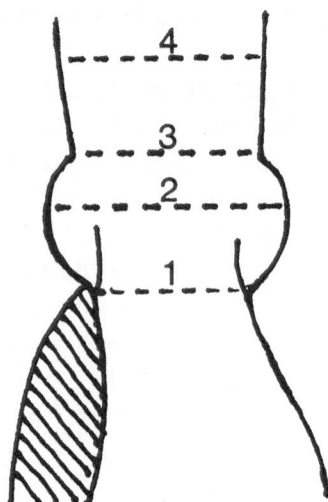

Figure 3. The levels chosen for diameter measurements. Level 1: Just below the aortic valve (the annulus). Level 2: The largest diameter of the Sinus of Valsalva. Level 3: Just distal to the sinus of Valsalva. Level 3: 2 cm distal to the sinus of Valsalva.

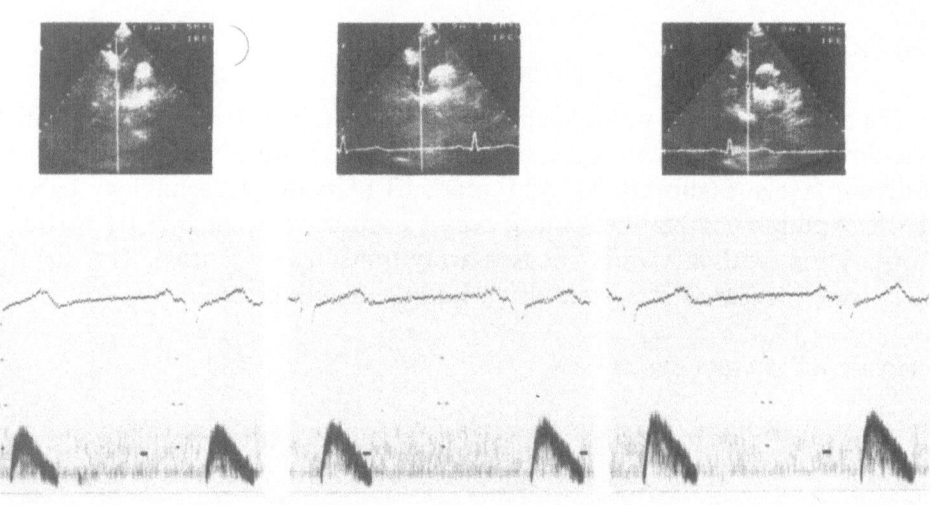

Figure 4. Velocity measurements in the ascending aorta. Left: Velocity recording at the outer curvature. Middle: Centerline velocity recording. Right: Velocity recording at the inner curvature.

ultrasound beam and the direction of flow was close to zero (Figure 4). The Irex III B instrument was used which allows pulsed and continuous wave Doppler recordings to be made simultaneously with imaging.

RESULTS

The smallest diameter was in all patients found at level 1 (mean 2.09 cm, ± 0.36 cm (± 1 SD)). The next smallest diameter, found at level 3, was 0 to 18 mm larger (mean 2.61 cm, ± 0.58 cm (± 1 SD)), giving up to 3 times larger cross sectional area than the area at level 1. The largest diameter was found at level 2 (mean 3.02 cm, ± 0.69 cm (± 1 SD)), while the diameter at level 4 was somewhat larger than the diameter at level 3 (mean 2.76 cm, ± 0.65 cm (± 1 SD)). Table I shows per cent increase in diameters from level 1 to levels 2, 3 and 4.

The criteria for making velocity measurements in the ascending aorta were met in 6 patients. The highest velocity was in all recorded at the inner curvature, and the integral of the velocity curve was 8–22% higher than the integral of the centerline velocity curve. The lowest velocity was measured at the outer curvature.

Table 1. Per cent increase in diameters at levels 2, 3, and 4 compared to level 1.

	Level 2	Level 3	Level 4
Range	14-86 %	0-75 %	10-88 %
Mean	45 %	25 %	34 %
	$p < 0.001$	$p < 0.001$	$p < 0.001$

DISCUSSION

Most experimental studies on the velocity profile in the ascending aorta conclude on a 'flat, but skewed' profile [6–8]. This means that the velocities increase steadily from one side of the aorta to the other. This was also found in 6 patients in this study. Seed and Wood [7] found that the centerline velocity was representative for the cross sectional mean velocity. In our patients, calculated CO was from just slightly higher (about 8% as in the paitent shown in Figure 4), and up to 22% higher when the highest velocities were integrated compared to when centerline velocities were integrated. Since the degree of skewing is different in different patients, and experimental findings indicate a variable skew when the contractility of the heart

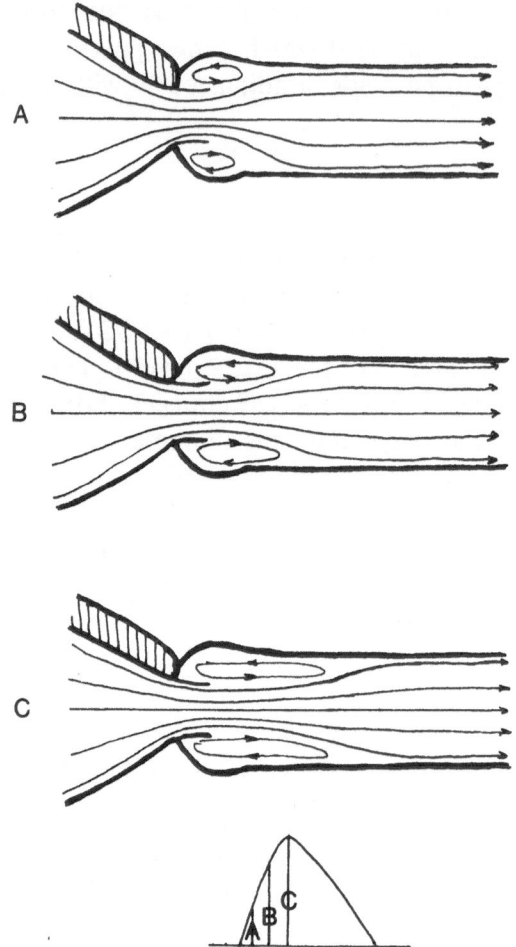

Figure 5. Expected flow patterns in the aortic root when there is a dilation of the aorta compared to the annulus. The patterns are indicated for three different parts of systole.

changes [8], this overestimation is impossible to correct for, except to use a combined echo/Doppler instrument and record centerline velocities. However, in our experience it was very difficult to adequately visualize the ascending aorta in adults.

Since the presence of a skewed profile explains only a fraction of the overestimation of CO we made when we first tried the method, we had to seek other explanations.

According to our diameter measurements, which showed that the smallest diameter was found at the aortic annulus and the largest at the Sius of Valsalva, there is in many patients a sudden expansion of the cross sectional flow area distal to the annulus. Therefore, flow patterns as indicated in Figure 2B and 2C is expected in these patients. The downstream extension of the central core of flow depends on the velocity of flow, and, accordingly, varies in pulsatile flow. In Figure 5 the expected flow patterns in a simplified (straight) model of the ascending aorta is shown. In a curved model the flow pattern is complicated by the skewing of the velocity profile. The highest velocities are found in the proximal aortic root, and will be similar to the velocities at the annulus. Theoretically then, if the highest velocities in the ascending aorta are recorded, only the cross sectional area of the annulus can be expected to give a good estimate of CO. This suggestion is supported by the findings of Ihlen [9]. The overestimation we experienced in estimating CO noninvasively, can now be explained. Since we originally used the diameter at level 3 to calculate CO, the overestimation should be proportional to the increase in cross sectional flow area from level 1 to level 3, which in this series was up to 206%.

One should note that these findings do not preclude CO estimations by velocity and diameter recordings distal to the aortic annulus. However, it then appears necessary to make the measurements at a level distal to the jet-like flow in the aortic root.

It can be concluded that the ascending aorta exhibits geometrical features that will have significant influence on the velocity profile. The velocity profile at all levels in the ascending aorta can therefore not be expected to be flat in an unselected group of patients.

REFERENCES

1. Magnin PA, Stewart JA, Myers S, von Ramm O, Kisslo JA: Combined Doppler and phased-array echocardiographic estimation of cardiac output. Circulation 63:388–392, 1981.
2. Goldberg SJ, Sahn DJ, Allen HD, Valdes-Cruz LM, Hoenecke H, Carnahan Y: Evaluation of pulmonary and systemic blood flow by 2-dimensional Doppler echocardiography using fast Fourier transform spectral analysis. Am J Cardiol 50:1394–1400, 1982.
3. Huntsman LL, Stewart DK, Barnes SR, Franklin SB, Colocousis JS, Hessel EA: Noninvasive Doppler determination of cardiac output in man. Clinical validation. Circulation 67:593–602, 1983.
4. Alverson DC, Eldridge M, Dillon T, Yabek SM, Berman W: Noninvasive pulsed Doppler determination of cardiac output in neonates and children. J Pediatr 101:46–50, 1982.
5. Hatle L, Angelsen B: Doppler ultrasound in cardiology (2nd ed.), pp 18–19, Chpt 2, Lea & Febiger, Philadelphia, 1985.
6. Farthing S, Peronneau P: Flow in the thoracic aorta. Cardiovasc Res 13:607–620, 1979.
7. Seed WA, Wood NB: Velocity patterns in the aorta. Cardiovasc Res 5:319–330, 1981.
8. Falsetti HL, Carrol RJ, Swope RD, Chen CJ: Turbuluent flow in the ascending aorta of dogs. Cardiovasc Res 17:427–436, 1983.
9. Ihlen H, Amlie JP, Dale J, Forfang K, Nitter-Hauge S, Otterstad JE, Simonsen S, Myhre E: Determination of cardiac output by Doppler echocardiography. Br Heart J 51:54–60, 1984.

6. Convenient monitoring of cardiac output and global left ventricular function by transcutaneous aortovelography – an update

L.H. LIGHT, G. CROSS, J.M. RAWLES and NEVA HAITES

INTRODUCTION

Doppler instrumentation is now widely used in cardiac diagnosis – often in association with echocardiography – by specialists in so-called 'Doppler Echocardiography'. A very different, but equally important, application of non-invasive Doppler technology is in circulatory patient monitoring and optimization of cardiac output, where beside measurements may be required at all hours of the day to follow changes in cardiac output and other variables reflecting cardiac function. A much less demanding technique is required in the latter application, as the measurement must be quick to perform by equipment which gives reliable results in the hands of the nurse or resident in immediate charge of the patient.

This chapter outlines applications of a Doppler 'non-echocardiographic' technique – Transcutaneous Aortovelography (TAV) – which has been developed specifically for this purpose [1]. Unlike some derived techniques, it was designed with the ergonomics of the bedside situation uppermost in mind: This implies recording 'blind' (i.e. without imaging facilities) a variable which can be measured reproducibly without requiring high precision in the aim of the ultrasound beam. The highest flow velocity present at any one time within the aortic curvature satisfies this requirement: When continuous wave ultrasound is used, the envelope of the spectrum automatically indicates this variable as long as the region of fastest flow ('mainstream' flow) is somewhere within the beam [2]. Using this principle, a wide beam can be advantageously used to provide tolerance in aim; it is also apparent from a display of the full spectrum (particularly the 'crispness' of the envelope) whether the above condition for a valid measurement has been satisfied [3]. This approach thus maximises the reliability and ease of measurement and in addition avoids the problems associated with pulsed Doppler ultrasound (velocity ambiguities, extra controls to be adjusted). On the other hand, although the transverse velocity profile is known to be fairly blunt throughout the thoracic aorta [4–6], the highest local – velocity, as given by the spectral envelope, will differ somewhat from the ideal (but formidably difficult) measurement – that of the spatial average speed of blood flow across the whole vascular cross-section. This is one of the several reasons why it is necessary to ascertain whether measurements by TAV – as indeed by any other technique – reflect volumetric blood flow sufficiently closely in practice for their intended applications.

Exhaustive studies have shown that the spectral envelope obtained from the aortic arch indeed tracks instantaneous flow rate and also cardiac output in any one subject with adequate accuracy: Results of multi-centre comparisons with serial invasive cardiac output measurements under a wide variety of circumstances are summarised below. Additional validation was provided by studies of interventions with known haemodynamic effect. Perhaps the most important practical evidence of reliability of the measurement, however, came from critical assessment, on a broad front, of the correspondence between the blood velocity measurements on one hand and patients' condition and progress on the other.

The results suggest that in spite of theoretical reservations [7], this simple technique (1) gives reliable and reasonably accurate quantitative information on serial changes in cardiac output, (2) allows the time-course of global left ventricular contraction to be visualised, (3) permits quantitation of moderate and severe aortic regurgitation and further (4) appears to give on its own (i.e. without knowledge of an adult patient's aortic diameter) a measure of the adequacy of his cardiac output. This unexpected finding seems to result from a developmental process which, as briefly discussed below, adjusts aortic dimensions throughout childhood to match the individual's growing cardiac output.

The technique is thus valuable in the emergency room and anaesthesia [8] as well as in intensive and coronary care. A further application, currently being studied with promising results, is the use of imposed and spontaneous hemodynamic perturbations, e.g. stress tests [9], arrythmias [10, 11], to assess left ventricular function. More than a decade's experience has now been gathered in various fields [12].

CLINICAL CONSIDERATIONS

Undesirable consequences of depressed cardiac output and peripheral hypoxia include (a) increased sympathetic tone, with its arrhythmogenic effect, (b) byproducts of anaerobic metabolism, which further depress cardiac function and (c) slowing of venous flow, with consequent tendency to

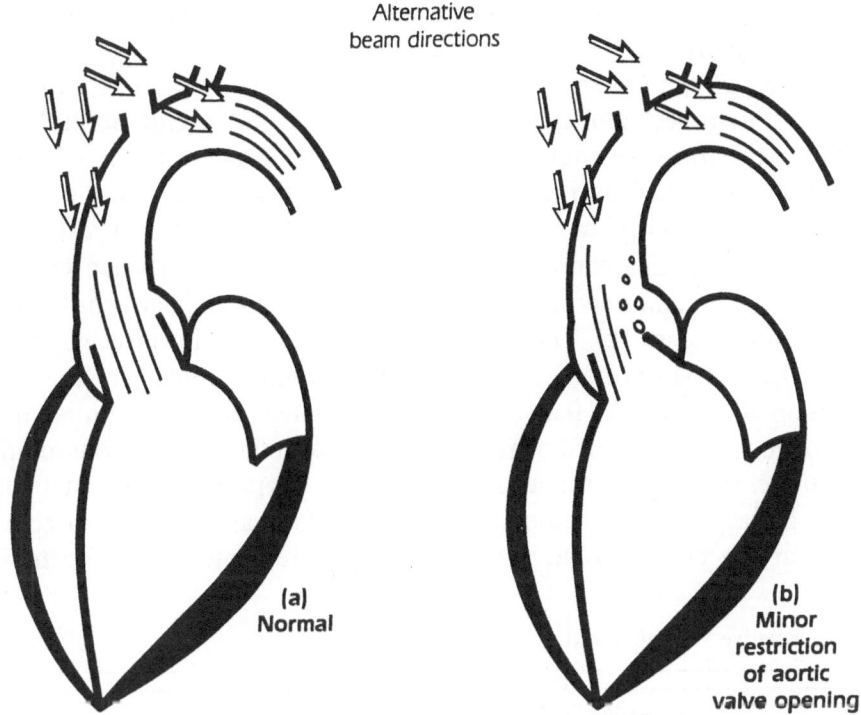

Figure 1. Assymetry of aortic valve opening can distort the normally blunt transverse velocity profile in the ascending aorta (a) into a near-trangular one (b). Doppler measurements in the aortic arch, where a blunt velocity profile is largely restored, yield velocity values which are more reliably representative of flow.

venous and sometimes also pulmonary thrombosis. Manipulation of cardiac output to keep it relatively high is feasible even after recent infarction [13]. This reduces morbidity and mortality; but cannot be safely employed without flow-orientated monitoring because of the unpredictability of individual response to interventions. Unless these involve volume expansion, success in raising cardiac output automatically leads to reduced pulmonary capillary pressure and alleviation of pulmonary oedema. Cardiac output monitoring is also valuable in intensive care (particularly when positive pressure ventilation is used), and in vascular surgery, where avoidance of low flow conditions can reduce the incidence of early graft failure by clotting. Unfortunately, established measurement techniques are invasive, costly, restricted to short-term use and require skilled handling to avoid complications and to give even moderately reliable results [14]. Their use is therefore confined to a minority of those who could benefit.

Transcutaneous Aortovelography was developed not only to meet the monitoring requirement fully, but also to permit assessment of global cardiac function, studies of circulatory physiology and the natural history cardiovascular disease.

The preferred site for measuring mainstream blood velocity is extracardiac (so as to reflect global ventricular function and useful output) and arguably in the *transverse* aorta: This is generally simplest and avoids both patient discomfort and problems due to complexities of the flow pattern in the ascending aorta [15]. In particular even a small asymmetrical restriction in aortic valve opening can convert the normally blunt transverse velocity profile in the *ascending aorta* (Figure 1a) into a near-triangular profile, with eddy shedding (Figure 1b). The highest velocities present, towards which the ultrasound beam is normally aimed, are then unrepresentative of the total flow within the lumen so that this is overestimated. Whether similar flow profile distortions result from asymmetric (diskinetic) contractions of the left ventricle, requires examination. As they can alternate with normal contractions in patients with regional ischemia, coronary artery spasm or ectopic foci, varying errors would result from measurements in the ascending aorta.

Table 1. Quatitative validation trials against reference techniques

TRIAL	DEVIATION from exact agreement or proportionality (s. d. as % of mean)	TOTAL RANGE COVERED	TRIAL CENTRES
REPRODUCIBILITY – (4 trials) within – observer agreement between – observer agreement	6·6 % 7·3 %	42 subjects, aged 3-67 yrs. 14 observers, including 8 inexperienced.	Brompton Hosp./C.R.C. Bristol Royal Infirmary Sefton G. Hosp., Liverpool, England.
Proportionality against acetylene CARDIAC OUTPUT during exercise	11 %	C.O. = 7-22 l/min (13 normal/athl. subjects)	Field Physiol. Lab, N.I.M.R. England
Proportionality against intra-aortic BLOOD VELOCITY measurement	6 %	Vpk = 48 to 120cm/s (8 IHD patients)	Northwick Park Hosp. /C.R.C. England
Proportionality against green dye measurement of STROKE VOLUME	13 %	S.V. = 20 to 160 ml. (20 IHD patients)	Northwick Park Hosp. /C.R.C.
Proportionality against thermo-dilution CARDIAC OUTPUT (reproducibility = 5% S.D.)	9·7 %	C.O. = 2.5 to 10 l/min. (14 critically ill patients)	Whipps Cross Hosp. (I.T.U.) London, England
Proportionality against thermo-dilution CARDIAC OUTPUT	11·8 %	C.O. = 2.9 to 9 l/min. (5 cardiomyopathy pts.)	Clinica Fisiologia. Pisa, Italy.
Proportionality against thermo-dilution CARDIAC OUTPUT	8·9 %	C.I. = 1.7 to 3.7 l/min/m^2 (11 IHD patients)	Univ. Hospital, Munich F.D.R.

By the time flow reaches the distal part of the arch (where near-inline insonation is again practicable), such flow disturbances are decaying and the normal blunt profile is largely restored. In addition to yielding better consistency, signal acquisition in the arch is also often easier and free of discomfort for the patient, while turbulence persisting to the arch points to more significant flow obstruction. Despite potential variations in the ~20% flow loss to head and arms, arch measurements have shown very acceptable correlation with cardiac output (Table 1) over a wide range of clinical conditions.

Flow in the aortic arch can be insonated from the suprasternal notch in >90% of subjects, with an angle shallow enough to give quantitative velocity information with good reproducibility (5-7% s.d.) [14, 16]. A brief description of the technique [17] is followed by a summary of its validation as a measure of cardiac output and indications in clinical practice.

THE TECHNIQUE

A relatively broad ultrasound beam is directed from the suprasternal notch to intersect flow in the distal part of the aortic arch near-tangentially. This is achieved with the help of the Doppler sounds and the appearance of the real-time recordings, which present a grey-scale spectral analysis (sonogram) of all the Doppler shifts present in the signal backscattered by blood moving anywhere in the beam. A crisp envelope to the spectrum of *negative* Doppler shifts [1] (which originate in blood *receding* from the transducer and thus exclude signals from the carotid and subclavian arteries) indicates quantitatively the instantaneous value of the highest velocity present anywhere in the lumen of the transverse aorta (= 'mainstream aortic blood velocity'). The potential accuracy is $\pm 5\%$ providing that the minimum angle between beam and flow is less than 26° – a condition which seems to be satisfied in practice.

For convenience and to provide clinical documentation, the instrument produces on-line hard copy grey-scale recordings of the spectrum on inexpensive paper (Figure 2). A filter bank with 32 analogue channels is currently used in the direction-resolving spectral analyser, but FFT or chirp-Z techniques [18] could equally well be employed. As is desirable in a technique for routine use by a variety of personnel, such recordings confirm that the signals picked up are adequate and give visual discrimination between aortic signals and artefacts. After typically two hours of training, medical and paramedical staff have found it simple to produce trustworthy measurements in the majority of patients. (With alternative forms of signal processing and display, much greater demands are made on the operator and interpreter to obtain valid data).

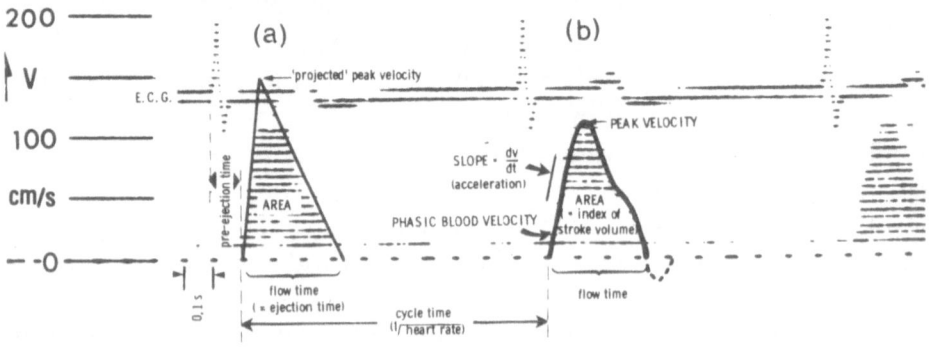

Figure 2. Normal TAV blood velocity recording from aortic arch, with corecorded ECG. Some hemodynamic variables which can be extracted by triangular approximation (a) or curve following (b) are indicated.

Figure 2 shows a normal recording of arch flow velocity by Transcutaneous Aortovelograph, with co-recorded ECG. Only negative Doppler shifts (from receding flow) are displayed on the range shown. (An alternative bidirectional range is used for showing reverse velocities in aortic regurgitation). A distinct outline to the complexes verifies that mainstream flow has indeed been insonated and shows its instantaneous velocity. The area of a complex (the systolic velocity integral) equals 'stroke distance' (the axial distance travelled by mainstream flow during a beat) and is a measure of stroke volume [19]. 'Minute distance', the product of stroke distance and heart rate, provides a measure of cardiac output: an alternative measure (equal to minute distance $\div 60$) is mean (time-averaged) velocity, the area divided by cycle time.

Quantitative data extraction is conveniently performed on a dedicated digitizer/microprocessor combination, which is programmed to accept triangular approximations (a) or curve-following (b). Its print-out gives average and beat-by-beat values for the above measures as well as peak velocity, early systolic acceleration (mean gradient of up-slope), heart rate, systolic time intervals and three waveform shape indices which characterize the time-course of left ventricular volumetric contraction and offer diagnostic information [27].

The utility of the direct hard copy presentation for dynamic investigations is illustrated in Figure 3. This shows (a) an atypical 'diving reflex' response: instead of the usual progressive bradycardia, one subject reacted to ice-cold water sprayed on his face with the arrhythmia shown, which culminated in 4 seconds' asystole. Figure 3 (b) illustrates stroke volume changes during the Valsalva manoeuvre: Beat-to-beat changes in stroke distance are shown in 5 young adults. The continuous hard-copy recordings produced by the instru-

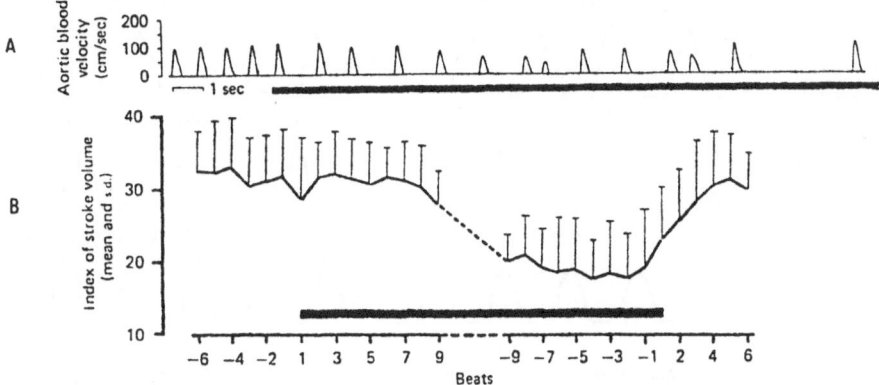

Figure 3. Dynamic studies: Beat-by-beat changes resulting from the diving reflex in one individual (a) and stroke distance changes (in cm) during the Valsalva maneuver in 5 students (b) are shown. Bars indicate duration of maneuvers.

ment are valuable also in studies of arrythmias (see Section 9) and the dynamics of drug action.

QUANTITATION OF CARDIAC OUTPUT TRENDS

A number of studies, in which stroke distance and minute distance (or its equivalent, mean indicated velocity) were compared with reference measurements of stroke volume and cardiac output respectively (Table 1), have confirmed that the measured blood velocity is a good index of volumetric blood flow in the systemic circulation in any one subject over a wide range of conditions [20–23]. The results (s.d. from exact proportionality with other measurements of cardiac output = 9–13%) suggest that TAV allows ratios of serial cardiac output values to be measured with an accuracy which is of the same order as that of invasive techniques in clinical use: Cardiac output changes ~15% should be detectable with >95% confidence. (Even closer correlation may be expected with blood flow into the descending aorta, often the most direct determinant of survival).

In spite of systematic errors, such as those introduced by measuring in the aortic arch *, these results do not seem inferior to multicentre experience with much more demanding Doppler techniques applied to the ascending aorta. This may result from the intrinsically high reproducibility of TAV measurement and the simpler flow conditions in the aortic arch, which may

---

* This error is often overestimated; thus, a 20% in the proportion of flow going to head and arms will cause only 5% misestimation of change in cardiac output.

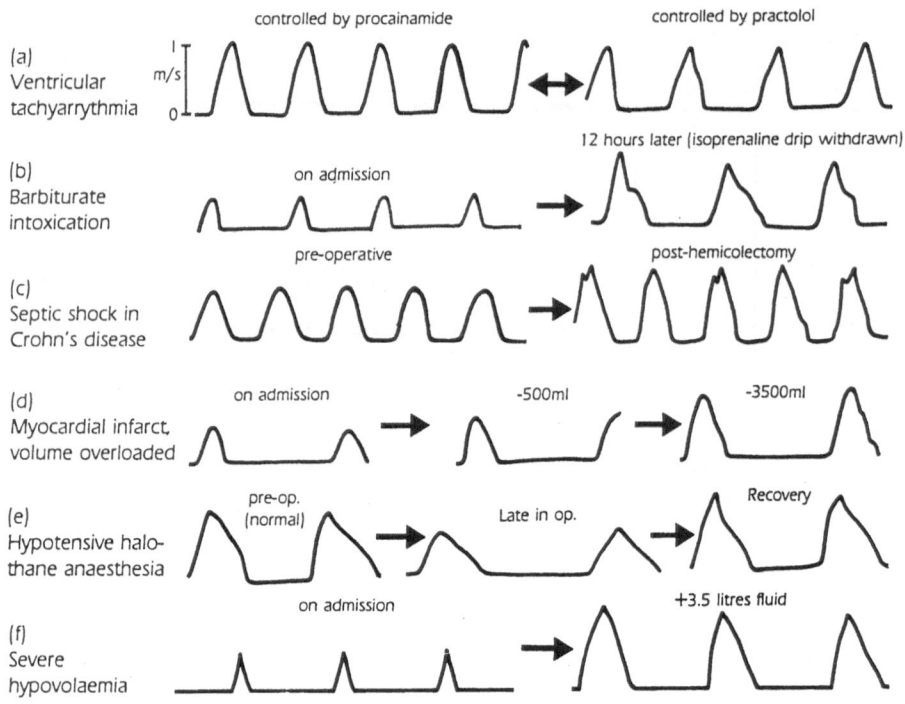

Figure 4. Serial TAV recordings in six patiens, illustrating applications in cardiology, intensive care and anaesthesia. (a) Anti-arrhythmic therapy: Minimum effective doses of two anti-arrhythmic agents used alternately are seen to produce different degrees of myocardial depression. (b) Barbiturate overdose: Initial and final recordings from patient who arrived moribund. Isoprenaline dosage was repeatedly readjusted during recovery in the light of TAV readings. (c) Late septic shock: Waveform in deteriorating patient suggested toxemia – other signs were masked by steroids. Improved cardiovascular state and responsiveness to inotropes after major eleventh-hour surgery. (d) A.M.I., volume overload: Cautious TAV-monitored withdrawal of 0.5 l blood increased stroke distance noticeably (~ 15 %). Further improvement (also in pulmonary oedema) after overnight withdrawal of 3 l fluid by dialysis. (e) Deep halothane anesthesia: Low acceleration and stroke volume resulting from myocardial depression without reflex sympathetic arousal during deep halothane anesthesia. (f) Severe hypovolemia: Normal circulatory state restored by 3.5 l infusion over 5 hours. (Courtesy of Drs. G.C. Hanson, Whipps Cross Hospital and D.C. White, Northwick Park Hospital).

offset the theretical advantages gained by measuring in the ascending aorta and painstakingly finding the optimum measurement point there.

In principle, the accuracy with which flow changes can be measured should be improved if simultaneous echosonic measurements are taken of vascular cross-section (or at least vessel diameter). It is far from clear, however, that this complication is worthwhile. The dimensional variations are often much smaller in practice than the reproducibility with which they can be measured at the bedside. Our own angiographic study thus suggests that the reduction in aortic arch diameter for a 45 mm fall in blood pressure rarely exceeds 5% in adults (Wilkins and Light, unpublished). The inclusion of the dimensional measurement may therefore actually decrease accuracy while greatly detracting from the otherwise excellent effort/benefit ratio of the primary blood velocity measurement.

Transcutaneous aortovelography has indeed been found to be of particular value in guiding therapy in intensive/coronary care, where it has allowed drug dosage, blood volume, pacing rate and settings of ventilators or balloon pumps to be optimised [17, 24–28]. Figure 4 illustrates by serial recordings from six patients with different conditions how the shape and size of complexes gives feedback on the effect of therapy on the manner of left ventricular contraction and on stroke volume respectively. This allows assessment of the appropriateness and volumetric effect of interventions, and opens the way to therapy which – though perhaps not widely applicable – can be seen to benefit the individual patient (Figure 4d). The initial waveform, which was normal only in (e), further often gives clues to the underlying abnormality and suggests the degree of circulatory depression [severe in the low-output conditions (b), (d) and (f)].

In contrast to catheter techniques, Doppler gives flow-directed information from first contact with the patient through perhaps protracted treatment to long-term follow-up.

ABNORMALITIES IN ABSOLUTE CARDIAC OUTPUT

Unexpectedly, clinical users found that the blood velocity recordings on their own (i.e. without reference to aortic dimensions) appeared to reflect the degree of depression or elevation of cardiac output. (This – rather than its absolute value – is the information required clinically when the severity of circulatory disturbance is to be assessed). Thus, in Figure 5 mean stroke distances from groups of patients with anaemia, hypertension, uncomplicated myocardial infarction, atrial fibrillation, cardiac failure or who were pregnant are compared with age-matched normal values [29]. The diagnosis of patients in different groups were 'pure', i.e. patients in the atrial fibrillation group did not have hypertension or cardiac failure. Myocardial infarction patients were convalescing after an uncomplicated course and had normal ejection fractions where measured. Most of the patients with hypertension were being treated with beta-blocking drugs. The differences in minute distance from normal are in the same direction and of the same magnitude as would be expected of a measure of cardiac output, and the results are fully consistent with previously published work where volumetric cardiac output has been measured by conventional invasive techniques in patients with these diagnoses. The compensatory effect of increased heart rate in the

82

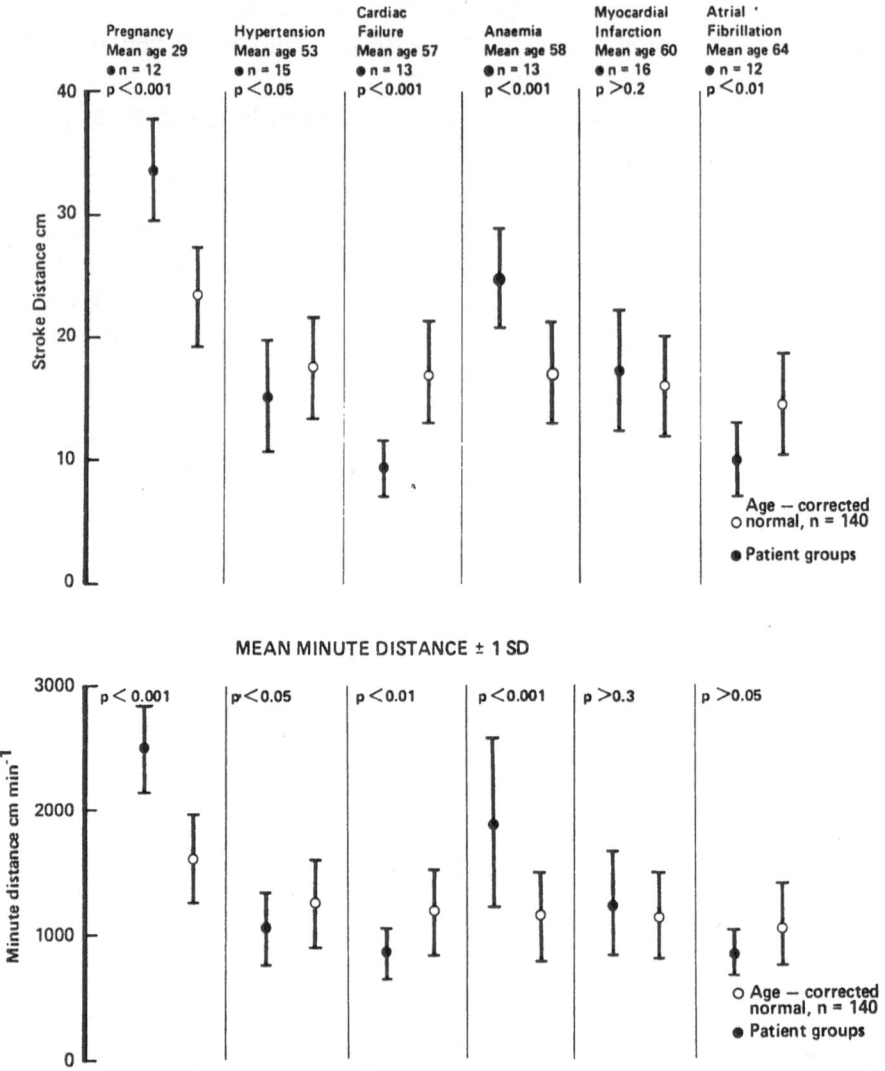

MEAN STROKE DISTANCE ± 1 SD

Figure 5. Stroke distance and minute distance in 6 patient groups for which mean ages are given, compared with age-matched normal values. The diagnoses of patients in different groups were 'pure', i.e. patients in the atrial fibrillation group did not have hypertension or cardiac failure. Myocardial infarction patients were convalescing after an uncomplicated course and had normal ejection fractions where measured. Most of the patients with hypertension were being treated with beta-blocking drugs. The compensatory effect of heart rate in the two low-stroke volume conditions is evident from a comparison of the two diagrams. (Mean heart rates in the 6 patient groups were 74, 68, 91, 75, 71, and 84 respectively).

two conditions with the lowest stroke distances, heart failure and atrial fibrillation, is evident from a comparison of the two diagrams. Thus, in heart failure there is a 43% reduction of stroke distance compared with

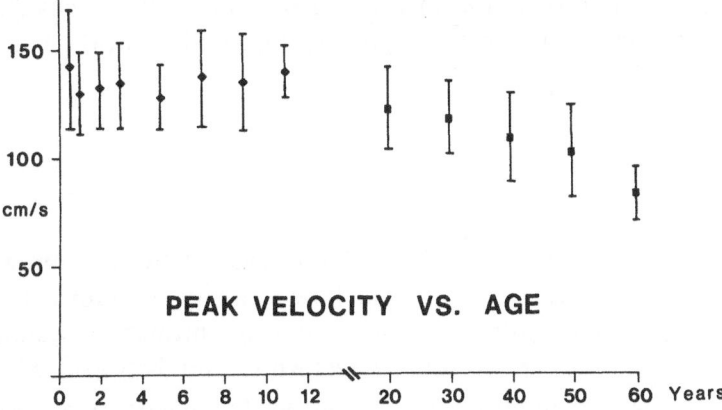

Figure 6. Peak systolic blood velocity (mean ± s.d.) in normal supine resting children and adults as a function of age. (Children's results by courtesy of Drs. J. Beardshaw and E. Shinebourne, Brompton Hodspital, London).

age-adjusted normal values, but the reduction of minute distance is only 28% because of an increase of the mean heart rate to 91. Stroke distance therefore reflects left ventricular function, and minute distance provides a measure of overall cardiovascular function including the ability of the circulatory reflexes to increase heart rate to compensate for reduced stroke volume.

What is the rationale of this finding that stroke volume/cardiac output abnormality can be derived from aortic blood velocities without knowledge of the individual's vascular cross-section? In searching for an explanation, we have found much evidence for a growth-controlling mechanism which continuously and sensitively increases aortic cross-sectional area throughout the individual's development period so that his resting cardiac output, be it large or small, is carried within the same, relatively narrow, normal range of velocities. Thus peak mainstrem velocity is virtually constant with age in normal children between ½ and 12 years and has a spread of only 14% s.d. [17, 30] (Figure 6). This adaptive process has the effect of biologically 'normalising' young adults' basal blood velocities – particularly peak velocity – into a relatively tight range. With maturation, however, this capacity for adaptation seems largely or entirely lost, with the effect that both acute and relatively chronic departures from normal cardiac output are marked in adults by corresponding departures of blood velocity from the normal range for the appropriate age [19, 27]. The gradual progressive decrease in normal blood velocities throughout adult life is largely attributable to passive aortic dilatation [37], and is shown in Figure 6 for peak velocity and in Figure 9 for mean velocity and minute distance; this must be borne in mind when assessing the degree of abnormality in adults. *In children*, caution is required in the interpretation of other than acute velocity changes, as the time-scale on which the above regulatory mechanism works has not been established.

INFORMATION IN THE PULSATILE WAVEFORM

If, as is normally the case, all the blood ejected by the contracting left ventricle enters the aorta, the aortic flow velocity waveform reflects the time-course of global ventricular volume change throughout systole. Differences between flow and velocity waveforms, and between those in the ascending aorta and in the transverse aorta, are relatively small. Studies, which have become practicable for the first time with the development of this non-invasive tool, have shown that the waveform varies considerably with physiological state and over the spectrum of disease [27]. Indices derived from the whole waveform are often more informative than isolated variables, such as early systolic acceleration or left ventricular ejection time. These can of course also be derived from the waveform, but need cautious interpretation because of their high sensitivity to sympathetic tone [7]. Figure 4 gives several examples of abnormal waveforms. Initial observations often provide diagnostic clues, while shape changes supplement those of stroke distance in providing feedback on the circulatory effect of interventions.

All the waveforms illustrated show a smooth outline, indicating that flow is laminar or minimally disturbed. The duration of major flow disturbances, as seen for example in aortic stenosis, is indicated by irregularity of the spectral envelope [27]. Excess backflow, allowing quantitative estimation of regurgitant fraction [23, 27], is evident on a bi-directional range in aortic regurgitation of greater than mild degree. (The distorted transverse velocity profile, with which *low* rates of backflow are often carried, probably accounts for sporadic failures to assess minor degrees of regurgitation).

PHYSIOLOGICAL STUDIES

Twenty-four hour studies over 12 subject-days have shown that minute distance in fit young men is raised after meals by some 24% [31]. Waveform changes indicating changes in inotropic state after meals and during night rest were also seen. The effect of ventilatory manoeuvres and of some neurocirculatory reflexes has been examined [32] (Figure 8).

The response to isometric exercise (Vpk ↓, Vav ↑) [33] differs from that to dynamic exercise (Vpk ↓, Vav ↓). In supine bicycling with progressively increasing workload, stroke distance rises to a plateau 23 ± 7 (s.d.) % above control already at fairly low loads (~ 75 W) [34]. Cardiac output variations throughout normal and twin [35] pregnancies are under study, as is the effect of recumbent posture in late pregnancy [36].

LEFT VENTRICULAR FUNCTION

Major abnormality of left ventricular function is sometimes apparent from inspection of the waveform at rest. Pronounced rounding of the normally near-triangular complexes and/or a shift of the peak to the right indicate incoordinate contraction or more diffuse impairment of contractility. If function is severely depressed, resting stroke distance usually becomes subnormal. The potential contribution of extra-cardiac factors which influence ventricular function must however always be borne in mind [7]: thus, electrolyte disturbance, circulating toxic factors, inotrophic agents and hypovolemia also affect the waveform and/or stroke distance. While they sometimes result in characteristic waveform patterns (e.g. the short, sharp spikes of uncomplicated hypovolemia, Figure 4e), the operation of extrinsic factors will generally be evident from the clinical context.

To demonstrate and evaluate *lesser* degrees of abnormality, perturbation of the circulatory state is generally required [7]. Of the various imposed stress tests, evaluation of the response of stroke distance and other velocity variables to supine dynamic exercise has progressed furthest. As shown in another chapter, depression of the above-mentioned normal response of stroke distance to exercise correlates well with ejection fraction in coronary artery disease [34] and indeed provides primary evidence of organ failure to cope with a normal stress. These findings may well lead to a test of mechanical function complementary to stress electrocardiography. The response to changing pacing rate and the contribution of timely atrial contraction to stroke volume [28] is also examined elsewhere in this volume. Here we shall outline a method of analyzing the beat-to-beat changes occurring in atrial fibrillation which yields particularly detailed information on left ventricular function:

ANALYSIS OF SEQUENTIAL RECORDINGS IN ATRIAL FIBRILLATION

Atrial fibrillation can be considered as a naturally occurring stress test in which wide beat-to-beat alterations in ventricular rate result in dissociated changes of pre-load, after-load and contractility to which the left ventricle responds with a variable stroke volume and stroke distance. Multiple regres-

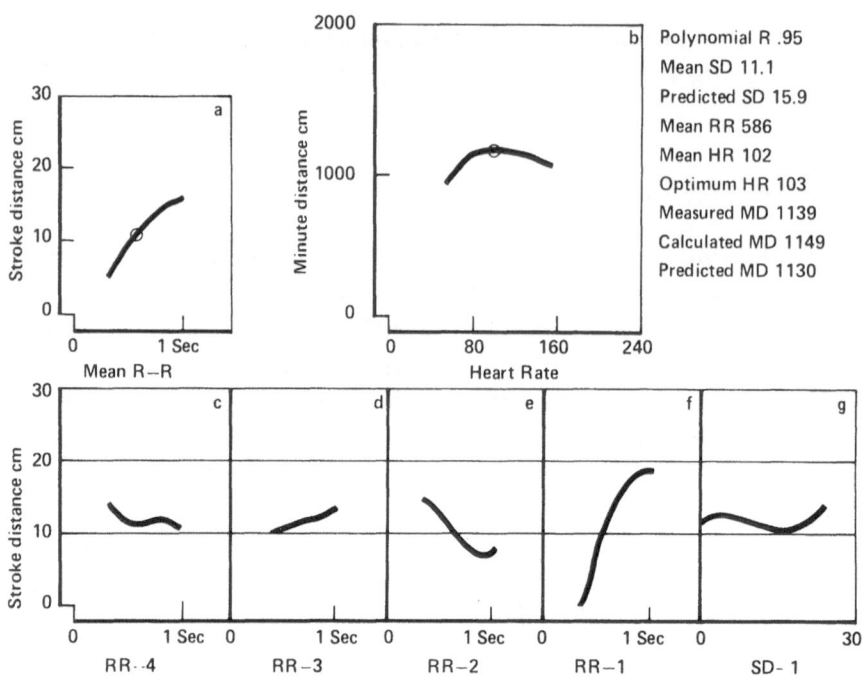

Figure 7. Computer plot of multiple regression analysis of Doppler ultrasound recording from a patient with atrial fibrillation and good left ventricular function.

sion analysis of a sequence of 2–300 heart beats recorded by aortovelography together with the ECG, enables the beat-to-beat variation of stroke distance to be described mathematically in terms of the previous stroke distance and 4 previous R-R intervals [11]. The unique multiple regression equation that results can be considered as an expression of left ventricular function, which may be manipulated to yield hemodynamic information.

Figure 7 shows a computer plot derived from multiple regression analysis of 200 heart beats from a patient with atrial fibrillation and good left ventricular function. This multiple correlation coefficient is 0.95 indicating that most of the variation in stroke distance can be described in terms of preceding events. The lower part of the figure, (c) to (g), relates stroke distance to previous stroke distance (SD-1), and 4 previous R-R intervals (RR-1 to RR-4), each section of the graph showing the independent effect of altering the determinant over the range of values encountered, the other 4 determinants being assigned mean values in the multiple regression equation. The independent relationship between stroke distance and the previous stroke distance (SD-1, Figure 7g) reflects the sensitivity of the left ventricle to afterload, which in this case is not significant. The relationship between

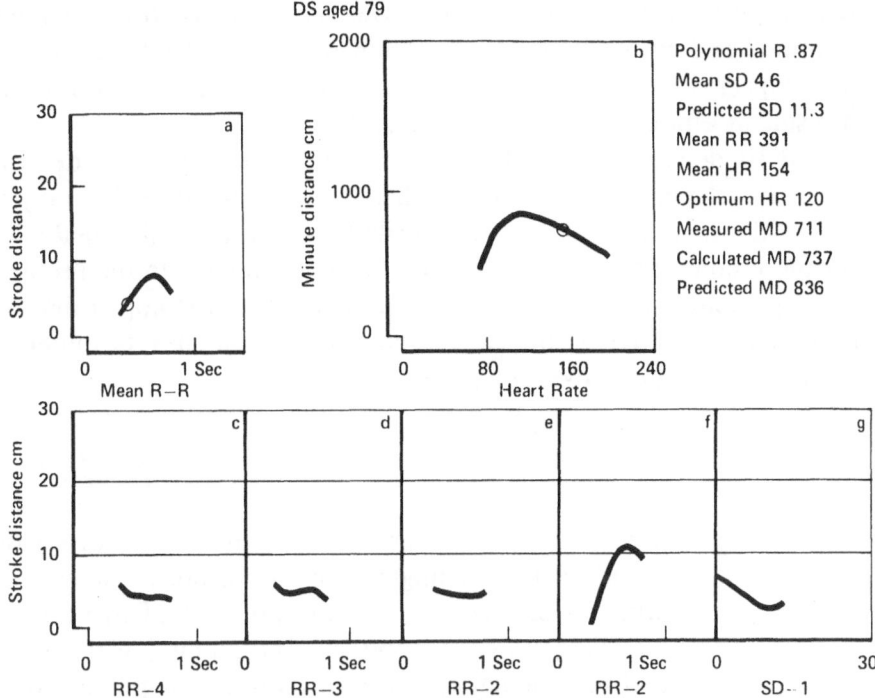

Figure 8. As Figure 7 from patient with poor left ventricular fucntion.

stroke distance and the previous R-R interval, related to left ventricular filling time and preload, effectively maps the Frank-Starling relationship (RR-1, Figure 7f), while the relationship to the second previous R-R interval (RR-2, Figure 7e) is related to changes in contractility mediated by the force-frequency effect.

If all 4 R-R intervals are altered simultaneously within the multiple regression equation this is equivalent to altering the mean R-R interval. The effect of this on stroke distance is seen in Figure 7a, and this is replotted in Figure 7b to show the predicted effect of a change of heart rate (HR) on minute distance (MD). This patient's mean ventricular rate, indicated by the small circle, is optimal for maximizing minute distance (cardiac output) which is normal at 1139 cm compared with an age-adjusted value for sinus rhythm of 1130 cm. Mean stroke distance is substantially below the predicted normal value, but increased ventricular rate provides perfect compensation.

Figure 8 is a similar computer plot from an older patient with poor left ventricular function. That the left ventricle is sensitive to afterload is shown by the negative slope of Figure 8g, and there is no increase of contractility with shortening of the R-R interval in Figure 8e. Mean stroke distance is only 41 % of predicted and in spite of a tachycardia, minute distance is not restored to the predicted normal value. However, mean ventricular rate is supra-optimal and reduction to the optimum rate of 120 beats per minute would be expected to normalize output though any further reduction of rate would result in a precipitous fall of minute distance.

The analysis described above besides providing a mathematical description of left ventricular function suggests therapeutic approaches that may be of value in the management of atrial fibrillation. However, the method is perhaps more noteworthy as an example of a new approach to the problem of obtaining hemodynamic information noninvasively; it is hoped that the technique may be adapted so that similar information may be obtained from patients with sinus rhythm.

LIMITATIONS

Quantitation is not reliable when a ragged outline over much of systole shows sustained flow turbulence, as might result from aortic stenosis or aortic dissection. Caution is also required in the presence of mediastinal tumors which can cause progressive compression and kinking of the aorta. In a small percentage of the population noninvasive access is prevented by the protrusion of lung into the path of the beam. The alternative atraumatic approach by oesophageal transducer is particularly suitable during anaesthesia and in unconscious patients.

CONCLUSIONS

Transcutaneous Aortovelography, a noninvasive Doppler ultrasound technique of measuring mainstream flow velocity in the aorta, has made available a variety of flow-related data on the central circulation by a procedure which is no more difficult than the inflated-cuff measurement of blood pressure in most subjects. Several features of the technique, such as the grey-scale spectral recorder and wide-beam probe make the acquisition of trustworthy data relatively undemanding: inadequate recordings are plainly visible.

In trials TAV has been shown to provide reliable and relatively accurate measurements of fractional changes in central flow and to give a useful indication of the degree of depression or elevation of an adult's cardiac output. These are the two purposes for which clinical cardiac output measurements are performed outside the pediatric field. Indeed, cardiac output, *as such,* is never required for clinical decision making. Normalization, is, for example, attempted by calculation of cardiac index, is essential. TAV conveniently and accurately satisfied the commoner requirement for which cardiac output is currently measured – that for quantitating (as a ratio) serial changes in stroke volume and cardiac output – and thereby facilities precise direction of therapy. The remaining indications for cardiac output measurement are to assess (1) whether symptoms originate in excessive flow demands on the heart (anemia, thyrotoxicosis, vasodilator shock) and (2) the seriousness of low output conditions and urgency for intervention. For these latter purposes, the ratio between the patient's present cardiac output and his normal, basal value should ideally be known. Thanks to the developmental normalization of mainstream blood velocities, which was discovered during the above studies, a useful estimate of the degree of cardiac output abnormality is obtained by recording a newly admitted adult's blood velocity and comparing his minute distance with the normal range for his age. Note that this approach eliminates the need for echosonic measurement error – and yet seems to yield useful quantitative information on cardiac output. In contrast to the conventional procedure, in which cardiac index must be derived after calculation of cardiac output from velocity and diameter information, no adjustment for body size is required. The biological normalization process eliminates, as it were, the need to calculate cardiac index in order to make some approximate compensation for body size.

Although both clinical requirements are thus satisfied by ratios obtainable by TAV, the absence of a quotable value for cardiac output in litres/minute may be thought to present problems in communicating results to others. An acceptable alternative is to quote measured velocity values and other 'linear' measures such as stroke and minute distance. When quantitative Doppler observations become more frequent in the literature – as they surely will – their implications will become generally understood [14, 27]. The close agreement between the normal velocity statistics obtained in three centres in the U.K. with different TAV instruments demonstrates that reproducible population norms exist (Figure 9). Some differences may however be expected between values obtained with different Doppler techniques because of variations in sample volume and details of signal processing. The possibility of ethnic variation in the normal range must also be explored.

The pulsatile waveform, which reflects the global (volumetric) manner of left ventricular contraction, often conveys information on myocardial condition and the effect of extrinsic influences on the myocardium. Diagnostic information is also given on certain cardiac lesions, and moderate/severe aortic regurgitation can be quantitated. Quantitative assessment of the response to various stimuli or stresses has applications in grading global myocardial function. The technique thus complements echocardiography which primarily gives information on regional function. In practical patient management, TAV has provided valuable feedback of response to therapy and has allowed this to be optimized.

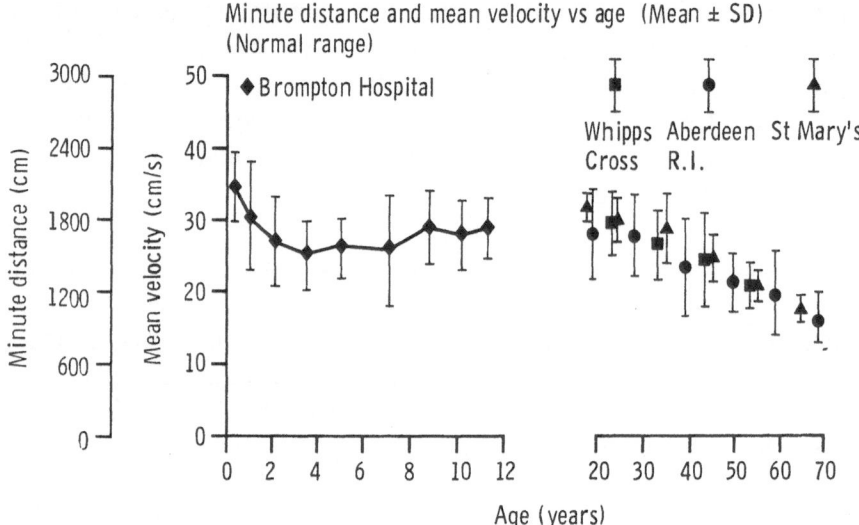

Figure 9. Minute distance and time-averaged mainstream blood velocity – in normal supine children and adults as a function of age. The St. Mary's results (n = 66, courtesy Dr. M. Salmasi) were obtained by triangular approximation, those from Whipps Cross Hospital (n = 120, courtesy Drs. A. Buchthal and G.C. Hanson) and Aberdeen Royal Infirmary (n = 140) by curve-following.

We conclude that TAV largely satisfies the clinical need for flow-orientated information on the central circulation. In addition, the wide applicability of this noninvasive technique and the relative ease with which it gives physiological and pathophysiological data on central blood flow should do much to advance our knowledge in this vital field.

ACKNOWLEDGEMENTS

We thank the many clinicians who have helped in the trials and have contributed greatly to the interpretation of TAV observations.

REFERENCES

1. Light LH, Cross G: In: Blood flow measurement. Roberts C (ed.), Sector Publishing, London, 60 1972.
2. Light LH: Non-invasive ultrasonic technique for observing flow in the human aorta. Nature 224:1119, 1969.
3. Light LH: In: Cardiovascular applications of ultrasound. Reneman RD (ed.), North Holland Publ, Amsterdam, pp 335, 1974.
4. Schultz DL, Tunstall Pedoe DS, Lee G de J, Gunning AJ, Bellhouse BJ: In: Circulatory and

respiratory mass transport. Wolstenholme GEW, Knight J (eds.), J & A Churchill Ltd., London, p 172, 1969.

5. Nerem RM: In: Cardiovascular flow dynamics and measurements. Hwang NHC, Normann NA (eds.), Univeristy Park Press, Baltimore, p 191, 1977.

6. Farthing S, Peronneau P: Cardiovascular Research 13:607, 1979.

7. Light LH: British Heart Journal 38:433, 1976.

8. Newman B: Anaesthesia 37:270, 1982.

9. Salmasi SNA et al.: Proceedings of the third meeting of the world federation for ultrasound in medicine and biology, Brighton, 1982.

10. Rawles J, Haites N, Barclay R, Krikler D, Rowland E: European Heart J 4:Suppl E, 97, 1983.

11. Rawles J, Haites N: Proc. 6th Nordic Meeting on Med & Biol Eng Biological Engineering Society, London, 1984.

12. Rawles J, Haites N: British J of Hospital Medicine 31:292, 1984.

13. Forrester JS, Dimond GA, Swan HJC: Am J Cardiol 39:137, 1977.

14. Haites NE, McLennan FM, Mowat DHR, Rawles JM: Lancet 2:1025, 1977.

15. Skjaerpe T: Influence of the geometry of the ascending aorta upon the velocity profile. In: Cardiac Doppler Diagnosis, vol II. Spencer MP (ed.), Martinus Nijhoff, Dordrecht, p 65, this volume, 1986.

16. Fraser CB, Light LH, Shinebourne EA, Buchtal A, Healy MJR, Beardshaw JA: European Journal of Cardiology 4:181, 1976.

17. Cross G, Light LH: Biomedical Engineering 9:464, 1974.

18. Klepper J: in Volume 1.

19. Mowat DHR, Haites NE, Rawles JM: Cardiovascular Research 17:75, 1983.

20. Sequeira RF, Light LH, Cross G, Raftery EB: British Heart Journal 38:443, 1976.

21. Brotherhood J, Cross G, Hanson GC, Light LH, Sequeira RF: Journal of Physiology 281:4, 1978.

22. Distante A, Moscarelli E, Rovai D, L'Abbate A: Journal of Nuclear Medicine and Allied Sciences 24:171, 1980.

23. v Arnim T, Bolte HD: Zeitschrift fur Kardiologie, 71, 596, 1982.

24. Buchthal A, Hanson GC, Peisach AR: British Heart Journal 38:451, 1976.

25. Bilton AH, Hanson GC: In: Doppler Ultrasound in the Study of the Central and Peripheral Circulation. Woodcock JP, Sequeira RF (eds.), Bristol Univeristy Pringing Unit, Bristol, p 39, 1978.

26. Sequeira RF: ibid, p 30.

27. Light LH, Sequeira RF, Bilton A, Hanson GC: J Nuclear Med and Allied Sciences 23:137, 1979.

28. Moscarelli E et al.: British Journal of Radiology 55:481, 1982.

29. Haites NE, McLennan FM, Mowat DHR, Rawles JM: British Heart Journal. In pres.

30. Light LH: Journal of Physiology 285:17, 1978.

31. Appelhoff J, Fentrop T, Hartung S, Light LH, Stelling R: Journal of Physiology 289:26, 1979.

32. Light LH, Low HS: J Physiol 315:19, 1981.

33. Bloom DS, Light LH: In: Cardiac Dynamics. Baan J, Arntzenius AC, Yellin EL (eds.), Martinus Nijhoff, The Hague, p 381, 1980.

34. Salmasi A-M: Chapter 7, this volume.

35. Campbell DM, Campbell AJ, McLennan FM, Haites NE, Rawles JM: Acta Genetici et Gemellologiae. In press.

36. Newman B, Derrington C, Dore C: Anaesthesia 38:332, 1983.

37. Furukawa et al.: Jap Heart J 17:468, 1976.

7. Exercise Doppler cardiography

ABDUL-MAJEED SALMASI

INTRODUCTION

Electrocardiographic stress testing is one of the most important non-invasive cardiac investigations mainly to diagnose ischemic heart disease. Although Bousfield was the first to detect ECG changes during stress in 1918 [1], Master and Jaffe [2] introduced this idea as a diagnostic tool in 1941. Since then this technique has been in increasing use, with modifications, in order to increase its value for the diagnosis of coronary artery disease. Information on myocardial performance is of value in evaluating the prognosis of a disease process, especially in coronary artery disease. Recent emphasis has been to the study of myocardial function during exercise. Several attempts have theefore been made using different non-invasive methods [3, 4] but these were either expensive to run and involved complicated technologies, difficult to repeat or impossible to pursue during exercise [5].

THE TECHNIQUE

The continuous-wave Doppler technique of transcutaneous aortovelography (AV) has been in clinical cardiological use since its introduction in 1972 by Light and Cross [6]. The signals obtained (Figure 1) are the spectrogramic representation of the aortic blood flow and the wave outline is the instantaneous blood velocity in the systolic phase. Recordings are made with the transducer in the suprasternal notch and the ultrasound beam is directed downwards laterally and backwards until the maximum Doppler signal is obtained.

The characteristic wave forms obtained in various clinical conditions have made this technique of value in the diagnosis and follow up of patients

94

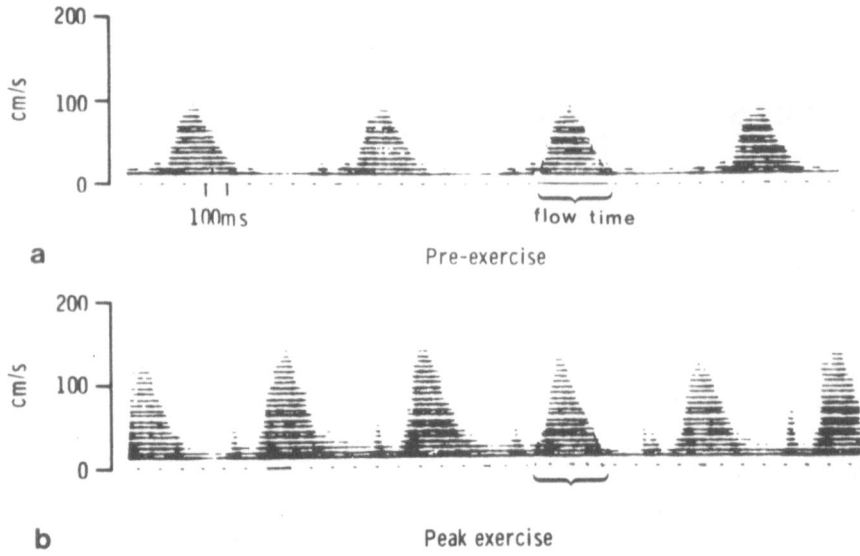

Figure 1. Typical recordings by transcutaneous aortovelography a) at rest and b) during exercise, in normal subject. The envelope of the dark near-triangle complexes (which show the spectral frequency content of the Doppler signal returned by moving red blood corpuscles) indicates quantitatively the time-course of mainstream blood velocity in the aortic arch. Stroke distance – the axial distance travelled by the blood per cycle, and thus a measure of stroke volume in any one subject – is given by the area of the corresponding complex, i.e. the systolic velocity integral. In all the normal subjects stroke distance increased with exercise. Paper speed = 5 cm/second.

suffering from cardiomyopathies, shock, aortic valvular disease and myocardial infarctions [7]. Changes in the area under the curve (which represents the distance travelled by the blood per beat and termed the stroke distance) were said to be highly proportional to changes in the cardiac output [8, 9, 10]. I have, therefore, investigated the use of the Doppler TAV technique during exercise to study left ventricular function. Exercise was carried out on a supine bicycle ergometer according to a technique previously described by Salmasi and co-workers [11]. Doppler recordings were carried out after 5 minute supine rest and also at maximum-tolerated supine exercise. In the normal individuals exhaustion was the limiting factor while in the patients, chest pain, dyspnoea, exhaustion or ST depression of 4 mm were the reasons for stopping exercise. None of the patients developed arrhythmias during exercise.

From the TAV complexes (both resting and peak exercise) various indices were derived including peak velocity (Pv), stroke distance (Sd; distance travelled by the blood per cycle or index of stroke volume) and minute distance (Md; distance travelled by the blood per minute or index of cardiac output).

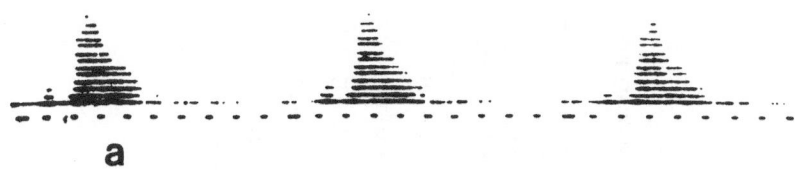

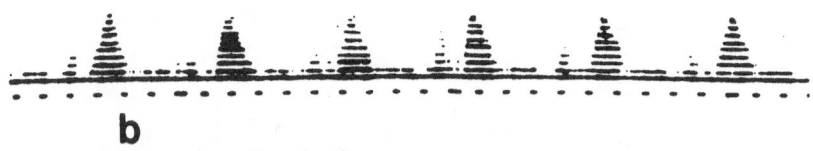

Figure 2. TAV recording at rest (a) and peak exercise (b) in a patient with three vessel coronary disease and resting ejection fraction (obtained from left ventriculography) of 18%. Note the obvious decrease in the area under the curve (i.e. stroke distance) at peak exercise; a typical finding in patients with coronary artery disease and ejection fraction below 60%.

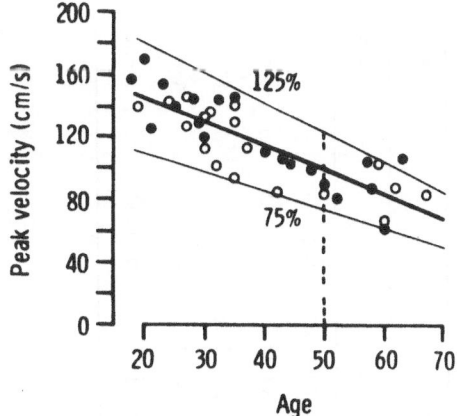

Figure 3. Effect of age on resting peak velocity (Pv) in 40 normal subjects. Pv decreases by 1.1% per year. The spread is almost entirely contained within the faint line $Pv = 175 - 1.52 \times age$

O males
● females

THE INITIAL EXPERIENCE

In order to investigate the differences in the Doppler profile between normal individuals and patients with coronary artery disease, an initial study was carried out on 40 normal subjects (18 males and 22 females) whose age ranged between 18 and 67 (mean 39.6 ± 14.3) and who were not athletic (Group 1). Their TAV recordings both at rest and at maximum-tolerated

Table 1. Comparison of TAV parameters (resting and peak exercise) between 40 normal individuals (Group 1) and 60 patients with coronary artery disease (Group 2). ss = statistical significance, ns = non-significant.

TAV paramter	Pre exercise			Peak exercise			SS Group 1 pre & peak exercise
	Group 1	Group 2	SS	Group 1	Group 2	SS	
Stroke distance	18.9± 3.3	18.7± 4.7	NS	22.8± 4.2	18.5± 6.4	p=0.0001	p<0.0001
Minute distance	1451 ±399	1291.6±442	p<0.04	1717 ±609	1848.7±715	p=0.0000	p<0.001
Peak velocity	99.4± 13.6	101.2± 24.8	NS	128 ± 21	105 ± 31.5	p=0.0000	p<0.0001
Flow time	371 ± 36.2	374 ± 74	NS	349 ± 32	348 ± 73	NS	p<0.0001
Heart rate	75.6± 10.5	69.5± 14.9	p<0.02	116.6± 15.2	101.3± 21.6	p=0.0001	p<0.0001

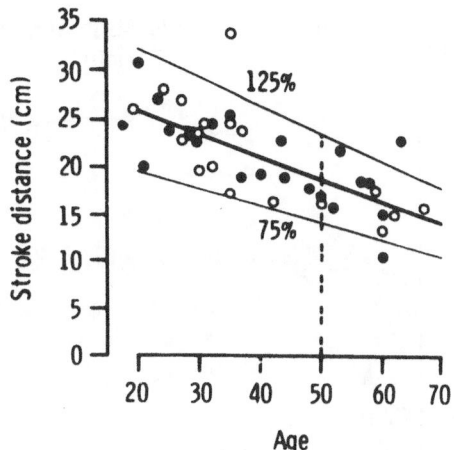

Figure 4. Effect of age on stroke distance (Sd) in resting adults. The values are in cm. The regression line is Sd = 30.3 − 0.23 × age.

○ male

● female

supine exercise (Figure 1) were compared with that of 60 consecutive patients (Figure 2) who had presented with angina pectoris and had angiographically proven coronary artery disease (Group 2). They were 58 males and 2 females whose ages ranged between 27 and 69 (mean 50.5 ± 9). History of myocardial infarction (at least six months prior to the study) was present in 21 of the 60 patiens, 31 were receiving beta-adrenergic blockade at the time of the study.

The Pv profile in Group 1 confirmed previous reports that Pv declines with age [12, 13]. It falls by a factor of 1.1 % per year (Figure 3) and the Sd falls by 1 % per year [14] (Figure 4).

The response to exercise was very remarkable with a substantial increase in the Pv, Sd and Md, while a shortening in the flow-time is shown in Tables 1 and 2. From 10 subjects in Group 1, it was noticed that both Pv and Sd rose progressively and significantly for the first three minutes, then a plateau value was reached (Figure 5). The increase in the Sd resulted from a 30 % increase in the Pv offset by 6 % reduction in the flow-time.

The variation with age (expressed as percentage of the mean) for the Pv and Sd in the normal subjects was virtually the same in the resting and exercising states; hence percentage changes with exercise of these variables are age-independent.

The experience with patients with coronary artery disease was different. The percentage change in the Sd with exercise (% Δ Sd) in Group 2 ranged widely between 47 % and 39 %. This contrasts with Group 1 in whom Sd increases consistently with exercise (Figure 6). Good correlation was ob-

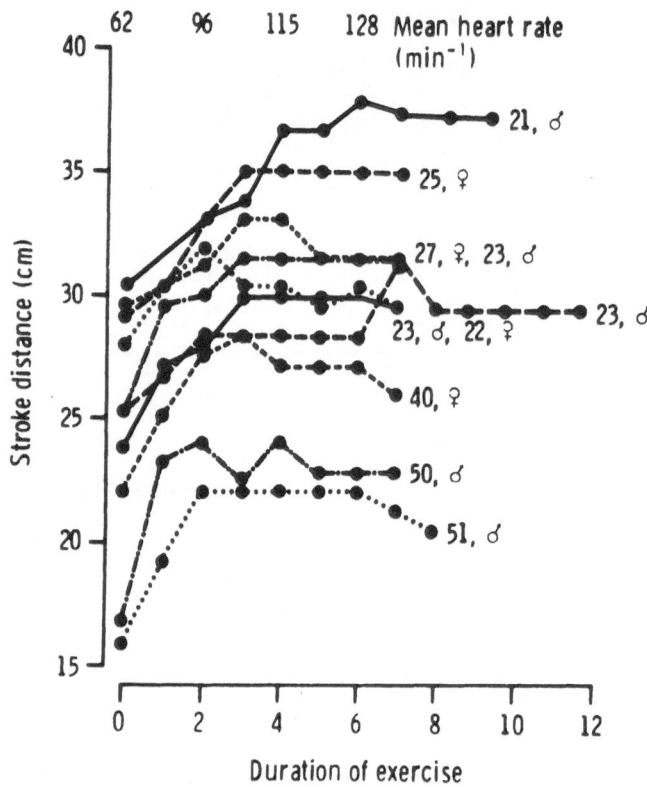

Figure 5. Variation in stroke distance with exercise duration in 10 normal subjects from Group 1 throughout the step-wise increasing workload protocol described by Salmasi and associates [11]. Mean heart rate is shown at two minute intervals. The ages and sex are indicated against the individual curves.

served between % Δ Sd in Group 2 and their resting ejection fraction (as measured by left ventriculography) (Figure 7). An ejection fraction of < 60% is regarded indicative of impairment in left ventricular function [15, 16]; accordingly 33 patients in Group 2 had impaired left ventricular function in whom the Sd increased at peak exercise. None of these 33 patients had a

Table 2. Comparison of the percentage changes in some TAV parameters with exercise between Group 1 (normal subjects) and Group 2 (patients with coronary artery disease).

	Group 1	Group 2	SS *
% Δ Sd	20.9± 7.8	− 2.0±19.9	p<0.0001
% Δ Md	88.2±28.5	44.9±43.3	p<0.0001
% Δ Pv	28.6±10.7	4.4±21.7	p<0.0001

* SS = statistical significance.

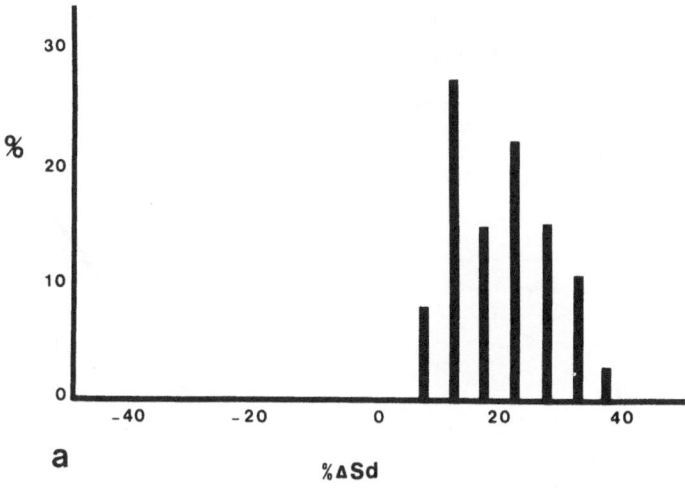

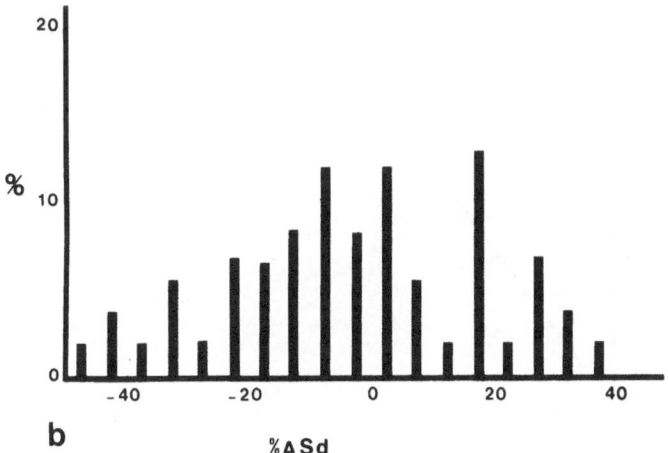

Figure 6. Histogram distribution of the % *Δ* Sd (percentage change in stroke distance) amongst 40 normal subjects (a) and 60 patients with coronary artery disease (b). Note the wide variation in % *Δ* Sd is always in the positive side, i.e. the Sd increases with exercise.

% Δ Sd above the zero. Whereas no significant difference is observed in the resting Pv or Sd between the normal subjects and the patient group, at peak exercise they are significantly lower in patients with coronary artery disease. These findings therefore suggest a reduction in the stroke volume at peak exercise in patients with coronary artery disease and impaired left ventricular function. This finding is in agreement with previous work of Sharma and associates carried out by left ventriculography during exercise [17]. This has also been further confirmed using radionuclide ventriculography [18]. The

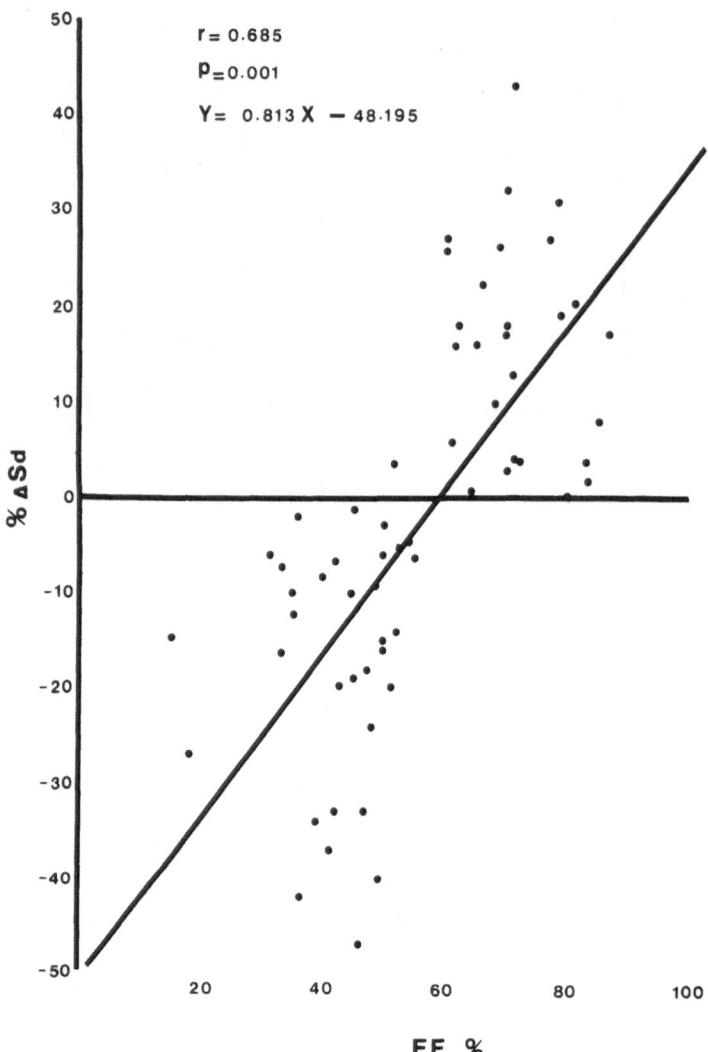

Figure 7. Scattogram of the % Δ Sd in the patient group against the resting ejection fraction calculated from the left ventriculographies. All 33 patients with ejection fraction lower than 60% have a negative % Δ Sd.

parameter % Δ Sd with exercise thus provides an important measure of left ventricular function.

The approach to study global left ventricular performance by Doppler during exercise is easier, cheaper, safer and highly reproducible [14, 19], and should prove more useful than other methods. Therefore, this technique can be used repeatedly to assess the progress and prognosis of a disease in response to various therapeutic procedures.

EFFECT OF PREVIOUS MYOCARDIAL INFARCTION

The effects of previous myocardial infarction on left ventricular function was ascertained; in 21 patients the $\% \Delta$ Sd with exercise was significantly lower than in patients without previous infarct (p<0.001) [19]. However, the Sd both at rest and with exercise was significantly lower in patients with such a history (p<0.001) and much lower when they were receiving beta-adrenergic blockade (p<0.02) [19, 20]. On the other hand, in non-infarct patients, the Sd both at rest and with exercise, was higher in patients who were receiving beta-adrenergic blockade than patients without such medication. These findings may have been due to the stimulating effect of the beta-blockade on the ischaemic myocardium as suggested previously [21, 22]. In a heart with an infarction scar on the other hand, such an effect is much less because of the presence of a dead myocardial tissue; the net result of which will be a weaker response to the stimulant action of the beta-blockade which is much more dependent upon the availability of ischaemic myocardial tissue.

EFFECT OF NUMBER OF CORONARY ARTERIES WITH SIGNIFICANT STENOSIS

Although relatively few, the observations which suggest a significant linear effect of the number of diseased vessels are a lower $\% \Delta$ Pv and $\% \Delta$ Sd as well as ejection fraction with increasing number of diseased vessels (Table 3).

Table 3. Distribution of some TAV parameters which significantly vary according to the number of vessel disease.

| TAV parameter | Group 1 | | Patients (Group 2) | | | | Statistical significance of linear trend |
| | | | No. of diseased vessels | | | | |
	Mean	Sd	1 Mean	2 Mean	3 Mean	Pooled SD	
% Δ Pv	28.6	10.7	17.1	5.4	1.2	21.3	p<0.05
% Δ Sd	20.9	7.8	12.4	− 1.9	− 5.5	16.9	p<0.0001
EF (%)	−	−	64	62	54	12	p<0.02
Age	39	14	48	45	52	8	
Number	40		10	8	42		

Pv = peak velocity
Sd = stroke distance
SD = standard deviation
EF = ejection fraction

102

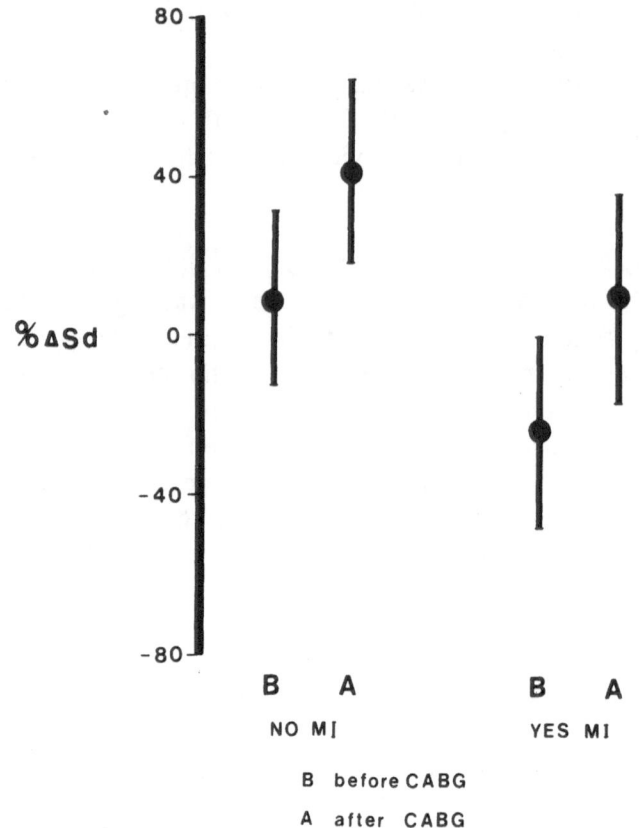

Figure 8. Comparison of the percentage change in stroke distance (% Δ Sd) between patients with and without history of myocardial infarction (MI) before and after coronary artery bypass grafting (CABG). Note that before CABG, the Sd in most of the patients without history of MI tended always to increase with exercise whereas it decreased in patients with previous infarct during exercise. After CABG, although the improvement in % Δ Sd was significant and similar in both groups of patients, yet the Sd tended to decrease following CABG in 5 out of 10 patients with previous infarct. The Sd in all patients without myocardial infarction increased with exercise.

EXERCISE DOPPLER CARDIOGRAPHY IN STUDYING THE EFFECT OF
CORONARY ARTERY BYPASS GRAFTING (CABG)

The operation of CABG is nowadays an established procedure for the treatment of angina pectoris. The effect of such a therapeutic procedure on left ventricular function is debatable. Taylor and associates [15] using radionuclide techniques reported improvement in exercise left ventricular performance following CABG.

Twenty-three patients (all males) of the age range 39 to 70 (mean 55.5±8.3) were studied by TAV with exercise before and six weeks after

Table 4. TAV variables that show significant differences before and after coronary artery bypass grafting in 23 patients. HR1 and Md1 are resting values for heart rate and minute distance. HR2, Pv2, Sd2 and Md2 are exercise values for heart rate, peak velocity, stroke distance and minute distance.

TAV variable	Before CABG	After CABG	p value
HR1	61.1 ± 10.2	82.9 ± 14.1	0.0001
HR2	99 ± 15.9	114 ± 16.4	0.001
Pv2	101 ± 26.8	131 ± 35.6	0.0007
Sd2	16.4 ± 6.2	20.5 ± 6.8	0.01
Md1	1055 ± 325	1309 ± 323	0.004
Md2	1609 ± 630	2324 ± 800	0.0007
% $\varDelta$ Pv	-0.8 ± 19.3	28.1 ± 25.5	0.0001
% $\varDelta$ Sd	-5.2 ± 27.1	27.3 ± 28.4	0.001
% $\varDelta$ Md	52 ± 41	78 ± 49	0.05

CABG [23]. Whereas improvement in their left ventricular function on effort following CABG was detected by TAV, no significant change in the resting TAV indices was observed following the operation (Table 4) [23]. This is in agreement with the findings of Taylor and associates (1983) [15]. Patients with a history of myocardial infarction on the other hand, though showing similar improvement on effort following CABG, tended to have left ventricular function inferior to patients without a history of infarction, both before and after CABG (Figure 8).

CONCLUSION

My experience suggests that Doppler cardiography during exercise is an invaluable tool to study patients with coronary artery disease, and to follow up their response to different therapeutic and surgical manipulation. The ranges for different indices of minute distance and stroke distance in normals and in this group of patients have already been established.

Patients with disturbed left ventricular function failed to increase their stroke distance and minute distance during exercise. Beta-adrenergic blockade therapy improved, though slightly, left ventricular function in patients with coronary artery disease, but in the presence of an infarct it induced severe depression in function, especially during exercise. Multiple-vessel coronary artery disease induced greater depression in left ventricular function than single-vessel disease.

Exercise Doppler cardiography proved invaluable in studying the immediate effect of coronary artery bypass grafting on myocardial function. Such an operation improved the left ventricular performance in the majority of the patients, especially patients without history of infarction. Patients with history of myocardial infarction behaved differently from those without infarction following the operation. Exercise Doppler technique is thus a very useful procedure to study and follow up patients following surgical therapy. It is suggested that in the long-term follow up, such group of patients should be assessed during exercise when myocardial performance is to be estimated. My experience with exercise Doppler cardiography has also shown that it has an application in studying and following up the effects of beta-adrenergic blockade [24] and calcium-channel blockers [25] on myocardial performance.

Doppler cardiography during exercise therefore proves a very useful technique to study the process of coronary artery disease and the effect of various therapies on such a process, as well as the prognosis. Its use in other fields such as sports medicine and even space medicine is feasible and may prove of value.

REFERENCES

1. Bousfield G: Angina pectoris – Changes in electrocardiogram during paroxysm. Lancet 2:457, 1918.
2. Master AM, Jaffe HL: The electrocardiographic changes after exercise in angina pectoris. J Mt Sinai Hosp 7:629, 1941.
3. Iskandrian AS, Hakki AM: Left ventricular function in patients with coronary heart disease in the presence or absence of angina pectoris during exercise radionuclide ventriculography. Am J Cardiol 53:1239, 1984.
4. Borer JS, Bacharach SL, Green MV et al.: Real-time radionuclide cine angiography in the non-invasive evaluation of global and regional left ventricular function at rest and during exercise in ptients with coronary artery disease. N Engl J Med 296:839, 1977.
5. Gibson D: Personal Communication.
6. Light LH, Cross G: Cardiovascular data by transcutaneous aortovelography. In: Blood Flow Measurement, Roberts C (ed.). Sector Publishing, London, pp 60–63, 1972.
7. Light LH: Transcutaneous aortovelography. A New window on the circulation. Br Heart J 38:433, 1976.
8. Sequeira RF, Light LH, Cross G, Raftery EB: Transcutaneous aortovelography – A quantitative evaluation. Br Heart J 38:443, 1976.
9. Buchtal A, Hanson GC, Peisach AR: Transcutaneous aortovelography – potentially useful technique in management of critically ill patients. Br Heart H 38:451, 1976.
10. Light LH, Sequeira RF, Cross G et al.: Flow-orientated circulatory patient assessment and management using transcutaneous aortovelography, a non-invasive Doppler technique. J Nucl Med All Sci 23:137, 1979.
11. Salmasi AM, Nicolaides, AN, Vecht RJ et al.: Electrographic chest wall mapping in the diagnosis of coronary artery disease. Br Med J, 287:9, 1983.
12. Mowat DHR, Haites NE, Rawles JM: Aortic blood velocity measurement in healthy adults using a simple ultrasound technique. Cardiovasc Res 17:75, 1983.
13. Distante A, Moscarelli E, Rovai D, L'Abbath A: Monitoring changes in cardiac output by transcutaneous aortovelography, a non-invasive Doppler technique: comparison with ther-

modilution. J Nucl Med All Sci 24:171, 1980.

14. Salmasi AM, Salmasi Sajida, Light LH et al.: Changes in aortic blood velocity, stroke distance and other determinants of cardiac output with exercise and age in normal adults. Submitted for publication.

15. Taylor NC, Barber RW, Crossland P et al.: Effects of coronary artery bypass grafting on left ventricular function assessed by multiple gated ventricular scintigraphy. Br Heart J 50:149, 1983.

16. Jones RH, McEwan P, Newman GE et al.: Accuracy of diagnosis of coronary artery disease by radionuclide measurement of left ventricular function during rest and exercise. Circulation 64:586, 1981.

17. Sharma B, Goodwin JF, Raphael MJ et al.: Left ventricular angiography on exercise. A new method of assessing left ventricular function in ischaemic heart disease. Br Heart J 38:59, 1976.

18. Slutsky RA, Mancini GBJ, Gerber KH et al.: Response to supine bicycle exercise in normal subjects and in patients with coronary heart disease. Am Heart J 105:802, 1983.

19. Salmasi AM, Salmasi Sajida, Light LH et al.: Non-invasive assessment of left ventricular function in coronary artery disease by continuous-wave Doppler. In preparation.

20. Salmasi SNA, Salmasi AM, Hendry WG et al.: Exercise-induced changes in stroke volume measured non-invasively in coronary artery disease. Acta Cardiol 6:337, 1983.

21. Marshall RC, Wisenberg G, Schelbert MR, Henze E: Effect of oral propranolol on rest, exercise and post exercise left ventricular performance in normal subjects and patients with coronary artery disease. Circulation 63:572, 1981.

22. Battler A, Ross J, Slutsky RA et al.: Improvement of exercise-induced left ventricular dysfunction with oral propranolol in patients with coronary heart disease. Am J Cardiol 44:318, 1979.

23. Salmasi AM, Salmasi Sajida, Light LH et al.: Evaluation of the effect of coronary artery bypass grafting on myocardial performance by continuous wave Doppler. In preparation.

24. Salmasi AM: Comparison between the effects of penbutolol and atenolol on myocardial performance in coronary artery disease. A study by continuous-wave Doppler. In preparation.

25. Salmasi AM: Non-invasive evaluation of the effect of nisoldipine on left ventricular function in coronary artery disease. In preparation.

8. Value of real-time two-dimensional Doppler flow imaging in cardiology *

Y. NIMURA, K. MIYATAKE, M. OKAMOTO, S. IZUMI, N. KINOSHITA, H.
SAKAKIBARA

INTRODUCTION

The introduction of the pulsed Doppler technique became a clue of non-invasive approach to intracardiac blood flows [1–5]. This technique was combined with two-dimensional echocardiography, so that it became possible to detect blood flow conditions at a desired site in the cardiac chamber [6, 7]. However, in conventional Doppler echocardiography, the sampling site for the blood flow Doppler signal has been usually only a single point in the cardiac chamber. Therefore, in order to assess the whole aspect of intracardiac flow topography, Doppler searching should be done from point to point in the cardiac chamber, so that it has been rather troublesome. Thus, it has been desired to image blood flows in the cardiac chamber together with the cardiac structures on the echocardiogram.

Noninvasive visualization of the intracardiac blood flow was first reported by Stevenson et al. [8]. In their report, the blood flow Doppler signals were displayed in the color-coded mode on the monochrome M-mode echocardiogram. The two-dimensional display of the intracardiac blood flow was reported by Bommer et al. [9], although this report was a brief communication.

Independently from these reports, Namekawa and Kasai developed a new technique to display the intracardiac flow Doppler signal in the color-coded mode two-dimensionally on the monochrome image of the cardiac structures [10, 11]. It has been assessed from the medical point of view by Omoto et al. [12] and the present authors' laboratory [13]. In the present paper, general trends of new informations obtained by this new technique on the intracardiac blood flow will be presented.

* This study was supported in part by the Grant-in-Aid for Scientific Research B of the Ministry of Education, Science and Culture of Japan in 1984 (No. 58480247).

OUTLINE OF THE REAL-TIME TWO-DIMENSIONAL DOPPLER FLOW IMAGING TECHNIQUE

In the present technique, the pulsed Doppler mechanism is incorporated in a real-time echo-imaging system. A wide-angle phased array transducer is simultaneously used for the two-dimensional echogram and the Doppler. At the present stage, the frequency of ultrasound is 2.5 MHz and the pulse repetition rate is 4 kHz, so that the measurable depth is 18 cm. Each cross section is composed of 32 beam directions and in each beam direction 8 ultrasound pulses are successively transmitted. It takes 66 ms to make one sector scan.

The reflected pulses are composed of the components reflected from the cardiac structures and those from the intracardiac blood. They are separated into 2 parts in the circuit. One of the two parts is used for imaging the conventional two-dimensional echocardiogram in the monochrome mode. In the conventional echocardiogram, the blood itself does not appear, because the amplitudes of the components reflected from the blood are very small in comparison with those from the cardiac structures.

The reflected pulses with small amplitude are mostly from the intracardiac blood, so that they have blood flow information within. They are extracted from the above-mentioned other part of the reflected ultrasound pulses through a comfilter and are processed by the high-speed autocorrelation principle [10, 11]. Through this process, flow informations, such as mentioned in the following, are calculated.

The present equipment is designed to give the following 5 modes of display by switch-over:

(1) Cine-mode: The flow data, i.e. the magnitude and direction of spatial mean velocity and the velocity variance, at each area in the cardiac chamber are displayed in the color-coded mode at the same area in the cardiac image in the sector field which is composed of 16,000 small areas, in real time, or, strictly speaking, with an allowance of time delay of 2 ms. The sector scan rate is 15 a second, so that the successive images appear as a moview. The flow direction toward the transducer is represented by reddish color and that away from the transducer by bluish color. The magnitude of velocity is represented by the brightness of color. It is measurable up to 2 kHz at the pulse repetition rate of 4 kHz, which means that the measurable magnitude of velocity is 60 cm/s in the beam direction. It the velocity is higher than measurable range of velocity, color reversal arises in the color-coded display. The measurable range is divided into grades at steps of 250 Hz. These grades are represented by increasing the brightness of color at 8-step scale beginning from the lowest grade which is not colored on the screen. The Doppler frequency variance, indicating flow turbulence, is expressed by

adding green to each color, i.e. red shifts to yellow and blue to cyan. Strictly speaking, the present technique does not visualize the blood itself, but images the flow velocity wave. The data obtained are usually stored by a videotape and displayed on the color-television screen.

(2) Gated mode: The ECG-gated still picture is obtained at any desired frame in one cardiac cycle.

(3) M-mode: The M-mode display similar to that of Stevenson et al. [8] is also obtained in the present equipment. The beam direction for the M-mode display is indicated in the two-dimensional image.

(4) Conventional two-dimensional echocardiogram: It is alone obtained in the monochrome mode, stopping the Doppler mechanism.

(5) Conventional Doppler frequency spectrogram: It is also obtained at any desired site in the visual field by the fast Fourier transformation analysis (abbreviated as FFT analysis in the following).

Details on the present technique is presented in another chapter in this monograph.

CLINICAL APPLICATIONS

(a) *Normal flow pattern in the left ventricle*

The apical and parasternal approaches are advantageous for assessing normal flow patterns in the left ventricle.

In systole, the ejection flow is imaged in blue over the left ventricular cavity from the apical approach (Figure 1). However, at this time it should be emphasized that the velocity displayed on the screen by the present technique is not a flow velocity as a whole, but the component on the beam direction, according to the principle of the Doppler. If the flow is perpendicular to the beam direction, it is not colored on the screen, because it has no velocity component on the beam direction.

In early diastole, the mitral rapid inflow spreads through the maximally opened mitral orifice over the left ventricular cavity (Figure 1).

In presystole, the inflow is a narrow flux, reflecting the semiclosure of the mitral valve. This feature has never been clearly disclosed until it is visualized by the present technique.

(b) *Valvular diseases*

In mitral stenosis, the mitral inflow jet runs down as a bel-like flux toward the apex and sustains through diastole (Figure 2). However, it does not necessarily run toward the apex, but it often goes anteriorly or posteriorly. In about 10% of the cases the inflow jet spurts simultaneously into two different directions. Such findings become easily noted at the first time

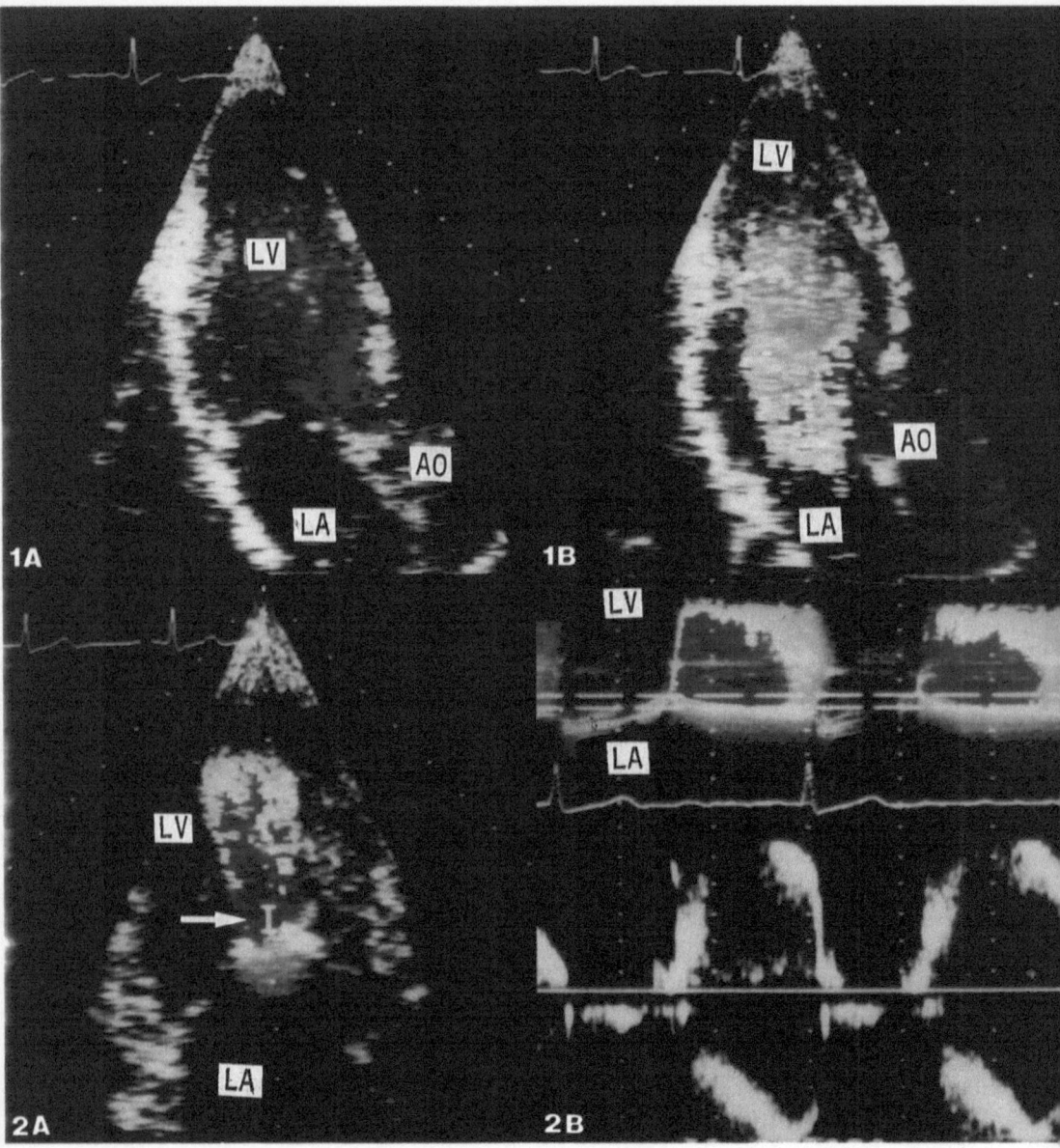

Figure 1. Normal flow patterns in the left ventricular cavity in the apical long-axis view. A. The ejection flow is expressed by bluish color in systole. The flow velocity appears faster in the outflow tract than in the major part of the left ventricle. B. The mitral inflow appears to spread from the mitral valve to the major part of the left ventricular cavity in early diastole. LA = left atrium; LV = left ventricle; AO = aorta.

Figure 2. Mitral stenosis in the apical long-axis view. A. The mitral inflow flux appear band-like from the mitral orifice toward the apex. Its central zone is bluish, being caused by 'aliasing' in the equipment. The arrow indicates the sample volume of the Doppler signals for the right panel. B. M-mode image and frequency spectrogram by the fast Fourier transform analysis. The color reversal in the M-mode image is coincident with the aliasing in the spectrogram. LA = left atrium; LV = left ventricle.

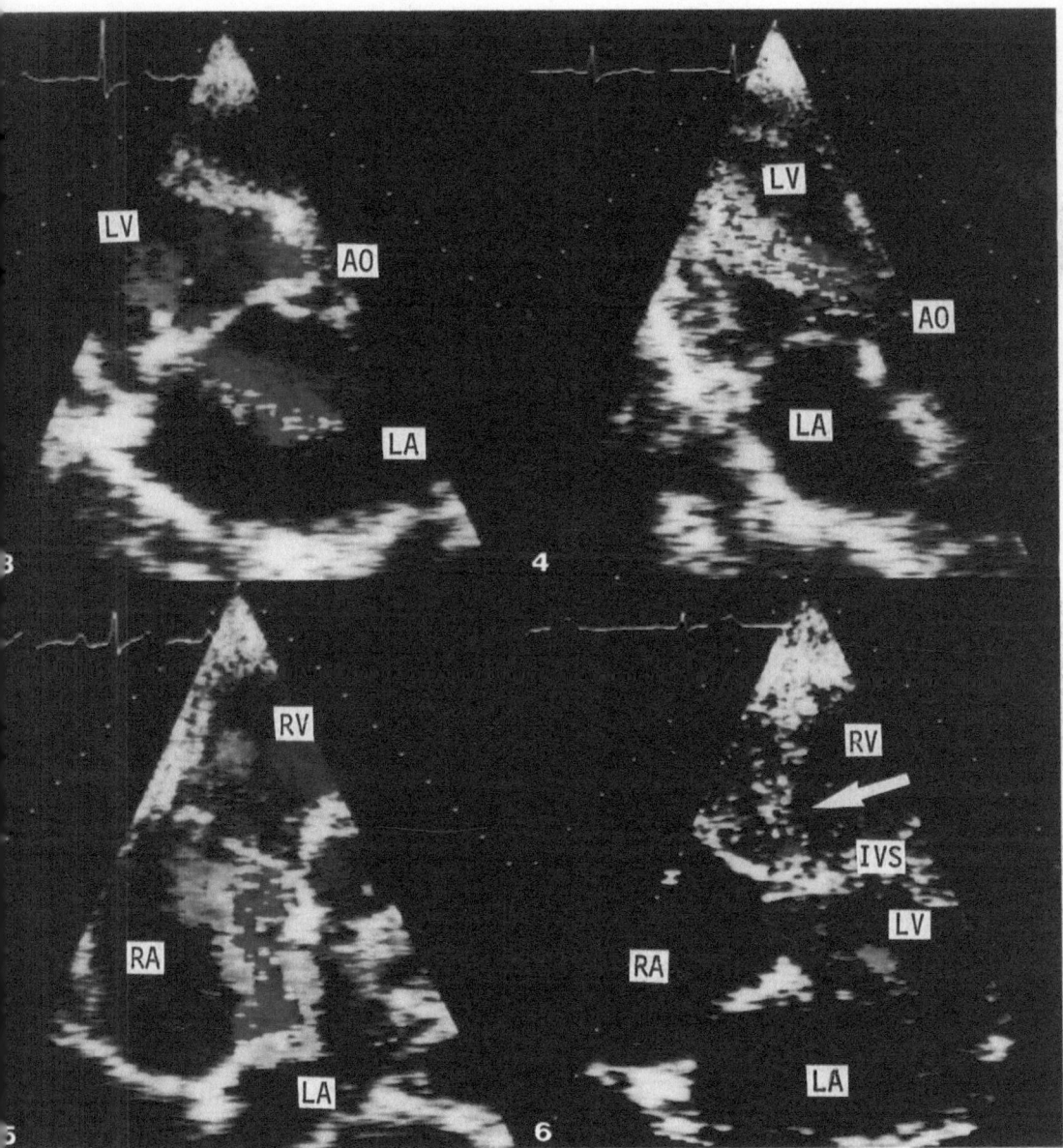

Figure 3. Mitral regurgitation in the lower parasternal long-axis view. Blue signals are noted from the mitral orifice into the left atrial cavity. The central zone of the signal area appears to be mosaic, indicating that the regurgitant flow is so speedy in this zone that 'aliasing' arises. LA = left atrium; LV = left ventricle; AO = aorta.

Figure 4. Aortic regurgitation in the apical long-axis view. The aortic regurgitant flow runs from the aortic orifice posteroapically. It exhibits bluish color in the outflow tract, indicating a color reversal because of very high velocity near the aortic orifice. LA = left atrium; LV = left ventricle; AO = aorta.

Figure 5. Atrial septal defect in the parasternal four-chamber view. Left-to-right shunt flow widely spreads from the left atrial cavity into the right atrial cavity. The central zone of the shunt flow is bluish, indicating a color reversal because of a high velocity. LA = left atrium; RA = right atrium; RV = right ventricle.

Figure 6. Ventricular septal defect in the short-axis view at the level just above the tricuspid

by the present technique, showing one of the advantages of the two-dimensional display.

In case from the apical approach, the mitral inflow jet is displayed in reddish color. However, the central zone of the inflow jet is often colored in blue, while the peripheral zone in reddish color (Figure 2). This blue color is not interpreted to indicate a flow away from the transducer at the apex, but to be a color reversal corresponding to the 'aliasing' in the frequency spectrogram based on the FFT analysis, because the inflow jet is too much accelerated through the stenotic orifice [14]. 'Aliasing' is a problem to be solved not only in the FFT spectrogram, but also even in the present technique.

In mitral regurgitation, it is clearly demonstrated that unusual Doppler signals are noted over some range from the mitral orifice into the left atrial cavity in systole (Figure 3). The orientation and extent of regurgitation are easily judged spatially on the basis of the long-axis and short-axis cross sections. Such data are obtained even with conventional Doppler echocardiography, by searching the left atrial cavity from point to point for unusual Doppler signals, changing the beam direction and the site of sample volume [7]. However, while it has taken 30 minutes or longer to make such searching with the conventional technique, it takes only a few minutes by the present new technique.

The mitral regurgitant flow signals obtained from the apical approach are usually colored in mosaic of blue and orange in their central zone, while in blue in their peripheral zone (Figure 3). The FFT spectrogram sampled from the mosaic zone shows a bidirectional rough continuous spectrum. According to the present authors' other study, such a spectrogram is considered to be mainly resulted from multiple times of aliasing because of a very high velocity [14]. Therefore, the above-mentioned mosaic pattern is interpreted to show high velocity of the regurgitant flow because of a pressure drop from the left ventricle to the left atrium in systole.

The overall sensitivity of the Doppler flow imaging for mitral regurgitation is about 85% in reference to that of left ventriculography, although the latter is not necessarily a 'gold' standard.

The distance reached and area covered by the regurgitant signals are assumed to reflect the severity of regurgitation. Grading of the severity based on these items may be possible. However, the Doppler may fail to detect very mild cases documented by left ventriculography.

The Doppler flow imaging demonstrates a variety of topographic features of mitral regurgitant flow. The regurgitant flow sometimes exhibits complex features, e.g. peculiar course, twin regurgitant jets from different sites in the valve, those for different directions from the same site, and so forth. The regurgitant flow runs anteriorly from the mitral orifice mostly in posterior mitral valve prolapse, toward the central part of the left atrial cavity in rheumatic valvular disease and posteriorly in anterior mitral valve prolapse. These findings show that topographic features of regurgitation are very closely depending upon the anatomical conditions of the valve lesion. As in this case, the real-time Doppler flow imaging technique enables one easily to observe dynamic features of the intracardiac blood flow, connecting them with the morphological condition of the heart.

The direction of regurgitant jet may vary even during each systole. This is often in patients, the left atrium is markedly enlarged. It had never been clearly observed until the new technique was used. Such a finding shows another advantage of the new technique, that it demonstrates momentary changes of the intracardiac flow topography continuously.

Mitral regurgitation is often observed in patients after mitral valve replacement with a bioprosthetic valve. In some patients, mitral regurgitant jet appears to arise from the central part of the orifice, but in some other patients, it appears to arise from the valvular ring. The former is attributed to dysfunction of the cusps, and the latter to perivalvular leakage. It is considered to be also one of the advantages of the present new technique that the spot is precisely determined by this technique, where regurgitant jet arises showing a fine resolution of the technique.

The new technique is advantageous also for assessing dysfunctions of other valves. Tricuspid regurgitation is usually demonstrated from the lower parasternal approach. It is mostly functional, being secondary to the left-sided valve lesions. Tricuspid regurgitant jets are usually toward the posterior wall of the right atrium in parallel with the interatrial septum. It may hit against the interatrial septum in patients, in whom the septum domes into the right atrial cavity because of the marked enlargement of the left atrium.

Aortic regurgitation is well assessed by the new technique (Figure 4). It is clearly demonstrated by the new technique that the aortic regurgitant flow spurts from the aortic orifice into the left ventricular outflow tract. The overall sensitivity is about 85 % in reference to that of aortography. Grading of the severity of aortic regurgitation is also possible by similar ways to that of mitral regurgitation.

Aortic regurgitant jet exhibits a variety of directions of jet from the aortic orifice into the left ventricular outflow tract. Depending upon patients, it runs along the interventricular septum, in the central zone of the outflow tract or along the anterior mitral leaflet. Aortic regurgitation often accompanies mitral stenosis. In this case, aortic regurgitant flow is in parallel with mitral inflow in some patients, or joins the latter in some other cases.

The new technique is also very sensitive for pulmonary regurgitation. The sagittal section plane along the left sternal border demonstrates that pulmonary regurgitant jet is spurted from the coaptation point of three cusps into the right ventricular outflow tract.

(c) *Congenital heart*

Interatrial shunt flow in atrial septal defect is well observed in the horizontal plane from the parasternal approach. It spreads widely from the left atrial cavity toward the tricuspid valve through the defect on the interatrial septum (Figure 5). The shunt is prominent mainly from late systole to early diastole.

Atrial septal defect often accompanies tricuspid regurgitation. In such patients, it is often observed by the new technique that left-to-right shunt flow runs from the left atrial cavity toward the tricuspid valve through the anterior half of the defect and tricuspid regurgitant jet blows from the tricuspid valve by way of the right atrial cavity into the left atrial cavity through the posterior half of the defect, so that there are simultaneously two flows with opposite directions through the defect. It is assumed to be one of the mechanisms of bilateral shunt.

In cases of small ventricular septal defect, a thin flow of mosaic pattern composed of orange and blue colors is spurted from a spot on the interventricular septum into the right ventricular outflow tract in systole (Figure 6). In some patients, a flow entering into the defect is also observed in the left ventricular outflow tract in systole. In some other instances, the shunt jet in right ventricular outflow tract is observed even in diastole. In patients with a small defect, the site on the septum, where the shunt jet arises, is considered to indicate that of the defect, although the defect itself is not clearly imaged on the two-dimensional echogram. However, in this case, the searching should be carefully done from a variety of aspects, tilting and shifting the transducer little by little. A handy transducer and the monitoring with the real-time image are convenient for such a searching.

In case of large defect, it is clearly observed that the shunt flow goes there and back through the defect imaged on the echogram.

The sagittal and horizontal sections are advantageous to examine patent ductus arteriosus. The pulmonary trunk is irregularily filled by mosaic signals. In some patients, it is demonstrated that a shunt jet is spurted from a spot on the vessel wall, showing the site of the ductus, although the patent ductus itself is not observed in the two-dimensional echogram.

Aneurysm of the sinus of Valsalva is usually imaged on the two-dimensional echogram. However, as is well known, an echo interruption on the wall of the aneurysm does not necessarily mean a rupture, because if the ultrasound beam is in parallel with a part of the aneurysmal wall, this part is not imaged on the echogram. On the other hand, a rupture is not necessarily imaged on the echogram. Regardless the echo findings, rupture may be diagnosed on the basis of a shunt flow into the right heart chamber from a spot on the aneurysmal wall observed by the flow imaging.

CLINICAL SIGNIFICANCE AND PROSPECTS

The real-time Doppler flow imaging technique has various advantages in clinical use as follows:

(1) The new technique enables one to visualize the whole aspect of the intracardiac flow topography two-dimensionally. A lot of new findings which have not been obtained with previous examination techniques is obtained by the new technique, e.g. peculiar course of mitral regurgitant flow, simultaneous coexistence of a light-to-right and right-to-left shunts through a defect in atrial septal defect, and so forth. Semiquantitative grading of severity is noninvasively possible in mitral and aortic regurgitations.

(2) Unusual flow topography in the heart is interpreted in connection with abnormalities in analtomy: e.g. the direction of mitral regurgitant flow and its underlying condition.

(3) Momentary changes in flow topography are continuously observed.

(4) Observation of responses in flow topography to some physiological intervention becomes possible.

(5) Intracardiac searching is easy with a handy transducer, making reference to the real-time images, i.e., the site of defect on the interventricular septum is determined, although the defect itself is not necessarily visualized on the echogram.

(6) Examination time is shortened, and discomfort to examinee is reduced.

(7) The M-mode display and the FFT spectrogram may be convenient to study temporal relations between cardiac events and flow conditions. However, it should be necessary to make reference to the two-dimensional flow image for properly selecting the beam direction and the site of sample volume for these studies.

Since ultrasound was introduced into cardiology, 30 years have passed. In the first decade of cardiac ultrasound, there had been a variety of diagnostic techniques in progress, M-mode [15], CW-Doppler [16], C-mode [17], ultrasonocardiotomography [18] and so forth [19–21]. However, in this period, they were not brought to be routinely used in the world-wide base. This period should be called the dawn stage of cardiac ultrasound.

In the second decade, M-mode echocardiography became a routine technique. It might be called the first generation of routine cardiac ultrasound. In next decade, real-time two-dimensional echocardiography became widely

116

used in practice. It might be called the second generation of routine cardiac ultrasound.

Since a few years ago, the combination of two-dimensional echocardiography and the Doppler technique has allowed one to assess intracardiac blood flow topography noninvasively. However, in this period, the echogram and the Doppler should be separately recorded. This stage is considered to be a transitional period. The present new Doppler flow imaging technique raises epochally the diagnostic efficacy of cardiac ultrasound. The clinical concepts of major heart diseases are generally composed of 2 aspects, abnormalities in morphology and those in intracardiac blood flows. The new technique gives us informations on these two aspects simultaneously in real time. Therefore, it may be appreciated as a more essential approach to major heart diseases than the diagnostic procedures in the past. It will become widely used for routine cardiac diagnosis in future. It may become to be called the third generation of routine cardiac ultrasound.

REFERENCES

1. Baker DW: Pulsed ultrasonic Doppler blood flow sensing. IEEE Transactions on Sonics and Ultrasonics, Vol. SU-17, 3:170, 1970.
2. Peronneau P, Xhaard M, Nowicki A, Pellet M, Delouche P, Hinglais J: Pulsed Doppler ultrasonic flowmeter and flow patterns analysis. Blood Flow Measurement. C Roberts (ed.), pp 24–28, Sector Publishing Ltd, London, 1972.
3. Johnson SL, Baker DW, Lute RA, Dodge HT: Doppler echocardiography: the localization of cardiac murmurs. Circulation 48:810, 1973.
4. Stevenson JG, Kawabori I, Guntheroth WG: Differentiation of ventricular septal defects from mitral regurgitation by pulsed Doppler echocardiography. Circulation 56:14, 1977.
5. Kalmanson D, Veyrat C, Bouchareine F, Degroote A: Noninvasive recording of mitral valve flow velocity patterns using pulsed Doppler echocardiography. Application to diagnosis and evaluation of mitral valve disease. Brit Heart J 39:517, 1977.
6. Nimura Y, Matsuo H, Kitabatake A, Hayashi T, Asao M, Terao Y, Senda S, Sakakibara H, Abe H: Studies on the intracardiac blood flow with a combined use of the ultrasonic pulsed Doppler technique and two-dimensional echocardiography from a transcutaneous approach. In: Ultrasound in Medicine. D White and RE Brown (eds.), Vol 3B, pp 1279–1289, Plenum Publishing Corporation, New York, 1977.
7. Miyatake K, Kinoshita N, Nagata S, Beppu S, Park Y, Sakakibara H, Nimura Y: Intracardiac flow pattern in mitral regurgitation studied with combined use of the ultrasonic pulsed Doppler technique and cross-sectional echocardiography. Amer J Cardiol 45:155, 1980.
8. Stevenson JG: Multigate Doppler visualization of intracardiac flow disturbances in congenital heart disease. In: Cardiac Doppler Diagnosis. MP Spencer (ed.), pp 235–245, Martinus Nijhoff, Boston, 1983.
9. Bommer WJ, Miller L: Real-time two-dimensional colorflow Doppler: Enhanced Doppler flow imaging in the diagnosis of cardiovascular disease. Amer J Cardiol 49:944 (Abstr.), 1982.

10. Namekawa K, Kasai C, Koyano A: Real-time blood flow imaging system utilizing auto-correlation techniques. In: Ultrasound '82. RA Lerski, P Morley (eds.), pp 203–208, Pergamon Press, Oxford, 1983.

11. Namekawa K, Kasai C, Omoto R, Kondo Y, Katabaki T, Hidai T, Yoshioka Y, Tsukamoto M, Yokoto Y, Takamoto S, Koyano A: Real time two-dimensional blood flow imaging using ultrasound Doppler. J Ultrasound Med 2:Suppl 65, 1983.

12. Omoto R (ed.): Real-time two-dimensional Doppler echocardiography. Shindan to Chiryocha, Tokyo, (in Japanese), 1983.

13. Miyatake K, Okamoto M, Kinoshita N, Izumi S, Owa M, Takao S, Sakakibara H, Nimura Y: Clinical applications of a new type of real-time two-dimensional Doppler flow imaging system. Amer J Cardiol 54:857, 1984.

14. Nimura Y, Miyatake K: in preparation.

15. Edler I, Hertz CH: The use of ultrasonic reflectoscope for the continuous recording of the movements of the heart walls. Kungl Fysiogr Sallsk i Lund Forhandl 24:No 5, 1, 1954.

16. Satomura S, Nimura Y, Yoshida T: Ultrasonic Doppler cardiograph. Proceedings of the third International Conference of Medical electronics, pp 249–253, 1983.

17. Omoto R: Intracardiac scanning of the heart with the aid of ultrasonic intravenous probe. Jap Heart J 8:569, 1967.

18. Ebina T, Oka S, Tanaka M, Kosaka S, Terasawa Y, Unno K, Kikuchi Y, Uchida R: Ultrasono-tomography of the heart and great vessels in living human subjects by means of the ultrasonic reflection technique. Jap Heart J 8:331, 1967.

19. Wild JJ, Crawford HD, Reid JM: Visualization of the excised human heart by means of reflected ultrasound or echography. Amer Heart J 54:903, 1957.

20. Åsberg A: Ultrasonic cinematography of the living heart. Ultrasonics 5:113, 1967.

21. Carleton RA, Clark JG: Measurement of left ventricular diameter in the dog by cardiac catheterization. Validation and physiologic meaningfulness of an ultrasonic technique. Circ Res 22:545, 1968.

9. Development of real-time two-dimensional Doppler echocardiography and its clinical significance

RYOZO OMOTO, CHIHIRO KASAI, YUJI YOKOTE, SHINICHI TAKAMOTO, SHUNEI

KYO, KEISUKE UEDA, HARUHEKO ASANO, KOROKU NAMEKAWA, YUJI KONDO,

YOSHIHIRO YOSHIKAWA, AKIRA KOYANO

INTRODUCTION: RESEARCH STEPS TOWARD REAL-TIME DOPPLER BLOOD-FLOW IMAGING

One of the reasons why echocardiography has not replaced angiography is due to the poor resolution of intracardiac blood-flow images. Thus, a non-invasive method for real-time blood-flow imaging using ultrasound has long been required in the fields of both cardiology and cardiovascular surgery.

Contrast echocardiography has been developed in many ways by improving contrast material but, in general, its main objectives have been the application to the right heart system or the imaging of the right to left shunt. Still, this method is not completely noninvasive.

Although it has become an established practice to use the pulsed-Doppler technique combined with echocardiography, the so-called Doppler echocardiography [1, 2], this method provides information on blood flow only from a small sample volume along the ultrasound beam. Various multichannel pulsed-Doppler systems [3, 4] have been developed to record the on-line velocity profile along a beam line at discrete time intervals during one cardiac cycle. The color-coded Doppler system using pulsed-Doppler technique was developed for only M-mode display [5]. The use of a computer-based off-line system [6] has been attempted to obtain two-dimensional blood flow imaging, but it is still far from fulfilling the clinical requirement for real-time imaging of the intracardiac blood flow. It was not until 1982 that a new technique approaching real-time imaging of the intracardiac blood flow was developed and reported. In 1982, two research teams independently described real-time two-dimensional Doppler echocardiography. Bommer et al. [7] studied cross-sectional Doppler instrumentation, obtaining enhanced real-time blood-flow images using contrast agents in cases of tricuspid regurgitation. Namekawa et al. [8], the co-authors of this paper, reported on a real-time blood-flow imaging system with a new auto-correlation technique,

(1)   (2)   (3)

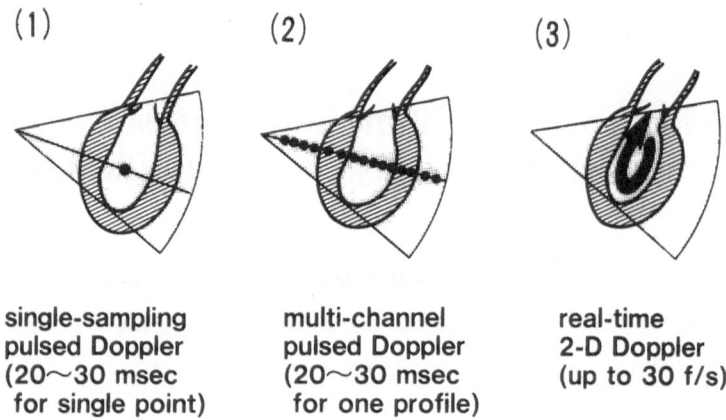

single-sampling
pulsed Doppler
(20~30 msec
for single point)

multi-channel
pulsed Doppler
(20~30 msec
for one profile)

real-time
2-D Doppler
(up to 30 f/s)

Figure 1. Steps to real-time color flow mapping: (A): single sampling; (B): velocity profile along a beam line; (C): two-dimensional imaging.

capable of producing, without enhancement, two-dimensional blood-flow images in real time in any chamber of a beating heart (Figure 1). In April of 1983, the authors first [9] described the clinical application of real-time two-dimensional Doppler echocardiography (hereafter abbreviated as '2-D Doppler' or 'color flow mapping') using the new device described above. The author's group [10] has confirmed the diagnostic effectiveness [8] in acquired valvular disease [11, 12], congenital heart disease [13–15] and aortic aneurysm [16, 17]. Since the introduction of practical 2-D Doppler systems, a number of vigorous studies on color flow mapping have been carried out in many cardiac centers [18–23].

It is genuinely believed that information on intracardiac blood flow, which can be repeatedly obtained quite easily by a fully noninvasive method, will undoubtedly exert influence on diagnostic steps in cardiology. An investigatin by 2-D Doppler may approach the correct diagnosis at the first outpatient examination, or in some cases permit diagnosis while omitting unnecessary ventriculography, or provide an indication for cardiac catheterization or X-ray angiography.

Continuous-wave Doppler [24, 25] (CW), though lacking range resolution, can measure the high velocity transvalvular flow without disturbance by aliasing. The pressure gradient across a valve can be calculated from the maximum velocity by the modified Bernouilli's formula [26–28].

$$P = 4V^2$$
P = pressure gradient
V = maximum velocity across a valve

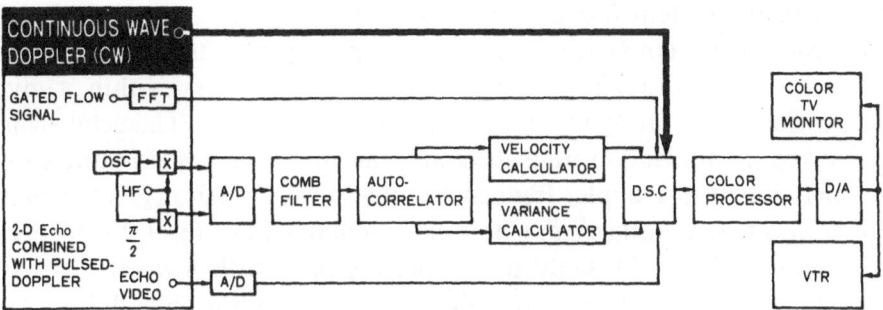

Figure 2. The block diagram of the new system. CW-Doppler device is added to 2-D Doppler system (Aloka 880).

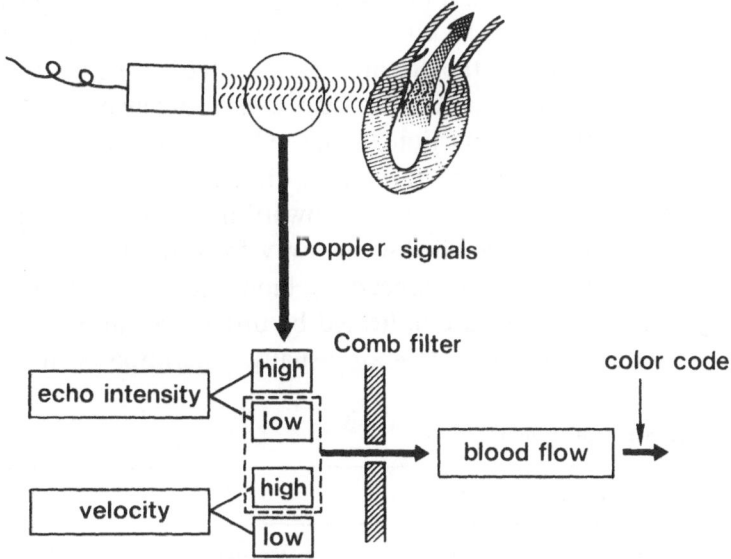

Figure 3. Schematic representation of comb filter to cancel the effects of wall motion.

Recently, we have added CW device to the 2-D Doppler system [26]. It is suggested that combined use of 2-D Doppler and CW may replace routine cardiac catheterization in acquired valvular diseases in some situations where coronary arterial lesions are ruled out.

INSTRUMENTATION

The 2-D Doppler system functions by calculating the two-dimensional distribution of various blood-flow velocities over the entire field of the 2-D image, producing color-coded blood-flow images in real time. The block diagram of the system (Aloka-880) is shown in Figure 2. In principle, the device combines a conventional pulsed-Doppler system and a newly developed auto-correlator [8, 27], in which blood-flow images within a given cross section of a beating heart are displayed in real time. The echo signals obtained by an ultrasound transducer are transmitted to a quadrature detector, where a pair of Doppler frequencies, that differ by 90° degrees in phase from each other, are obtained. Comb filter functions to cancel the effects or wall motions (Figure 3). Only the Doppler signals with low intensity and high velocity can pass through the filter as the signals from blood flow. This output is supplied to the auto-correlator, and is then written into a digital scan converter (DSC). The signals in the DSC are read out to a color converter where colors are assigned in accordance with the blood-flow direction and the extent of turbulence. Thus, with regard to the direction of blood flow, a red color is given to the blood flowing away from it. The velocity of blood flow is represented by the brightness of each color which is displayed in seven gradations. With regard to the degree of turbulence of blood flow, a green color is added in proportion to the extent of turbulence in sixteen gradations. Accordingly, as the turbulence increases, the color hue shifts from red to yellow for the blood flowing toward the transducer, and it shifts from blue to cyan for the blood flowing away from the transducer. Therefore, three kinds of information concerning blood flow, the direction, velocity and degree of turbulence are indicated by differences in color. The conventional B-mode echocardiograms are usually superimposed in black and

Table 1. Characteristics of system.

Characteristics of System (Aloka 880)	
Ultrasound frequency	2.5, 3.5 MHz
Pulsed repetion rate	4, 6, 8 MHz
Scanning angle for 2-D Doppler	27.5, 50, 90 degrees
for 2-D echo	90 degrees
Diagnostic range	6, 12, 15, 18, 21 cm
Frame rate	10–30 frames/sec
Display	B-mode, M-mode, FFT, (CW) ***
Transducer	phased array (13×10 mm, 48 elements)
Maximum detectable flow velocity *	120 cm/sec **
Minimum detectable flow velocity *	23 cm/sec (B-mode)
	6 cm/sec (M-mode)
Recording	VTR, 35 mm film, instant photo

* Assuming that beam angle to blood flow is 60 degrees.

** Images of blood flows with high velocities exceeding this range result in a wrap around of the top portion of Doppler frequencies (aliasing).

*** Optional.

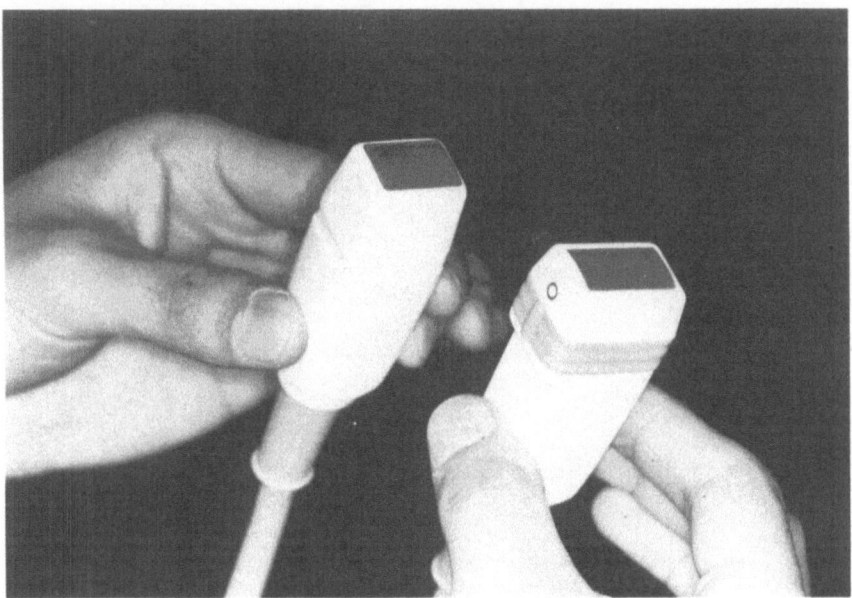

Figure 4. Transducers for a regular color flow mapping (left) and a combined use with CW (right).

white simultaneously with color-coded blood-flow images. Both M-mode and spectral analysis (fast Fourier transformation, FFT) displays are also available with this system. The characteristics of the regular system are briefly summarized in Table 1. Continuous wave ultrasound device can be added optionally to the system [26]. The probe with dual frequency transducer for the combined use is composed of phased array 48 elements for 2-D imaging (3.5 MHz) and two elements for CW transmitting/receiving (2 MHz). The distance between the center of phased array scanning and the CW elements is 10 mm (Figfure 4). The clinical use of 2-D Doppler system does not require special handling; rather it is used in the same manner as is conventional echocardiography (Figure 5). Actual findings of 2-D Doppler blood flow images in an adult normal heart are shown in Figure 6.

CLINICAL SIGNIFICANCE OF 2-D DOPPLER

Acquired valvular diseases

In the 2-D Doppler display, the regurgitant or stenotic blood flows were inlaid with red-and-blue mosaic patterns which were further superimposed with green color indicating the extent of turbulence. Investigations using

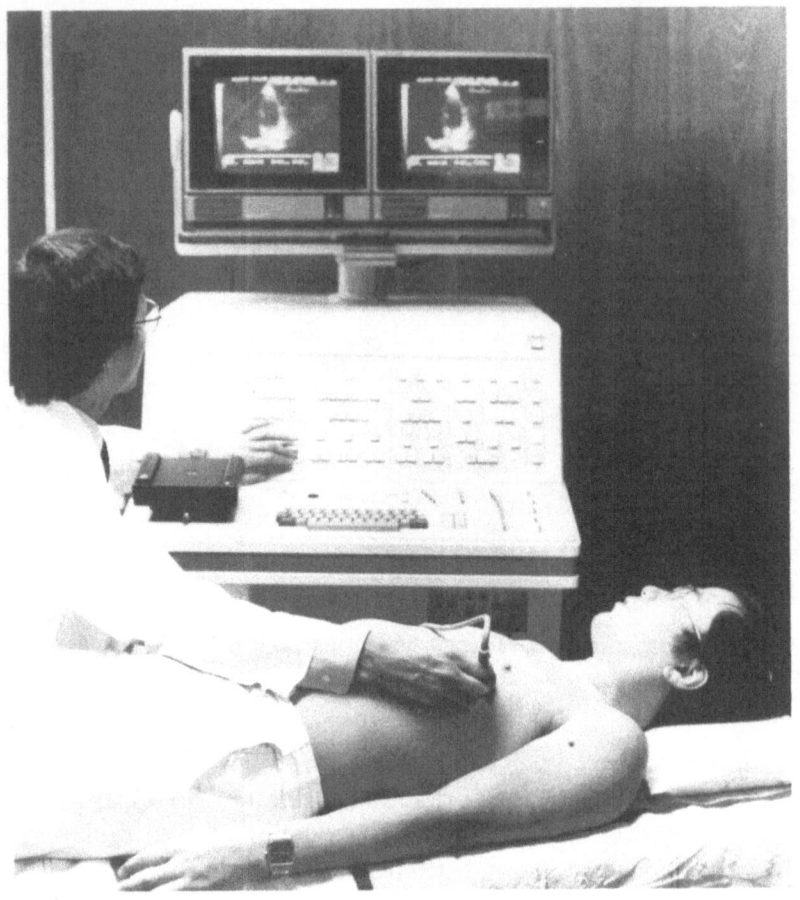

Figure 5. Clinical examination by 2-D Doppler.

Table 2A. Comparison of the grade of mitral regurgitation (MR) assessed by angiography (Angio) and 2-D Doppler (42 cases of MR). A significant correlation is noted.

Angio (0)	Doppler 2-D (I)	(II)	(III)	(IV)
0				
I	1	7		
II			15	3
III			1	12
IV				3

Grade	Criteria
(I)	RFIs are localized immediately posterior to the mitral valve in LA not exceeding the middle level between the mitral orifice and the valve ring.
(II)	RFIs reach almost the level of the mitral valve ring.
(III)	RFIs are present deep within 2 cm from the level of the mitral valve ring.
(IV)	RFIs are present deeper beyond the 2 cm from the level of the mitral valve ring, often visualized diffusely in the entire LA.

2-D Doppler clinically have shown that it is very useful in the detection of aortic, mitral and tricuspid regurgitations, and that it offers a favorable correlation with angiography or surgical findings in quantitative evaluation of severity of valvular regurgitation [10–12, 28]. The comparison of the grade of mitral regurgitation (MR) assed by angiography and 2-D Doppler in our 42 MR series [9] is shown in Table 2. Typical 2-D Doppler findings in mitral regurgitation (MR) associated with mitral stenosis (MS) are demonstrated in Figure 7. The appearance of acquired valvular diseases often coexists with two or more valvular lesions. 2-D Doppler has been found very sensitive and advantageous in diagnosing multivalvular diseases. Valvular stenosis can be adequately diagnosed with conventional echocardiography by the demonstration of the organic changes causing hemodynamic stenosis. In addition, quantification of pressure gradients across stenotic valves has become available by continuous-wave Doppler ultrasound (CW) [24, 25]. As described above, valvular regurgitation has been demonstrated accurately with 2-D Doppler and found to be highly correlated with the findings of angiography and/or surgery. Hence, it has been suggested that combined use of 2-D Doppler and CW can replace routine cardiac catheterization in some situations, such as where coronary artery disease is not suspected, or risks of cardiac catheterization are extremely high (Figure 8).

2-D Doppler is found also very sensitive in detecting a paravalvular leak. It is desirable to use a noninvasive technique in the follow-up study of valve replacement patients. In particular, when the replacement of the native valve by a mechanical valve has been performed in the aortic position, left ventricular angiography is not usually conducted due to the possible danger of damaging the leaflet of the mechanical valve. In this circumstance, 2-D Doppler serves to provide information which is not obtainable by any other noninvasive method.

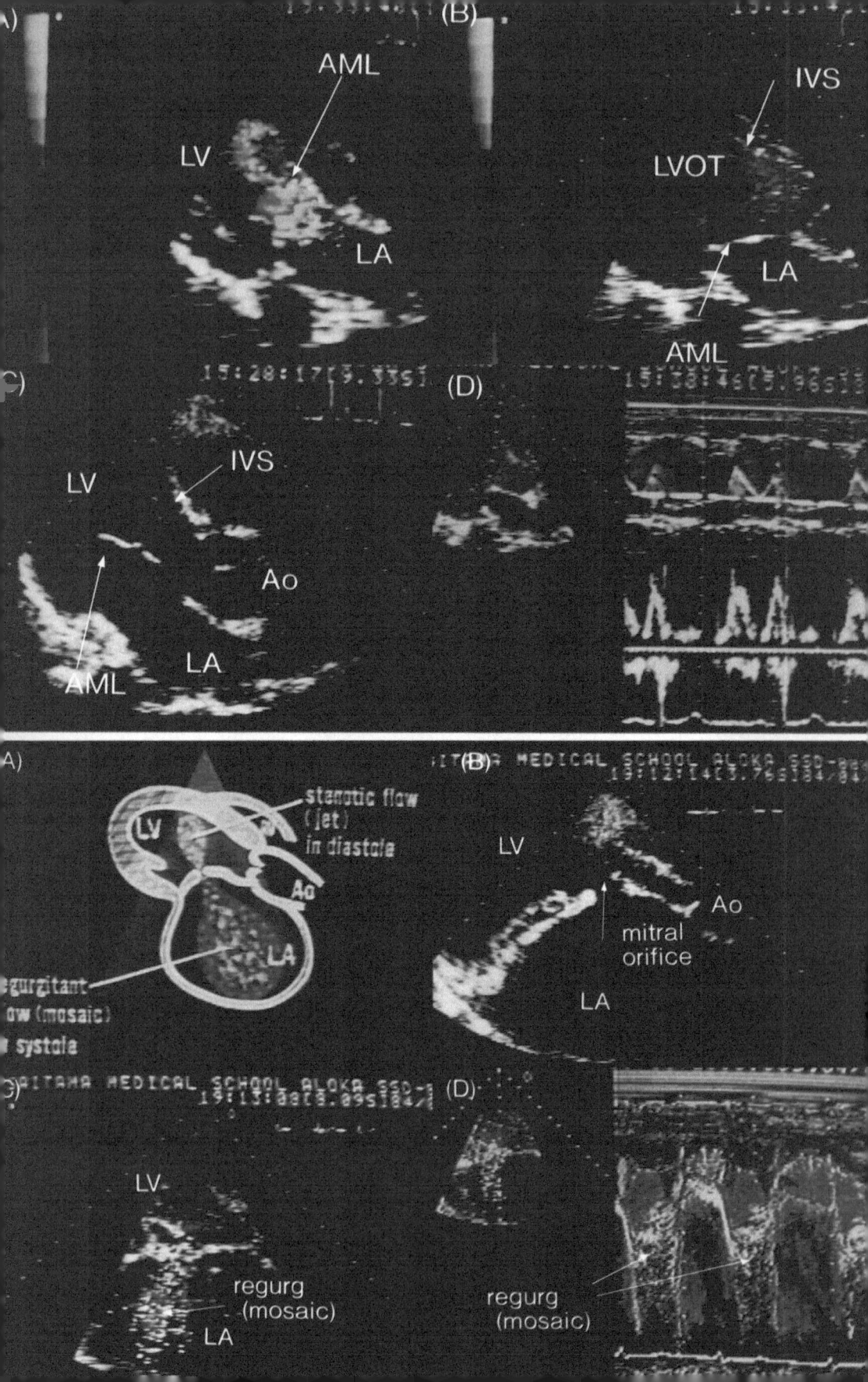

Figure 6. 2-D Doppler images in a normal heart: (A): 2-D Doppler (in diastole); (B): ditto (in systole); (C): B-mode (in diastole); (D): Simultaneous display of color flow-mapping M-mode and spectral analysis. AML: anterior mitral leaflet, IVS: interventricular septum, LVOT: left ventricular outflow tract.

Figure 7. 2-D Doppler images in a severely ill patient with MS MR. For this patient, 2-D Doppler findings alone determined cardiac surgery without catheterization: (A): schematic representation; (B): B-mode; (C): 2-D Doppler image (in systole). Severe MR is displayed in mosaic pattern: (D): color flow-mapping M-mode.

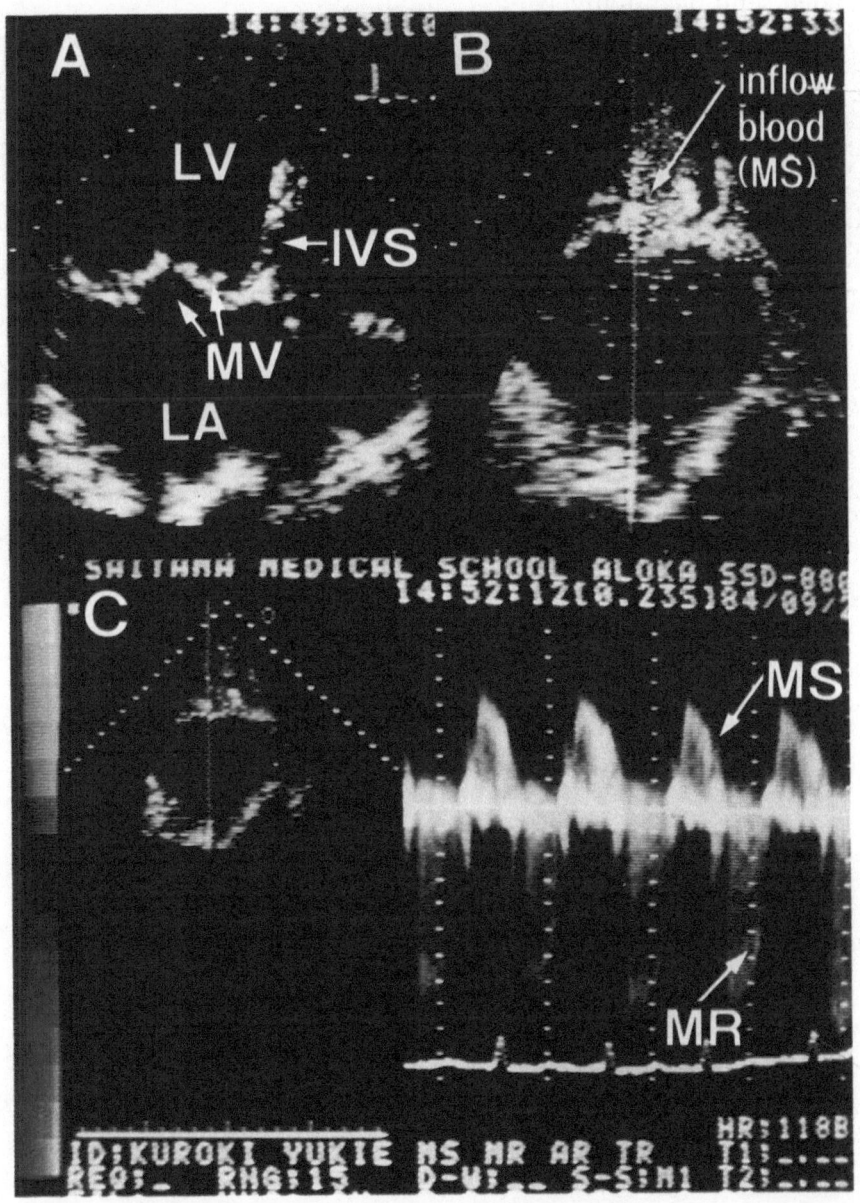

Figure 8. Combined use of 2-D Doppler and CW in a patient with MS MR: (A): B-mode; (B): 2-D Doppler; (C): Display by the combined use. Peak velocity across mitral valve in diastole is 2.2 m/sec. Pressure gradient (ΔP) is calculated as below: $\Delta P = 4 \times (2.2)^2 = 19$ (mm Hg).

Congenital heart diseases

The clinical significance of 2-D Doppler in congenital heart disease is that 2-D Doppler can visualize the intracardiac abnormal blood flow in real time. In 141 patients (97%) out of 145 patients with congenital heart diseases, abnormal blood flow with mosaic patterns (shunt flow, regurgitant flow and/or stenotic flow) was clearly visualized by 2-D Doppler [14], and also grade and severity of the abnormal intracardiac blood flow could be estimated semi-quantitatively.

The 2-D Doppler has been found very useful for determining good timing of palliative shunt surgery and in evaluating the effectiveness of shunt surgery, because 2-D Doppler is absolutely noninvasive and can be performed repeatedly [13]. The 2-D Doppler images of a patient with ventricular septal defect (VSD) in Eisenmenger syndrome are shown in Figure 9. In cases of VSD with Eisenmenger syndrome a bi-directional quadri-phasic shunt flow pattern was observed and it was consistent with the pressure gradient change between both ventricles observed by cardiac catheterization [15].

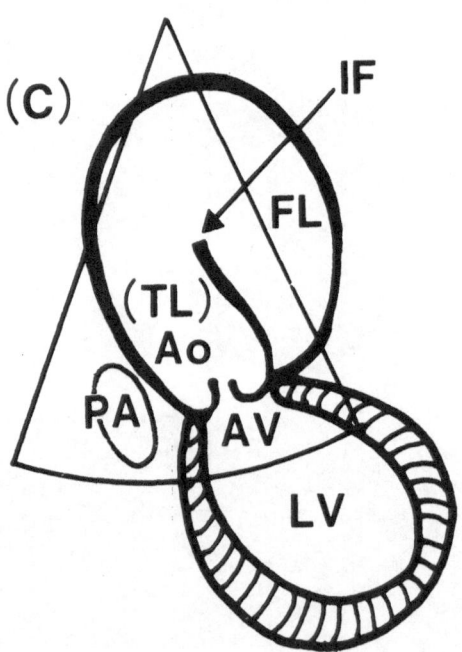

Figure 10C. Schematic representation; FL: false lumen, IF: intimal flap, TL: true lumen, AV: aortic valve.

Aortic aneurysms

In chronic dissecting aortic aneurysms, the entries in 3 out of 3 patients with DeBakey type-I and in 2 out of 6 patients with DeBakey type-III were demonstrated with 2-D Doppler [16]. An entry in the ascending aorta can be visualized easier than one in the descending aorta, where bone and air in the lung may prevent penetration by ultrasound. The detection of entries in dissecting aneurysms with 2-D Doppler is so far limited to DeBakey type-I [16]. Recently, intra-operative use of 2-D Doppler in the dissecting aortic aneurysm has been performed [17]. Intra-operative scanning of 2-D Doppler in the lung and short axis views gives almost complete three-dimensional informations about the structure and the blood flow very easily. The operation for dissecting aortic aneurysm is mainly aimed at closure of the entry and replacement of the dilated aorta and leaves large parts of the dissected aorta in situ. If the blood flow in the remnant dissected aorta is wrong, the operation cannot be successful. Therefore, it is very important to confirm that blood flow in the remnant aorta to the vital organs is well reestablished after the operative procedure. Intra-operative use of 2-D Doppler in dissecting aortic aneurysm has been found very effective in our clinical trials [17]. 2-D Doppler images in a patient with chronic DeBakey type-I dissecting aneurysm are shown in Figure 10.

CONCLUSIONS

The conclusions in this communication are summarized as follows:
(1) A real-time two-dimensional Doppler system for intracardiac blood-flow imaging (2-D Doppler or color flow mapping) has been successfully developed for wide clinical application.
(2) 2-D Doppler has been found to be very useful in detecting and estimating quantitatively the degree of valvular regurgitation.
(3) Combined use of 2-D Doppler and continuous-wave Doppler (CW) has been effective in evaluating quantiatively stenotic valvular lesions. It has been suggested that combined use of 2-D Doppler and CW may replace routine cardiac catheterization in some situations.
(4) 2-D Doppler can be a useful noninvasive diagnostic tool for congenital heart diseases, particularly useful for the evaluation of the severity of the disease. Under special circumstances, when a patient is critically ill, for instance, 2-D Doppler findings alone may decide the indication for cardiac surgery without examination by cardiac catheterization.
(5) The detection of entries in dissecting aneurysms with 2-D Doppler is so far limited to DeBakey type-I. Intra-operative use of 2-D Doppler in the surgery of aortic aneurysm seems to be promising.

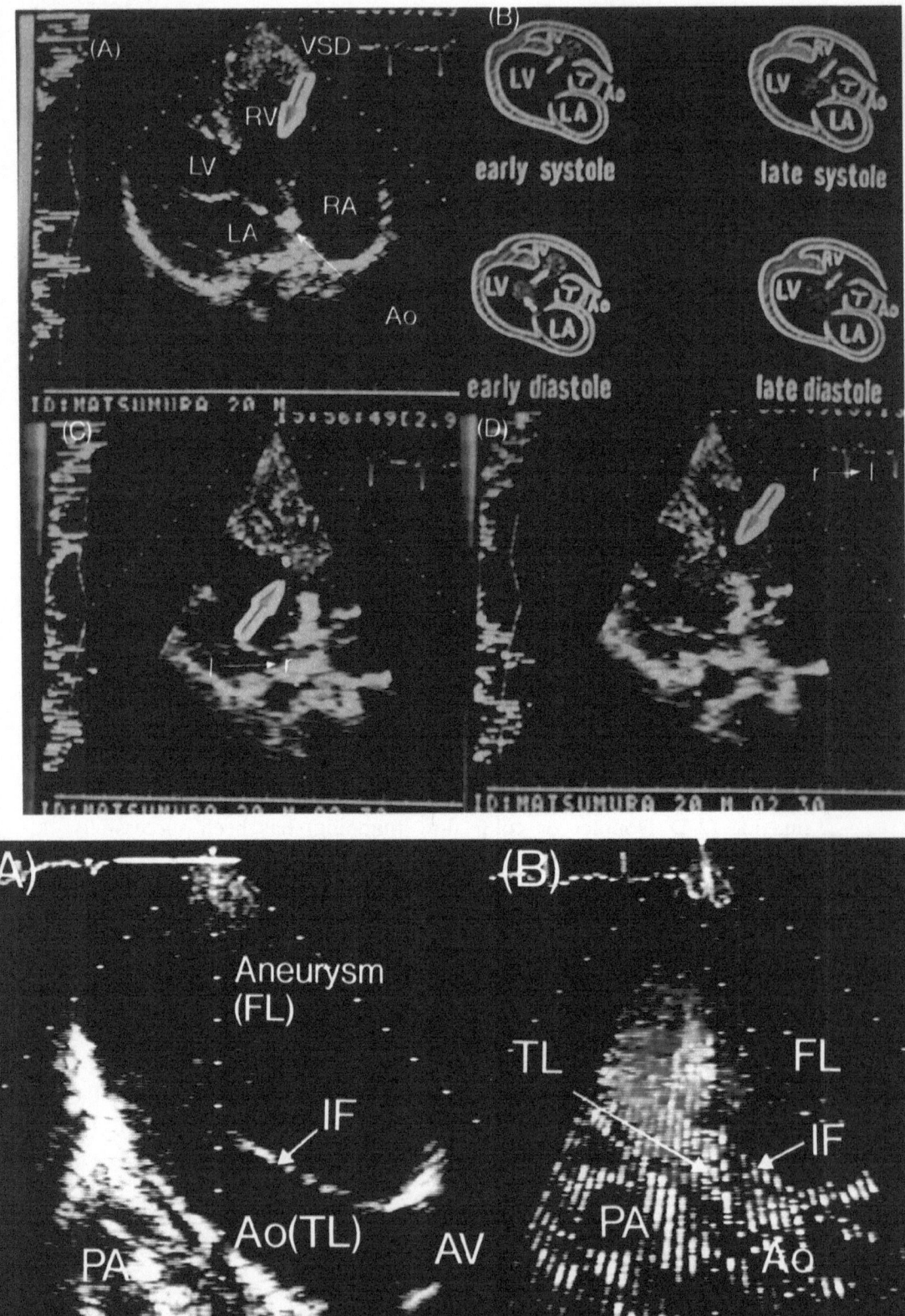

Figure 9. 2-D Doppler images in a patient VSD with Eisenmenger syndrome: (A): B-mode; (B): Diagrams of the VSD shunt flow pattern in early systole, late systole, early diastole and late diastole; (C): 2-D Doppler image in early systole (shunt flow: 1 → r); (D): 2-D Doppler image in late diastole (shunt flow: r → 1).

Figure 10A-B. 2-D Doppler images in a patient with dissecting aneurysm of the aorta (DeBakey type-I): (A): B-mode; (B): 2-D Doppler image.

←

REFERENCES

1. Baker DW, Rubenstein SA, Lorch GS: Pulsed doppler echocardiography. Principles and applications, Am J Med 63:69, 1977.
2. Goldberg SJ, Allen HD, Marx GR, Flinn CJ: Doppler echocardiography, Lea & Febiger, Philadelphia, 1984.
3. Fish PJ: Multichannel, direction resolving Doppler angiography, Abstracts of 2nd European Congress of Ultrasonics in Medicine 72, 1975.
4. Brandestini MA, Howard EA, Weile EB, Stevenson JG, Eyer MK: The Synthesis of echo and doppler in M-mode and sectorscan paper, No. 704: Proceedings of Annual Meeting of AIUM 125, 1979.
5. Stevenson JG, Kawabori I, Brandestini MA: Color-coded visualization of flow within ventricular septal defects: Implications for peak pulmonary artery pressure. Am J Cardiol 49:944, 1982.
6. Kitabatake K, Inoue M, Asao M, Mishima M, Tanouchi J, Masuyama T, Hori M, Abe H, Chihara K, Sakurai H, Senda S, Morita H, Matsuo H: Non-invasive visualization of intracardiac blood flow in human heart using computer-aided pulsed doppler technique. Clinical Hemorheology 1:85–91, 1982.
7. Bommer W, Miller L: Real-time two-dimensional color-flow Doppler: Enhanced Doppler flow imaging in the diagnosis of cardiovascular disease, (Abstract) Am J Cardiol 49:944, 1982.
8. Namekawa K, Kasai C, Tsukamoto M, Koyano A: Imaging of blood flow using autocorrelation, Ultrasound in Medicine & Biology 8:138, 1982.
9. Omoto R, Yokote Y, Takamoto S, Tamura F, Asano H, Namekawa K, Kasai C, Tsukamoto M, Koyano A: Clinical significance of newly developed real-time intracardiac two-dimensional blood flow imaging system (2-D Doppler), Japanese Circulation Journal 47:974, 1983.
10. Omoto R: Color atlas of real-time two-dimensional Doppler Echocardiography, Lea & Febiger, Philadelphia, 1984.
11. Omoto R, Yokote Y, Takamoto S, Kyo S, Ueda K, Asano H, Namekawa K, Kasai C, Kondo Y, Koyano A: The development of real-time two-dimensional Doppler Echocardiography and its clinical significance in acquired valvular diseases with special reference to the evaluation of valvular regurgitation. Japanese Heart Journal 25:325–340, 1984.
12. Omoto R, Yokote Y, Takamoto S, Ueda K, Emoto H, Hasegawa K, Tamura F, Asano H: Quantitative evaluation of valvular regurgitation in aortic, mitral and tricuspid regurgitatin with '2-D Doppler'. Japanese Circulation Journal 48:768–769, 1984.
13. Kyo S, Takamoto S, Ueda K, Emoto H, Tamura F, Asano H, Yokote Y, Omoto R, Takanawa E: Clinical significance of newly developed real-time two-dimensional doppler echocardiography (2-D Doppler) in congenital heart diseases with special reference to the assessment of the intracardiac shunts. Proceedings of the 43rd Meeting of Japan Society of Ultrasonics in Medicine 465–466, 1983.

14. Kyo S, Omoto R, Takamoto S, Takanawa E: Clinical significance of color flow mapping real-time two-dimensional doppler echocardiography (2-D Doppler) in congenital heart disease, (Abstract) Circulation 70:II-37, 1984.

15. Kyo S, Omoto R, Takamoto S, Yokote Y: Noninvasive analysis of bi-directional multiphasic intracardiac shunts by real-time two-dimensional doppler echocardiography, (Abstract) Circulation 70:II-365, 1984.

16. Asano H, Takamoto S, Kyo S, Ueda K, Emoto H, Yamada I, Yokote Y, Omoto R: Clinical assessment of the aortic disease by real-time two-dimensional Doppler Echocardiography. Proceedings of the 43rd Meeting of Japan Society of Ultrasonics in Medicine 171–172, 1983.

17. Takamoto S, Kondo Y, Yoshikawa Y, Kasai C, Koyano A, Kyo S, Yokote Y, Omoto R: The first clinical experiences of intra-operative real-time two-dimensional doppler echocardiography in the dissecting aneurysm of the oarta. J Ultrasound in Medicine 3 (Suppl):167, 1984.

18. Miyatake K, Okimoto M, Kinoshita N, Izumi S, Owa M, Takao S, Sakakibara H, Nimura Y: Clinical applications of a new type of real-time two-dimensional doppler flow imaging system. Am J Cardiology 54:857–868, 1984.

19. Sahn DJ, Swensson RE, Valdes-Cruz LM, Scagnelli S, Main J: Two-dimensional color flow mapping for evaluation of ventricular septal defect shunts: A new diagnostic modality, (Abstract) Circulation 70:II-364, 1984.

20. Yock PH, Segal J, Teirstein PS, Schnittger I, Popp RL: Doppler color flow mapping: utility in valvular regurgitation, (Abstract) Circulation 70:II-38, 1984.

21. Sewart WJ, Levine RA, King ME, Main J: Initial experience with color-coded two-dimensional doppler echocardiography, (Abstract) Circulation 70:II-405, 1984.

22. Yoshikawa J, Kato H, Yoshida K, Asaka T, Yanagihara K, Okumachi F, Shiratori K, Koizumi K: Real-time two-dimensional doppler echocardiographic diagnosis of aortic regurgitation in the presence of a mitral prosthesis, (Abstract) Circulation 70:II-39, 1984.

23. Sahn DJ, Valdes-Cruz L, Scagnelli S, Tomizuka F, Elias W, Covell J: Two-dimensional doppler color flow mapping for spatial localization and quantitation of aortic insufficiency: Validation of a new diagnostic modality using an open chest animal model, (Abstract) Circulation 70:II-38, 1984.

24. Hatle J, Brubakk A, Tromsdol A, Angelsen B: Noninvasive assessment of pressure drop in mitral stenosis by doppler ultrasound. Br Heart J 40:131–140, 1978.

25. Hatle L, Angelson B, Tromsdol A: Noninvasive assessment of aortic stenosis by doppler ultrasound. Br Heart J 43:284–292, 1980.

26. Omoto R, Yokote Y, Takamoto S, Kyo S, Asano H, Matsumura M, Kasai C, Namekawa K, Miura K, Kondo Y: Clinical significance of combined use of color flow mapping and continuous-wave doppler in acquired vasvular diseases, Proceedings of the 3rd International Cardiac Doppler Symposium (San Diego), 1985.

27. Namekawa K, Kasai C, Tsukamot M, Koyano A: Real-time blood flow imaging system utilizing autocorrelation techniques, Proceedings of the 3rd meeting of World Federation for Ultrasound in Medicine and Biology (Brighton), Pregamon Press, Oxford, 1982.

28. Sakakibara H, Miyatake K, Izumi S, Kinoshita N, Asonura H, Nimura Y: Assessment of mitral and aortic regurgitation by real-time two-dimensional doppler flow imaging system, (Abstract) Circulation 70:II-406, 1984.

10. Quantification of heart valve regurgitation by jet intrusion

BENGT WRANNE, PER ASK and DAN LOYD

INTRODUCTION

During the last few years a number of reports regarding the possibility to detect and quantify valve regurgitation with ultrasound doppler by measuring distance of intrusion of the regurgitant jet have appeared in the literature [1–4]. These reports are based purely on empirical data where ultrasound doppler and angiography are compared. The theory behind jet intrusion has not been considered. Some investigators, however, have failed to confirm the above findings [5–8]. This fact has led us to make model experiments and a theoretical analysis of the hydrodynamics of valve regurgitation in order to clarify the importance of different factors influencing the distance of jet intrusion [8]. One way to approach a complicated hydrodynamic problem is to present an application from common life.

AN ILLUSTRATIVE EVERYDAY EXAMPLE

Consider the man with the water hose, seen in Figure 1. The pressure in the water supplying main tube is supposed to be constant and equal in the two situations. Still, the water jet reaches much further for the man who has put a nozzle on his hose. We doubt that anyone would claim that more water comes out of the hose in situation A compared to B even though the jet reaches further. It has, however, in the main body of reports regarding valve regurgitation been claimed that the length of jet intrusion can be used as an estimate of volume flow in valve regurgitation. Understanding of the

* Supported by the County Council, County of Östergötland, Sweden, the Swedisch National Association against Heart and Chest Diseases and the Swedish Medical Research Council (Grant 07158).

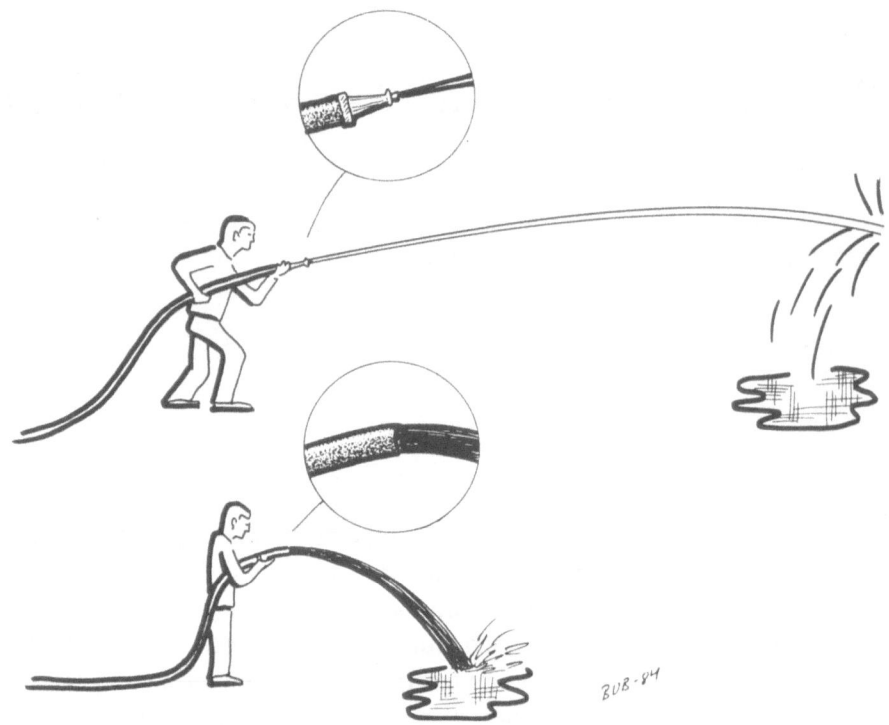

Figure 1. A man with a water hose with a nozzle of small area (A) and without a nozzle (B). When the nozzle area is decreased the volume flow is decreased and hence the pressure drop in the tubing is reduced. The higher pressure in the tubing just before the nozzle then increases the flow velocity at the nozzle and therefore also the length of the jet.

relation between driving pressure, flow velocity, orifice area, flow and length of the jet is essential both for the shown example and for the measurement of regurgitation with ultrasound doppler.

THEORY

The regurgitant flow through a heart valve can be modelled with the jet flow donwstream an orifice. At a certain distance x from the orifice this flow can be represented by velocity profiles as shown in Figure 2. In the general case the time depending flow, $\dot{Q}$, through such an orifice is given by

$$\dot{Q} = \int_A v_0 \, dA \qquad (1)$$

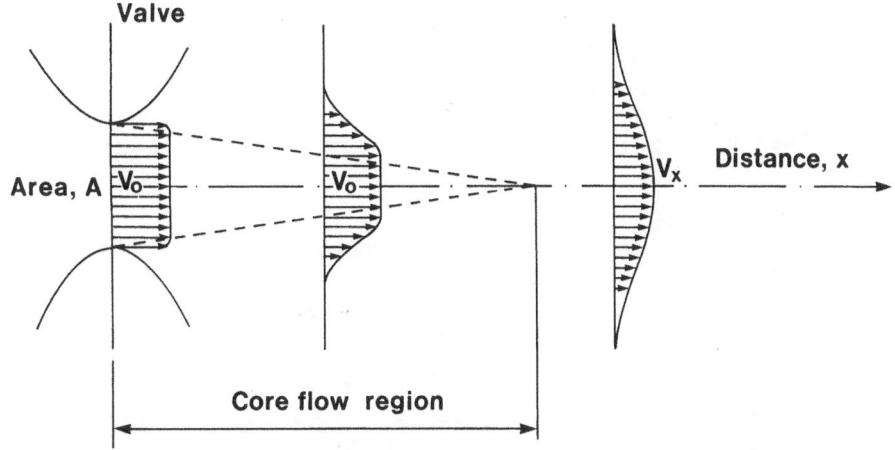

Figure 2. Velocity profile in the core flow region at a distance × from the orifice. v_0 is the flow velocity at the hole and v_x the velocity at a distance × from the hole. From Wranne et al., 1985.

where v_0 is the momentary value of the local flow velocity at the orifice and A the momentary area of the orifice. If the regurgitant flow is assumed to occur during a time period T_r the regurgitated volume is given by

$$V_r = \int_0^{T_r} \dot{Q}\, dt = \int_0^{T_r} \left(\int_A v_0\, dA \right) dt \tag{2}$$

We can simplify the calculations by assuming that the area of the hole and the driving pressure of the flow are constant during the regurgitation period. We can also instead of the local, time depending flow velocity v_0 use the average flow velocity, $\bar{v}_0$. Eq (2) then becomes

$$V_r = A\,\bar{v}_0\, T_r \tag{3}$$

and for a circular hole with the diameter, D

$$V_r = \frac{1}{4}\,\pi D^2\, \bar{v}_0\, T_r \tag{4}$$

For turbulent flow the velocity along the center line of the hole and at a distance x from that hole, the core flow region *not* included, is given by Hinze, 1959

$$v_x = \bar{v}_0\, \frac{k_1 D}{k_2 + x} \tag{5}$$

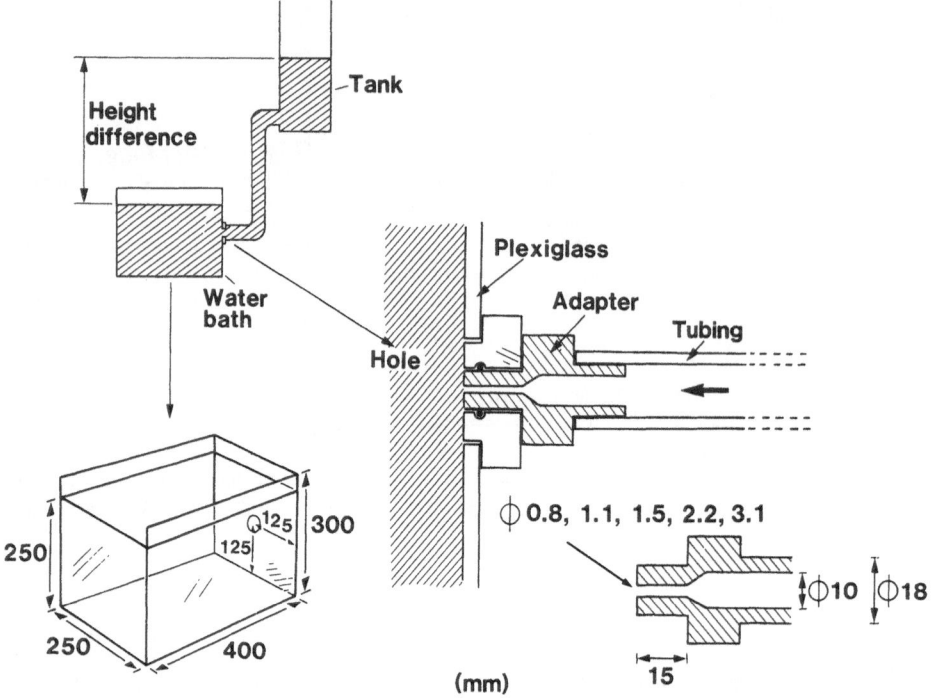

Figure 3. Diagram of the experimental set-up with water bath, water tank and adaptors with various hole diameters. From Wranne et al., 1985.

or

$$x = \frac{k_1 \overline{v}_0 D}{v_x} - k_2 \tag{6}$$

where k_1 and k_2 are constants.

By ultrasound doppler the distance x', where the flow velocity is reduced to a certain value, v_x' can be measured. By combining Eq (4) and Eq (5) the diameter is eliminated. The regurgitated volume can then be written as

$$V_r = \frac{\pi}{4} \cdot \frac{(v_{x_2}')^2}{k_1} (k_2 + x)^2 \frac{T_r}{\overline{v}_0} \tag{7}$$

MODEL EXPERIMENT

To investigate fluid jet intrusion, a water bath was used. Adaptors of various hole diameters (0.8, 1.1, 1.3, 2.2 and 3.1 mm) could be plugged into the end surfaces of the water bath as seen in Figure 3 [8]. The adaptors

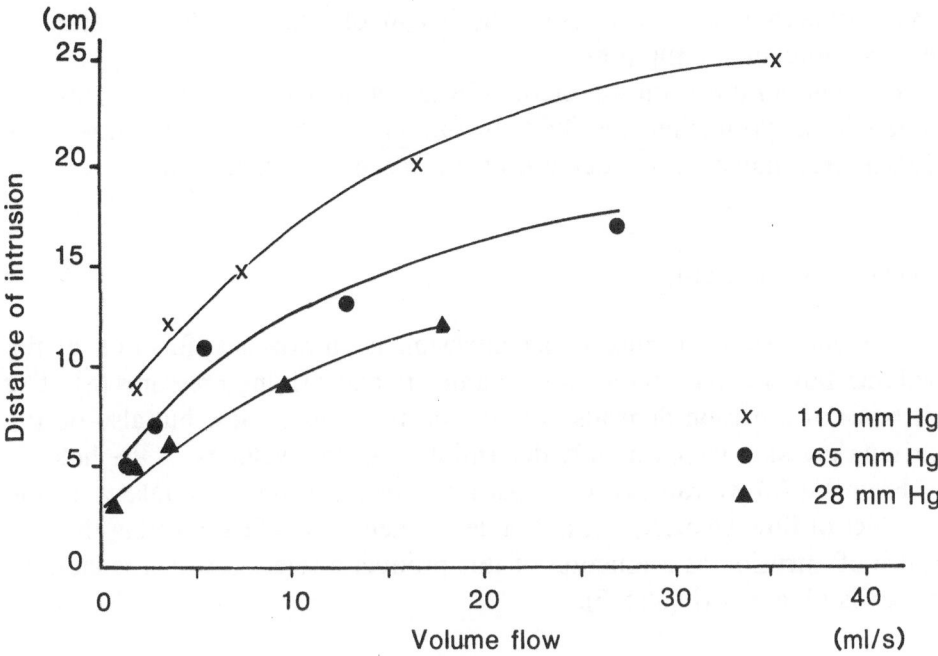

Figure 4. Distance of intrusion as a function of volume flow, shown for driving pressures of 28, 65 and 110 mm Hg. The lines show the best visual fits. From Wranne et al., 1985.

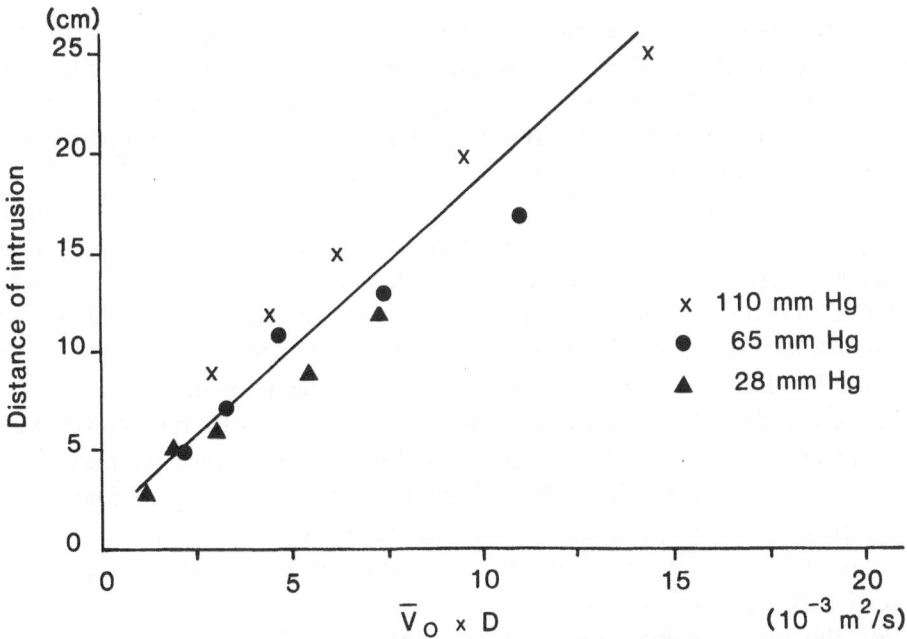

Figure 5. Distance of intrusion as a function of flow velocity $\bar{v}_0$, multiplied with hole diameter D. Data are plotted for driving pressures of 28, 65 and 110 mm Hg. The line with the equation $x' = 1.7 \cdot 10^3 \cdot (v_0 D) + 1.7$ was obtained using the method of least squares. The linear correlation coefficient was 0.97. From Wranne et al., 1985.

were connected to a water tank, the height of which could be varied to obtain different driving pressures.

The fluid jet intrusion was studied by injecting dye solution of methylene blue with a syringe into the fluid stream. The distance from the hole, to a visually estimated 90% reduction of the speed, was measured.

EXPERIMENTAL RESULTS

In Figure 4 the distance of jet intrusion is shown as a function of the volume flow for the various hole diameters and driving pressures [8]. The distance of intrusion depends not only on the volume flow but also on the driving pressure which mainly determines the flow velocity at the hole.

From Eq (6) we can expect the distance of intrusion to be related to the product of flow velocity, $\bar{v}_0$, and hole diameter, D. When plotting the distance of intrusion as a function of this product a relation which is close to linear is obtained (Figure 5).

DISCUSSION

The theoretical analysis shows that it is possible in the idealized model situation to estimate volume regurgitation if the following variables are known: distance of intrusion of the regurgitant jet, the regurgitation time and the mean flow velocity at the hole. The flow velocity is mainly determined by the pressure difference over the valve. All these variables can be estimated with ultrasound doppler. The analysis also shows that volume regurgitation in the general case cannot be estimated by measurement of distance of jet intrusion alone. Even in the idealized situation, it is only possible to estimate volume regurgitation by just measuring the distance of jet intrusion in the special case where the pressure difference over the valve and the friction loss in the orifice are constant and known.

Let us examine the pressure conditions present at the different valves. For the tricuspid valve, the driving pressure for the regurgitant jet may vary from 20 to more than 100 mmHg, which according to the approximate Bernoulli relationship corresponds to velocity values on the order of 2 to 5 m/s. The use of jet intrusion alone as a measure of regurgitation volume is indeed debatable in this case.

For the aortic valve, the diastolic pressure difference can vary from 100 mmHg in patients with diastolic arterial hypertension and mild regurgitation to 50 mmHg or less in patients with severe regurgitation. These pressure values correspond to approximate velocity values of 5 to 3.5 m/s, not taking into account viscous velocity losses that become important at very small holes Spencer and Arts [9]. For the mitral valve the pressure difference may vary from 180 to 80 mmHg corresponding to approximate flow velocity values of 6.5 to 4.5 m/s. Thus, the same criticism towards using jet intrusion alone for volume regurgitation is valid also for these valves although the misjudgments may not be as severe as for the tricuspid valve.

From the above it seems that the use of jet intrusion distance alone for estimation of regurgitation is at least not advisable for the tricuspid valve. Measurement of the width of the jet does not improve the method since the width of the regurgitant jet is to a large extent determined by the same factors as those determining jet intrusion distance Hinze [10]. Even in the case where flow velocity at the regurgitant valve hole or the corresponding pressure difference is known, it can be questioned if the regurgitant flow can be estimated from this information together with the measured distance of intrusion. Because in the real situation, the measured distance of intrusion is also determined by effects of the walls in the compartment into which the regurgitation occurs, the type of Doppler equipment used, size of sample volume, number of erythrocytes within the sample volume and patient selection. In addition to this inflow disturbances to the mitral valve may be caused by the chordae tendiniae and to the aortic valve by variations in anatomy and by the diastolic run off to the coronary arteries.

The situation is thus complex and further work is needed to determine to what extent a combination of measurement of velocity and jet intrusion will contribute tot the assessment of volume regurgitation.

REFERENCES

1. Quinones MA, Young JB, Waggoner AD, Ostojic MC, Riberio LG, Miller RR: Assessment of pulsed doppler echocardiography in detection and quantification of aortic and mitral regurgitation. Br Heart J 44:612–620, 1980.
2. Abbasi AS, Allen MW, Decristofaro D, Ungar L: Detection and estimation of the degree of mitral regurgitation by range-gated pulsed doppler echocardiography. Circulation 61:143–147, 1982.
3. Ciobanu M, Abbasi AS, Allen M, Hermer A, Spellberg R: Pulsed doppler echocardiography in the diagnosis and estimation of severity of aortic insufficiency. Am J Cardiol 49:339–343, 1982.
4. Miyatake K, Okamoto M, Kinoshita N, Ohta M, Kozuka T, Sakaibara H, Nimura Y: Evaluation of tricuspid regurgitation by pulsed doppler and two-dimensional echocardiography. Circulation 66:777–784, 1982.
5. Gacia-Dorado D, Falzgraf S, Almazan A, Delcan JL, Lopez-Bescos L, Menarguez L: Diagnosis of functional tricuspid insufficiency by pulsed-wave doppler ultrasound. Circulation 66:1315–1321, 1982.
6. Sgalambro A, Recusani F, Raisaro A, Cremaschi R, Tronconi L: Pulsed doppler diagnosis

of tricuspid insufficiency. G Ital Cardiol 12:270–277, 1982.

7. Wranne B, Marklund T: Diagnosis of tricuspid regurgitation. A comparison between pulsed doppler, jugular vein and liver pulse recording, contrast echocardiography and angiography. In: Cardiac Doppler Diagnosis, Spencer MP (ed.), pp 255–262, Martinus Nijhoff Publishers, Boston, 1985.

8. Wranne B, Ask P, Loyd D: Quantification of heart valve regurgitation: a critical analysis from a theoretical and experimental point of view. Clinical Physiology 5:81–88, 1985.

9. Spencer MP, Arts T: Continuous wave and pulsed doppler in acquired and congenital heart lesions. In: Cardiac Doppler Diagnosis, Spencer MP (ed.), pp 131–141, Martinus Nijhoff Publishers, Boston, 1983.

10. Hinze JO: Turbulence, pp 404–409, MacGraw-Hill, New York, 1959.

11. Quantitative evaluation of aortic and mitral stenosis by continuous wave Doppler echocardiography

JULIA W. WEN, R. BRAD STAMM, DONALD L. KAISER and ROVERT S. GIBSON

INTRODUCTION

M-mode and two-dimensional echocardiography (2DE) have become valuable assets in the noninvasive evaluation of valvular heart disease. By utilizing these techniques, the clinician can reliably identify the presence of abnormal valvular structure and indirectly demonstrate its hemodynamic significance through chamber enlargement or hypertrophy. However, neither technique can measure actual pressure gradients across stenotic valves and because of this, the clinician is often unable to distinguish aortic sclerosis from significant aortic stenosis, particularly in the setting of chronic hypertension. Moreover, the ability of 2DE to quantify mitral stenosis in patients with poor parasternal short-axis images is quite limited. This is especially true when assessing restenosis following commissurotomy since surgery frequently deforms the valve and submitral structures causing echo dropout of both the medial and lateral valve margins.

Since Doppler echocardiography can record the velocity and direction of blood flow within the heart, this comparatively new noninvasive technique offers the clinician the potential to measure pressure gradients across stenotic valves. Indeed, if doppler ultrasound proves feasible and reliable in this application, it would reduce the need for cardiac catheterisation since a better distinction among patients with significant lesions versus those with mild lesions could be made. Accordingly, the purpose of this report is to describe our experience with a variety of commercially available continuous wave doppler (CWD) instruments in 137 consecutive patients with suspected aortic or mitral stenosis. The specific objectives were: (1) to establish feasibility in a large consecutive series of adult patients; (2) to determine whether CWD can accurately quantify the pressure gradient across stenotic aortic valves using the modified Bernouilli equation [1], and if so, whether it correlates more closely with the peak-to-peak or, the peak-instantaneous gradient determined at cardiac catheterization; and, (3) to determine if CWD can estimate mitral valve areas, using Hatle's diastolic pressure half time equation [2, 3] in patients with denovo stenosis and those with suspected restenosis following commissurotomy.

Patient population

Eighty-four consecutive patients underwent CWD within 24 hours of diagnostic cardiac catheterization for suspected aortic stenosis. Three patients (4%) were eliminated when the aortic valve could not be crossed at the time of catheterization and an additional 6 (7%) were excluded because of technically inadequate doppler studies. Thus, the final study cohort comprised 75 patients including 50 men and 25 women, age 19–84 years (mean 63 ± 11). In this group, the average peak aortic valve gradient and cardiac index measured 74 mm Hg (range: 0–186) and $2.9 \, l/min/m^2$ (range: 1.3–4.6), respectively. Fifty patients subsequently underwent valve replacement for severe calcific aortic stenosis; the mean valve gradient and area in this group was 81 mm Hg and $0.6 \, cm^2$, respectively, and 18 patients had cath gradients between 75–186 mm Hg.

Doppler examination

The maximum doppler frequency shift and/or velocity was obtained from the cardiac apex (52%), right or left parasternal positions (21% and 1%), and suprasternal notch/right supraventricular fossa (25%) with the patient lying in the left lateral decubitus, right lateral decubitus or supine positions, respectively. During the examination, the ultrasound beam was maneuvered medial-laterally and anteroposteriorly until maximum velocity was identified by listening to the pitch of the audio signal and observing peak recorded velocity. Three commercially available instruments were used; namely, the Pedoff Doppler which was interfaced to an Irex II strip chart recorder, the Irex System III, and the Carolina Medical Electronics Sonacolor CD. A dedicated 2.0 MHz transducer was used for the first two instruments and a 2.5 MHz for the latter.

Catheterization and Doppler data

Figure 1 depicts a representative patient from our study cohort and illustrates the difference between peak-to-peak and peak-instantaneous catheter-

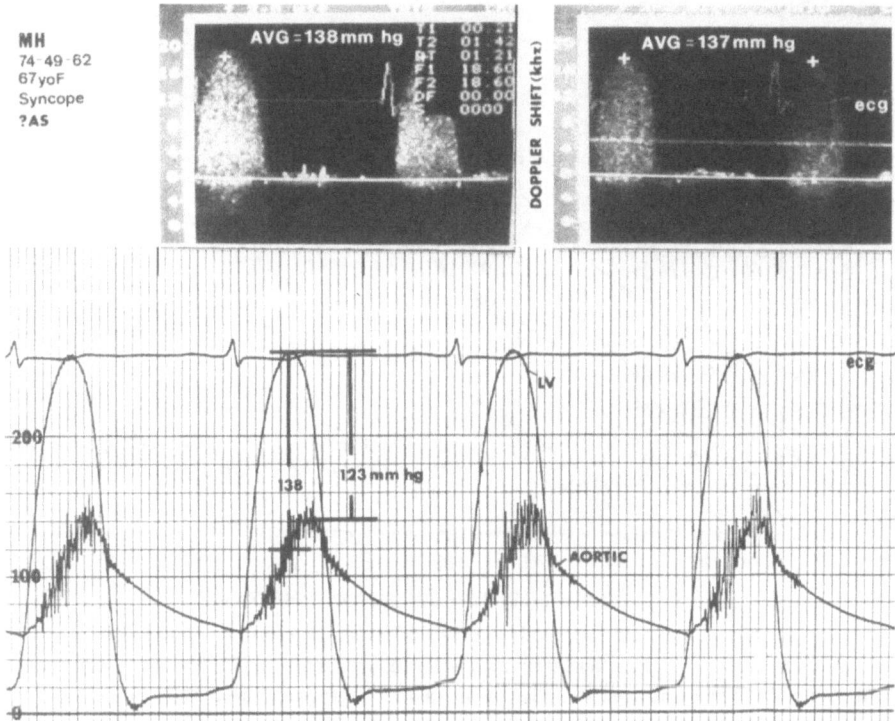

Figure 1. Severe aortic valvular stenosis. Top panel demonstrates an inverted display of the high velocity jet recorded from the cardiac apex. Notice the excellent signal to noise ratio and a peak frequency shift (F_1) of 18.6 kHz. Bottom panel shows the left ventricular (LV) and aortic pressure tracings obtained 18 hours after doppler. The peak-to-peak gradient measured 123 mm Hg and the peak-instantaneous or maximal gradient was 138 mm Hg. See text.

ization gradients. As can be seen, the maximal Doppler shift was 18.6 KHz and since a 2-5 MHz transducer was used, a peak Doppler derived gradient of 138 mm Hg was predicted. Thus, in this patient, the Doppler examination predicted very accurately the peak-instantaneous gradient, but overestimated the peak-to-peak gradient (i.e., 123 mm Hg) by 12%.

In our 75 patients, the correlation between maximal aortic valve gradient obtained by CWD and those measured at cardiac catheterization was excellent. Of interest, the correlations were equally good when CWD was compared with cath derived peak-to-peak and peak-instantaneous gradients (r = 0.90 and r = 0.89, respectively, p < 0.001). As might be expected from Figure 1, the CWD gradient overestimated by 4 ± 16 mm Hg the peak-to-peak aortic gradient. By comparison, the peak-instantaneous cath values were underestimated by 11 ± 16 mm Hg.

Neither the age of the patient nor left ventricular function appeared to

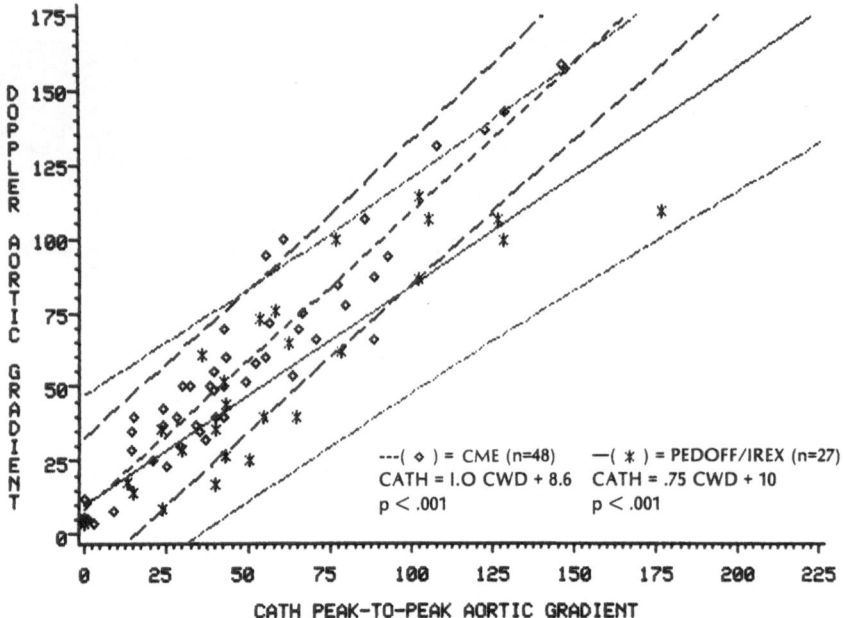

Figure 2. Comparison of peak aortic valve gradient derived by continuous wave doppler (CWD) and catheterization (CATH) measured peak-to-peak gradients in 75 patients with suspected aortic stenosis. Display format includes two separate regression lines, each bounded by 95% confidence intervals to illustrate the relationship between CWD and cath for the Carolina Medical Electronic (CME: dotted lines) Doppler and the Pedoff/Irex system (solid lines). See text.

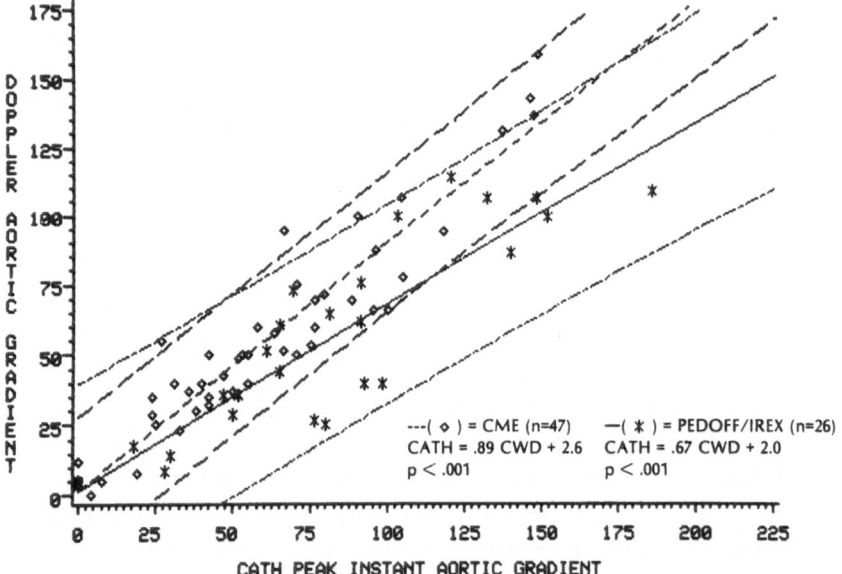

Figure 3. Comparison of peak aortic valve gradient derived by continuous wave doppler (CWD) and catheterization (CATH) measured peak-instantaneous (instnat) or maximal gradient in 73 patients with suspected aortic stenosis. Display format and abbreviations same as in Figure 2. See text.

affect our correlations. The r-value for patients under 50 years (n = 30) was 0.92, for those between 50–65 (n = 8) it was 0.89, and for the 37 patients who were greater than 65 years of age, the r-value was 0.93. For the 20 patients with cardiac indices of 2.2 $1/min/m^2$ or less, the correlation between CWD and the cath derived gradient was 0.85 (p<0.01).

Figures 2 and 3 illustrate the relationship between the CWD predicted gradients and those obtained at cardiac catheterization. The figures also show potential differences in the slopes of the prediction lines for the two instruments. While these slopes are not significantly different by test of Homogeneity of Slopes (p>0.1), there seems to be some inherent difference in the predictive relationships. More importantly, an identifiable difference in the variability for the two systems (peak-to-peak (Figure 2) F = 3.36, p = 0.002; and peak-instant (Figure 3) F = 2.94, p = 0.009) means that prediction of both peak-to-peak and peak-instantaneous cath gradients depends substantially on the instrument used, in addition to the expertise of the examiner.

MITRAL STENOSIS

Patient population

Fifty-three consecutive patients underwent CWD within 24 hours of diagnostic cardiac catheterization for suspected rheumatic mitral stenosis, including 19 (36%) with suspected restenosis following commissurotomy. Three patients (6%) were excluded because of technically inadequate doppler studies due to rapid atrial fibrillation. There were 14 men and 36 women in our study cohort, age 17–77 years (mean 51 ± 11). Thirty-seven of these patients subsequently underwent valve replacement or repair for severe mitral stenosis; the mean valve area in this group was $1.02 \, cm^2$.

Doppler examination

All patients were evaluated from the cardiac apex while lying in the left lateral decubitus position. Frequently, it was necessary to record multiple apical positions to identify both the maximum velocity during early diastole and a smooth flow-velocity profile. The same three commercial instruments as described above were used.

Catheterization and Doppler data

Figure 4 depicts a representative patient from our mitral stenosis cohort. As can be seen, the maximal doppler shift measured 6.1 KHz yielding a

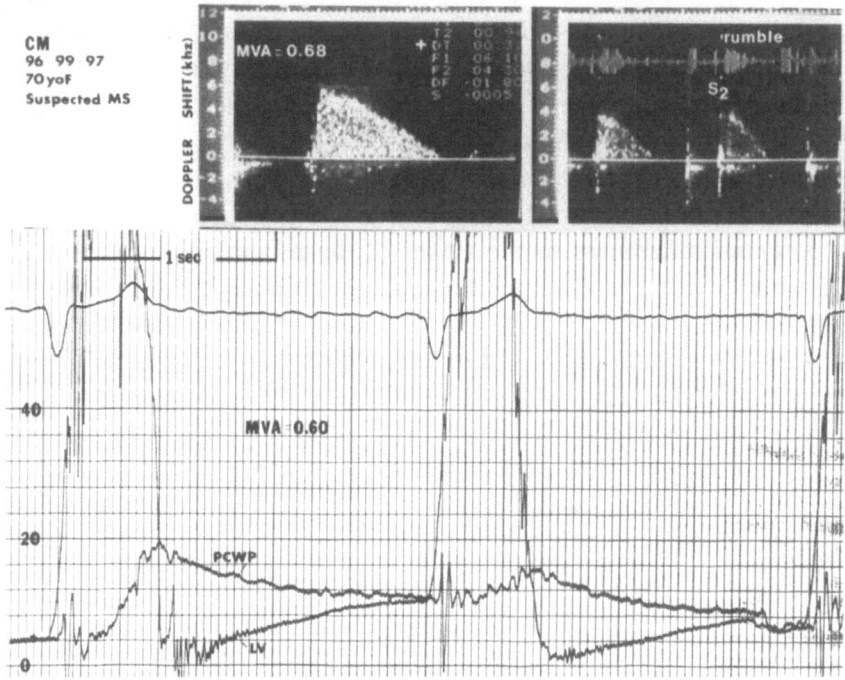

Figure 4. Severe rheumatic mitral stenosis. Top panel demonstrates the spectral output recorded from the cardiac apex. Since the patient was in a junctional rhythm, the flow profile is monophasic (i.e., no atrial contraction). During early diastole, the peak frequency shift (F_1) measured 6.1 kHz. Because a quadratic relationship exists between frequency and pressure, the transmitral pressure half-time was derived by first dividing F_1 by the square root of 2 to obtain F_2 (= 4.3 kHz) and then measuring the time in msec for F_1 to fall to F_2. Mitral valve area (MVA) is equal to 220 divided by this half-time value [2, 3]. Bottom panel shows the left ventricular (LV) and pulmonary capillary wedge pressure (PCWP) tracings obtained 6 hours after the doppler study. See text.

peak CWD derived gradient of 15 mm Hg during early diastole. This value and the measured half time of 320 msec correlated quite well with the catheterization results, as did the CWD derived mitral valve area of 0.68 cm².

In our 50 patients with suspected mitral stenosis, the correlation between mitral valve area obtained by CWD and that measured at cardiac catheterization was excellent ($r = 0.91$, $p < 0.001$). Since 19 of our patients (36%) underwent doppler-echocardiography 14 ± 4 years after mitral commissurotomy, we anticipated a stronger correlation with CWD derived mitral valve area and cardiac catheterization versus 2DE. Indeed, our results indicate this; specifically, the r-value for CWD was 0.91 versus 0.70 for 2DE ($p < 0.01$).

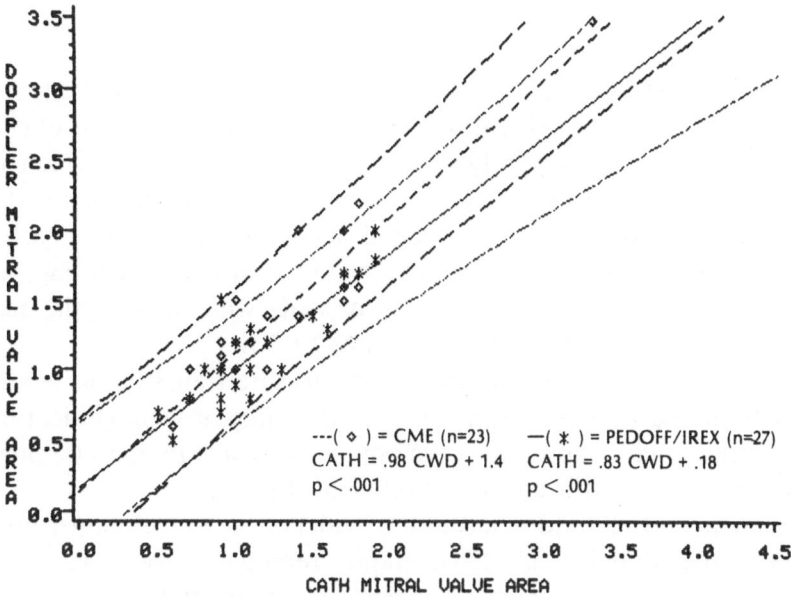

Figure 5. Comparison of mitral valve areas in 50 patients derived by doppler versus catheterization. Display format and abbreviations same as in Figure 2. See text.

Figure 5 shows the relationship between CWD predicted mitral valve area and that obtained at cardiac catheterization. In contrast to the findings for the aortic stenosis group described above, we found an appearance (from the regression lines) of more comparable predictive relationships for the two instruments, and no difference in variability by the type of CWD instrument used ($p > 0.1$).

DISCUSSION

Our results indicate that continuous wave doppler echocardiography can measure blood flow velocity across stenotic heart valves. By converting this information to pressure gradients, using the modified Bernoulli equation [1] (i.e., $\Delta P = 4V^2$), it can accurately predict the hemodynamic severity of aortic stenosis over a wide range of pressure gradients (20–186 mm Hg) and cardiac indices (1.3–4.6 l/min/m^2). Of interest, no significant difference in our correlation was found when we compared peak-to-peak and peak-instantaneous catheterization gradients to doppler derived data. Finally, mitral valve areas were accurately estimated using Hatle's diastolic pressure half time equation [2, 3] even in patients who had previously undergone commissurotomy. Indeed, our data indicate that doppler derived estimates are more accurate compared to two-dimensional echocardiography when a mixed clinical population of patients is evaluated.

Aortic stenosis

The diagnosis of aortic stenosis and an accurate assessment of its hemo-dynamic severity may be difficult to determine solely on the basis of clinical findings [4]. This is particularly true in the elderly patients, when other valvular lesions coexist or in the presence of left ventricular failure [5–8]. Unfortunately, most noninvasive studies including conventional echocar-diography, phonocardiography, and external carotid pulse recordings are of limited use, especially in distinguishing patients with mild aortic stenosis from those with severe valvular obstruction [9–13].

The use of doppler echocardiography to measure transvalvular gradients was first proposed by Holen et al. [4]. Subsequently, several clinical inves-tigators verified that continuous wave doppler was able to measure pressure gradients in patients with aortic stenosis [15–18].

The present study provides additional evidence, in a much larger number of patients, that doppler echocardiography represents a valuable tool for quantifying the severity of aortic stenosis. Successful studies were obtained in 93 % of our original cohort and unlike others [15], we found no difference in the strength of our correlation in elderly patients (i.e., ≥ 65 years) or those with left ventricular failure. Moreover, we demonstrated that CWD tends to overestimate peak-to-peak catheterization gradients. Although the magni-tude of this overestimation was slight, it was consistently observed. With this importat observation in mind, it thus appears that CWD represents a highly effective screening technique since very few patients with significant stenosis will be missed.

Mitral stenosis

Many investigators have examined the relationship of the 2DE mitral orifice size and the mitral valve area calculated from hemodynamic data [19–23]. All of these studies have shown good, if not convincing, cor-relations when both measurements could be obtained. However, other stu-dies have demonstrated that 2DE may provide erroneous information, par-ticularly when the valve and submitral structures are highly calcified and/or deformed [24]. Moreover, the difficulty in specifying the internal valve mar-gin in patients with poor parasternal short axis images and maintaining consistent contrast settings are recognized limitations.

Even when good quality images are available for analysis, the echocardio-graphic valve area tends to overestimate the hemodynamic area (i.e., under-estimate severity) by approximately $0.3 \, \text{cm}^2$ (range: 0.2–0.4) [19–23]. Ac-cording to Weyman [25], this occurs because 2DE records only the limiting valve orifice whereas the transvalvular catheterization gradient used in the

Gorlin formula includes all factors that contribute to left ventricular inflow obstruction; namely, the funnel shape of the valve, the decrease in orifice size and the resistance to inflow offered by thickened, fused chordae.

Our experience in 50 consecutive patients indicates that CWD offers a stronger overall correlation with catheterization quantification than is possible with conventional echocardiography. This result is not surprising since work by Hatle [3] has shown that the doppler-derived transmitral pressure half time permits accurate calculation of the mitral valve orifice area. Moreover, our study population included a sizeable number of post-commissurotomy patients whose mitral valve was quite deformed and difficult to evaluate with 2DE alone. Thus, in these patients and those with poor quality parasternal images, CWD represents a reliable noninvasive addition for assessing the severity of mitral stenosis.

REFERENCES

1. Hatle L, Angelsen B: Doppler ultrasound in cardiology-physical principles and clinical applications, p 24, Philadelphia, Lea-Febiger, 1982.
2. Libanoff A, Rodbards: Atrioventricular pressure half time, measure of mitral valve orifice area. Circulation 38:144, 1968.
3. Hatle L, Angelsen B, Tromsdol A: Noninvasive assessment of atrioventricular pressure half time by Doppler ultrasound. Circulation 60:1096, 1979.
4. Eddleman EE, Frommeyer WB, Lyle DP, Bancroft WH, Turner ME: Critical analysis of clinical factors in estimating severity of aortic valve disease. Am J Cardiol 31:687, 1973.
5. Finegan RE, Gianelly RE, Harrison DC: Aortic stenosis in the elderly: relevance of age to diagnosis and treatment. N Engl J Med 281:1261, 1969.
6. Davison ET, Friedman SA: Significance of systolic murmurs in the aged. N Engl J Med 279:225, 1968.
7. Roberts WC, Perloff JK, Costantino T: Severe valvular aortic stenosis in patients over 65 years of age: a clinicopathologic study. Am J Cardiol 27:497, 1971.
8. Braunwald E, Goldblatt A, Aygen MM, Rockoff SD, Morrow AG. Congenital aortic stenosis: clinical and hemodynamic findings in 100 patients. Circulation 27:426, 1963.
9. Bonner AJ, Sacks HN, Tavel ME: Assessing the severity of aortic stenosis by phonocardiography and external carotid pulse recordings. Circulation 48:247, 1973.
10. Weyman AE, Feigenbaum H, Dillon JC, Chang S: Cross-sectional echocardiography in assessing the severity of valvular aortic stenosis. Circulation 52:828, 1975.
11. DeMaria AN, Bommer W, Joye J, Lee G, Bouteller J, Mason DT: Value and limitations of cross-sectional echocardiography of the aortic valve in the diagnosis and quantification of valvular aortic stenosis. Circulation 62:304, 1980.
12. Gardin JM, Kaplan KJ, Meyers SN, Talano JV: Aortic stenosis: can severity be reliably estimated noninvasively? Chest 77:130, 1980.
13. Godley RW, Green D, Dillon JC, Rogers EW, Feigenbaum H, Weyman AE: Reliability of two-dimensional echocardiography in assessing the severity of valvular aortic stenosis. Chest 79:657, 1981.
14. Holen J, Aaslid R, Landmark K, Simonsen S: Determination of pressure gradient in mitral stenosis with a noninvasive ultrasound Doppler technique. Acta Med Scand 199:455, 1976.

15. Hatle L, Angelsen BA, Tromsdal A: Noninvasive assessment of aortic stenosis by Doppler ultrasound. Br Heart J 43:284, 1980.
16. Hatle L: Noninvasive assessment and differentiation of left ventricular outflow obstruction with Doppler ultrasound. Circulation 64:381, 1981.
17. Stamm RB and Martin RP: Quantification of pressure gradients across stenotic valves by Doppler ultrasound. J Am Coll Cardiol 2:707, 1983.
18. Berger M, Berdoff RL, Gallerstein PE, Goldberg E: Evaluation of aortic stenosis by continuous wave doppler ultrasound. J Am Coll Cardiol 3:150, 1984.
19. Henry WL, Griffith JM, Michaelis LL, McIntosh CC, Morrow AG, Epstein SE: Measurement of mitral orifice area in patients with mitral valve disease by real-time, two-dimensional echocardiography. Circulation 51:827, 1975.
20. Nichol PM, Gilbert BW, Kisslo JA: Two-dimensional echocardiographic assessment of mitral stenosis. Circulation 55:120, 1977.
21. Wann LS, Weyman AE, Feigenbaum H, Dillon JC, Johnston KW, Eggleton RC: Determination of mitral valve area by cross-sectional echocardiography. Ann Int Med 88:337, 1978.
22. Martin RP, Rakowski H, Kleman JH, Beaver W, London E, Popp RL: Reliability and reproducibility of two-dimensional echocardiographic measurement of stenotic mitral valve orifice area. Am J Cardiol 43:560, 1979.
23. Weyman AE, Wann LS, Rogers EW, Godley RW, Dillon JC, Feigenbaum H: Five year experience in correlating cross-sectional echocardiographic assessment of the mitral valve area with hemodynamic valve area determinations. Am J Cardiol 43:386, 1979.
24. Marino P, Zanolla L, Perini GP: Clinical assessment of two-dimensional echocardiographic estimation of mitral valve area in rheumatic mitral valve disease. Calcific deposits in the valve as a major determinant of the accuracy of the method. Eur Heart J 2:197, 1981.
25. Weyman AE: Cross-Sectional Echocardiography, p 156–157. Philadelphia, Lea-Febiger, 1982.

12. A new approach to noninvasive estimation of stenotic orifice area in semilunar valve stenosis by Doppler echocardiography

AKIRA KITABATAKE, KENSHI FUJII, HIROSHI ITO, JUN TANOUCHI, KEN

ISHIHARA, TOSHIO MORITA, YUTAKA YOSHIDA, MASATSUGU HORI and

MICHITOSHI INOUE

INTRODUCTION

In stenotic heart valve diseases, quantitative Doppler echocardiography provides the reliable estimation of the pressure gradient across the stenotic valve [1–9]. Although the pressure gradient is a practically useful parameter to evaluate the severity of stenotic valve lesions, it essentially depends on flow rate. For a given stenotic orifice, it may vary with the changes in the hemodynamic state of the heart, and not be simply regarded as an absolute measure of the obstruction.

Stenotic orifice area is another important consideration in evaluating the severity of stenosis [10–12]. The stenotic orifice area directly reflects the pathological changes of valve lesions and is expected to be constant independently of the changes in flow rate. In this chapter, we will introduce a unique Doppler method to estimate the stenotic orifice area based on 'equation of continuity' in hydraulics, and the preliminary application of this method to patients with semilunar valve stenosis.

THEORETICAL CONSIDERATIONS

The basic concept used for the calculation of stenotic orifice area is the 'equation of continuity' in hydraulics, which is based on the principles of the conservation of mass. Let us consider a one-dimensional steady flow of incompressive fluid in a cylindrical flow tract with a stenotic orifice (Figure 1). If there is no gain or loss of flow throughout the tract, the flow rate (Q), which is expressed as a product of cross sectional area and flow velocity, is constant at any cross section of the tract; that is described as:

$$Q = A_1 \cdot V_1 = A_2 \cdot V_2 \tag{1}$$

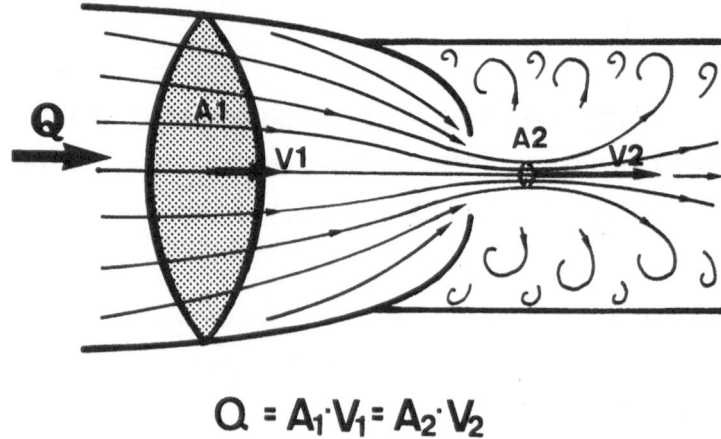

$$Q = A_1 \cdot V_1 = A_2 \cdot V_2$$

Figure 1. Schematic representation of the relationship between flow area (A) and flow velocity (V). Based on the 'equation of continuity' in hydraulics, flow rate (Q), which is expressed as a product of flow area and flow velocity, is constant throughout the flow tract. Abbreviations: see text.

where, A_1 and V_1 denote cross sectional area and flow velocity at a proximal portion of the orifice, A_2 denotes the effective stenotic orifice area, and V_2 denotes the maximal jet flow velocity. The effective stenotic orifice area represents the smallest cross setional area of the jet just distal to the orifice, where the flow velocity is at its maximum (at vena contracta). Therefore, the effective stenotic orifice area (A_2) can be determined from the measurements of A_1, V_1 and the jet flow velocity at the vena contracta by using the following equation as:

$$A_2 = A_1 \cdot V_1/V_2 \tag{2}$$

As shown in this equation, the calculated orifice area does not represent the actual geometric orifice area but the effective one. The ratio of effective orifice are (Ae) to the geometric orifice area (Ao) is defined as the discharge coefficient, Cd:

$$Cd = Ae/Ao \tag{3}$$

The Cd reflects the contraction of flow stream and the effect of friction at the orifice, and is thought to be relatively constant over a wide range of Reynolds number [11]. Its value, however, mainly depends upon the geometry of the orifice inlet; for example, the value of the Cd is 0.6 for sharp edged round inlet and close to 1.0 for a well rounded nozzle-like inlet [10]. The geometric orifice area can be determined by deviding the effective one by the Cd. It, however, cannot be a direct measure of stenosis, since the Cd may vary from orifice to orifice. On the other hand, the effective orifice area would be more preferable than the geometric one as a measure of stenosis, because it entirely determines the relationship between flow rate and flow velocity as shown in eq. (1).

In terms of the hydraulic loading to the heart, the mean orifice area over an ejection period seems to be as useful as the instantaneous one calculated directly by using eq. (2), because flow mode in cardiovascular system is not steady but pulsatile. Integration of both hands of eq. (2) over a ejection time (ET) yields the following expression as:

$$\overline{A}_1 \int^{ET} V_1 \, dt = \overline{A}_2 \int^{ET} V_2 \, dt \qquad (4)$$

where the bars over the symbols indicate an average over the ejection time. Since the left hand of eq. (4) represents the stroke volume (SV), the $\overline{A}_2$ is calculated by using another expression of eq. (4):

$$\overline{A}_2 = SV / \int^{ET} V_2 \, dt \qquad (5)$$

Thus, the mean effective stenotic orifice area can be determined from the measurements of the stroke volume and the instantaneous maximal jet flow velocity at the vena contracta, which can now be reliably measured by the Doppler echocardiography.

CLINICAL STUDY

Based on the theoretical considerations mentioned above, we attempted to calculate the stenotic orifice area in 11 patients with semilunar valve stenosis (eight with aortic stenosis and four with pulmonary stenosis) by the Doppler echocardiography. The feasibility and the reliability of our method was examined in comparison with a quantitative catheter technique. Doppler measurements required for the calculation of the orifice area are the stroke volume and the trace of instantaneous maximal jet flow velocity. The stroke volume was calculated from a cross sectional area and flow velocity in each ventricular outflow tract just proximal to the stenotic lesion by using two-dimensional pulsed Doppler echocardiography (Figure 2) [13]. Flow velocity, at the stenotic orifice, was recorded using a continuous wave Doppler technique from the cardiac apex in the cases of the aortic stenosis and from the precordium in the cases of the pulmonary stenosis (Figure 2), in which the maximal velocity was identified by listening to the highest and uniform pitch of audio outputs, and the Doppler incident angle was assumed to be 0. From these measurements, the stenotic orifice area was

154

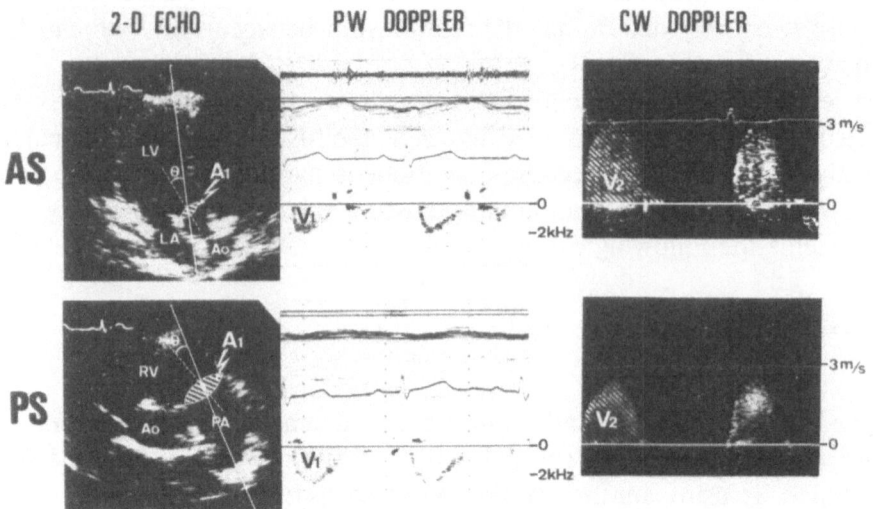

Figure 2. Doppler estimation of stenotic orifice area in semilunar valve stenosis. Cross sectional area (A_1) and flow velocity (V_1) are measured in each ventricular outflow tract just proximal to the stenotic lesion by two-dimensional pulsed Doppler echocardiography. The jet flow velocity (V_2) at the stenotic orifice is recorded by a continuous wave technique. The stenotic orifice area is calculated as a ratio of Doppler-determined stroke volume against the systolic integral of the jet flow velocity. Abbreviations: AS = aortic stenosis, PS = pulmonary stenosis.

obtained as a ratio of the stroke volume against the time integral of stenotic jet flow velocity trace using eq. (4). The stenotic orifice area was also determined from data obtained at catheterization by the Gorlin formula [14].

Doppler-derived stenotic orifice areas showed a good correlation with those by the catheter technique with a correlation coefficient of 0.76 ($p < 0.01$; $y = 0.86x + 0.06$).

CONCLUSION

The results of this study demonstrate that the quantitative Doppler method based on the 'equation of continuity' in hydraulics permits the accurate and reliable estimation of the effective stenotic orifice area in the patients with semilunar valve stenosis. Because the calculated orifice area directly indicates the extent of flow obstruction, the present method is quite useful in the management of patients with stenotic heart valve diseases as well as in the evaluation of the results of surgical treatments.

REFERENCES

1. Holen J, Aaslid R, Landmark K, Simonsen S: Determination of pressure gradient in mitral stenosis with a noninvasive ultrasound Doppler technique. Acta Med Sand 199:455, 1976.
2. Hatle L, Brubakk A, Trmosdal A, Angelsen B: Noninvasive assessment of pressure drop in mitral stenosis by Doppler ultrasound. Br Heart J 40:131, 1978.
3. Hatle L, Angelsen A, Tromsdal A: Noninvasive assessment of aortic stenosis by Doppler ultrasound. Br Heart J 43:284, 1980.
4. Hatle L: Noninvasive assessment and differentiation of left ventricular outflow obstruction with Doppler ultrasound. Circulation 64:381, 1981.
5. Stamm RB, Martin RP: Quantification of pressure gradients across stenotic valves by Doppler ultrasound. J Am Coll Cardiol 2:707, 1983.
6. Oliveira Lima C, Sahn DJ, Valdes-Cruz LM, Goldberg SJ, Vargas Barron J, Allen HD, Grenadier E: Noninvasive prediction of transvalvular pressure gradient in patients with pulmonary stenosis by quantitative two-dimensional echocardiographic Doppler studies. Circulation 67:866, 1983.
7. Stevenson JG, Kawabori I: Noninvasive determination of pressure gradients in children: Two methods employing pulsed Doppler echocardiography. J Am Coll Cardiol 3:179, 1984.
8. Berger M, Berdoff RL, Gallerstein PE, Goldberg E: Evaluation of aortic stenosis by continuous wave Doppler ultrasound. J Am Coll Cardiol 3:150, 1984.
9. Valdes-Cruz LM, Horowitz S, Sahn DJ, Larson D, Oliveira Lima C, Mesel E: Validation of a Doppler echocardiographic method for calculating severity of discrete stenotic obstructions in a canine preparation with pulmonary arterial band. Circulation 69:1177, 1984.
10. Holen J, Aaslid R, Landmark K, Simonsen S, Østrem T: Determination of effective orifice area in mitral stenosis from Noninvasive ultrasound Doppler data and mitral flow rate. Acta Med Scand 201:83, 1977.
11. Requarth JA, Goldberg SJ, Vasko SD, Allen HD: *In vitro* verification of Doppler prediction of transvalve pressure gradient and orifice area in stenosis. Am J Cardiol 53:1369, 1984.
12. Kosturakis D, Allen HD, Goldberg SJ, Sahn DJ, Valdes-Cruz LM: Noninvasive quantification of stenotic semilunar valve areas by Doppler echocardiography. J Am Coll Cardiol 3:1256, 1984.
13. Kitabatake A, Inoue M, Asao M, Ito H, Masuyama T, Tanouchi J, Morita T, Hori M, Yoshima H, Ohnishi K, Abe H: Noninvasive evaluation of the ratio of pulmonary to systemic flow in atrial septal defect by duplex Doppler echocardiography. Circulation 69:73, 1984.
14. Gorlin R, Gorlin SG: Hydraulic formula for calculation of the area of the stenotic mitral valve, other cardiac valves, and central circulatory shunts. I. Am Heart J 41:1, 1951.

13. Evaluation of left ventricular diastolic filling by a pulse Doppler flowmeter in patients with coronary artery disease

SHIGEHITO TAKAGI, MITSUHIRO YOKOTA, MASATSUGU IWASE, MASABUMI KOIDE, HU XIAO JING, HIROSHI HAYASHI and IWAO SOTOBATA

INTRODUCTION

Impaired left ventricular (LV) diastolic filling in patients with coronary artery disease (CAD) has been reported [1, 2], and in these reports, the rate of changes in LV volume is used for the assessment of LV diastolic filling. However, in CAD, the calculation of LV volume is sometimes difficult because of the regional abnormalities of LV wall motion. The transmitral blood flow during diastole is equal to the rate of changes in LV volume in the absence of regurgitation or shunt flow into the LV, which is independent of the regional LV wall motion.

For the evaluation of the LV diastolic filling in CAD, in the present study, transmitral blood flow velocity was measured by a pulse Doppler flowmeter and was correlated with cardio-hemodynamic parameters obtained from cardiac catheterization.

METHODS

The study population consisted of 37 patients with old myocardial infarction (OMI), 20 patients with effort angina pectoris (AP), and 15 normals. The OMI was divided into 2 groups; the one subgroup having an LV end-diastolic pressure (EDP) of less than 12 mm Hg (OMI-O) and the other group having an LVEDP of higher than 12 mm Hg (OMI-II).

The mean age of these groups was 55 yrs in OMI-I, 51 yrs in OMI-II, 55 yrs in AP and 52 yrs in normals. All the subjects except 5 normals were evaluated by cardiac catheterization, and coronary and left ventricular cineangiography (LVG).

158

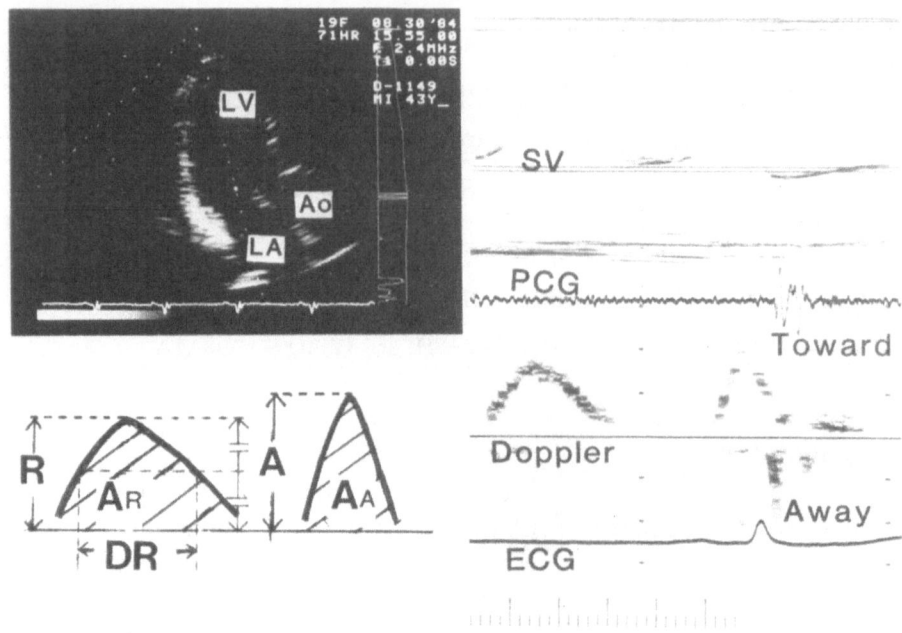

Figure 1. The measurement of transmitral flow velocity and the determination of Doppler parameters.

R = the peak velocity in the rapid filling phase

A_R = the area under the flow velocity curve in the rapid filling phase. A = the peak velocity due to atrial contraction, A_A = the area under the flow velocity curve in the atrial contraction phase. DR = the width of rapid filling wave at the level of one-half of the peak velocity.

Doppler examination

A pulse Doppler flowmeter combined with an electronic sectorscanning echocardiography (Toshiba SSH-11A and SDS-10A) was used with an ultrasonic frequency of 2.4 MHz and a pulse repetition rate of 4 or 6 KHz. The Doppler examination was performed with patients in the left semilateral position within 24 hours before cardiac catheterization.

After imaging the apical long axis view, the Doppler sampling volume was set at the center of the mitral ring. The transmitral flow velocity was calculated from shifted frequency using the Doppler equation (Figure 1). The transmitral flow velocity consisted of two components. The first component coincided in time with the rapid filling phase in early diastole, and the second one with the atrial contraction phase in late diastole.

The following parameters were obtained; (1) the peak velocity in the rapid filling phase (R), (2) the peak velocity in the atrial contraction phase

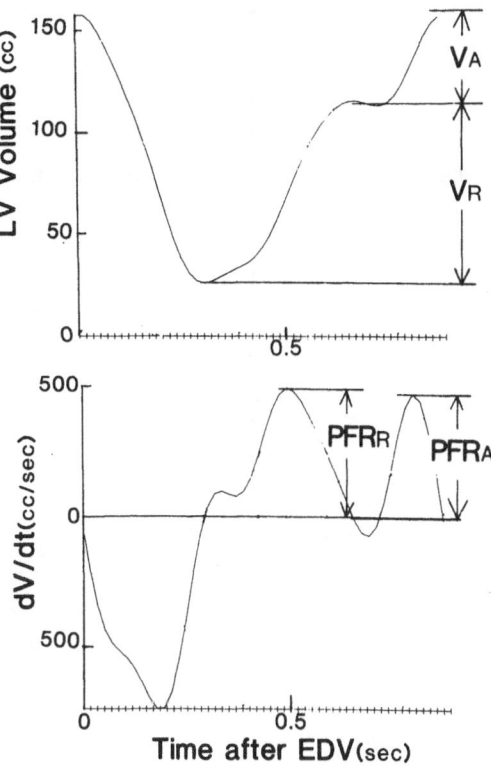

Figure 2. Left ventricular (LV) volume and dV/dt calculated from the single-plane cineangio-gram in a patient with effort angina pectoris. Fourier transformation (5th) was used for curve smoothing of the LV volume-time curve.
V_A = the increment in diastolic LV volume due to atrial contraction.
V_R = the increment in diastolic LV volume in the rapid filling phase.
PFR_R = peak filling rate in the rapid filling phase.
PFR_A = peak filling rate due to atrial contraction.

(A), (3) the ratio of A to R (A/R), (4) the ratio of the area under the flow velocity curve in the atrial contraction phase to that in the rapid filling phase (A_A/A_R), (5) the width of rapid filling wave at the level of one-half of the peak velocity as the duration of rapid filling (DR).

Cardiac catheterization

A catheter-tipped micromanometer or fluid filled catheter was used for the measurement of LV pressure. LV volume was calculated from single plane cineangiograms based on the area-length method. In 10 subjects without abnormal LV wall motion, the LV volume curve and its differential (dV/dt) curve in diastole were computed from the LVG (Figure 2). The

160

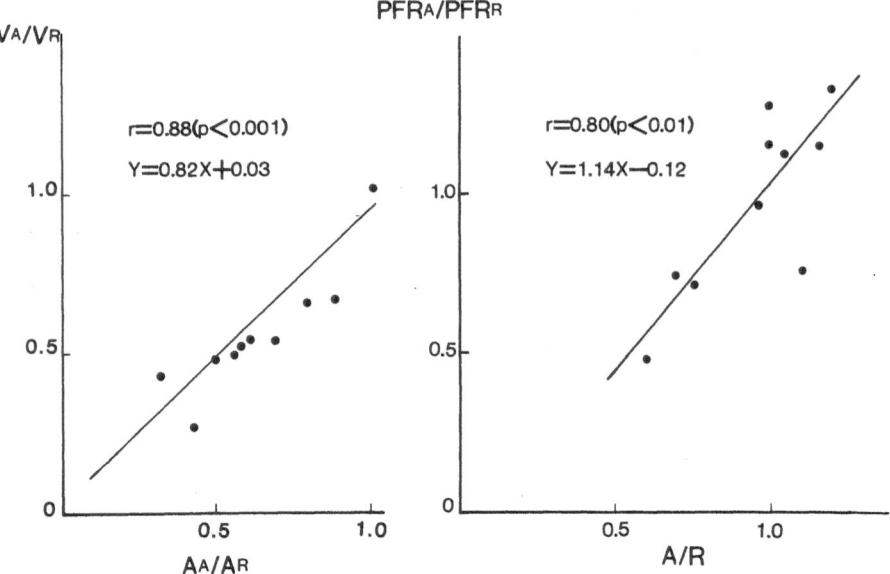

Figure 3. The correlation between the LV volume changes calculated from single-plane cinean-giograms and two parameters of transmitral flow velocity measured by a pulse Doppler flow-meter.

Transmitral blood flow velocity patterns

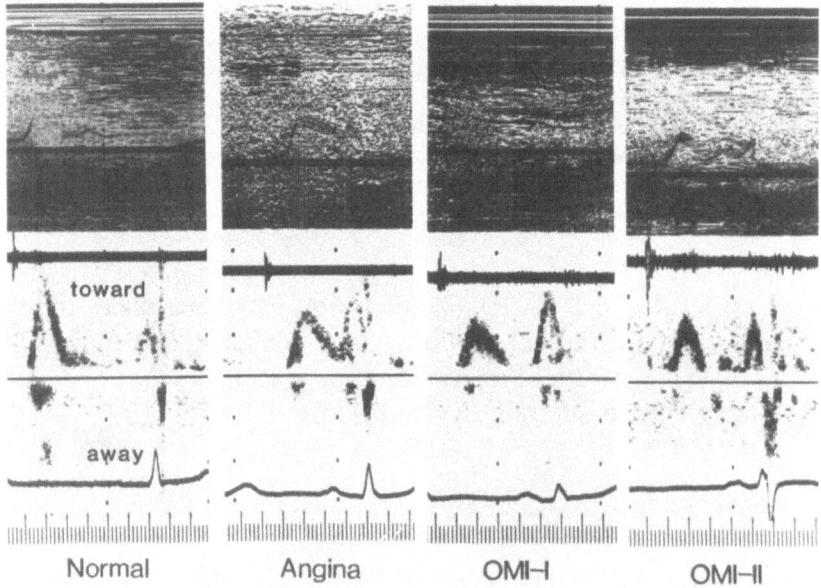

Figure 4. Representative patterns of transmitral flow velocity. As compared to normals, in AP, the peak velocity R decreased with a prolonged DR and the peak velocity A increased. In OMI-I, the flow velocity pattern was similar to that in AP. In OMI-II, the peak velocity R also decreased, but DR was not prolonged and the peak velocity A did not increase.

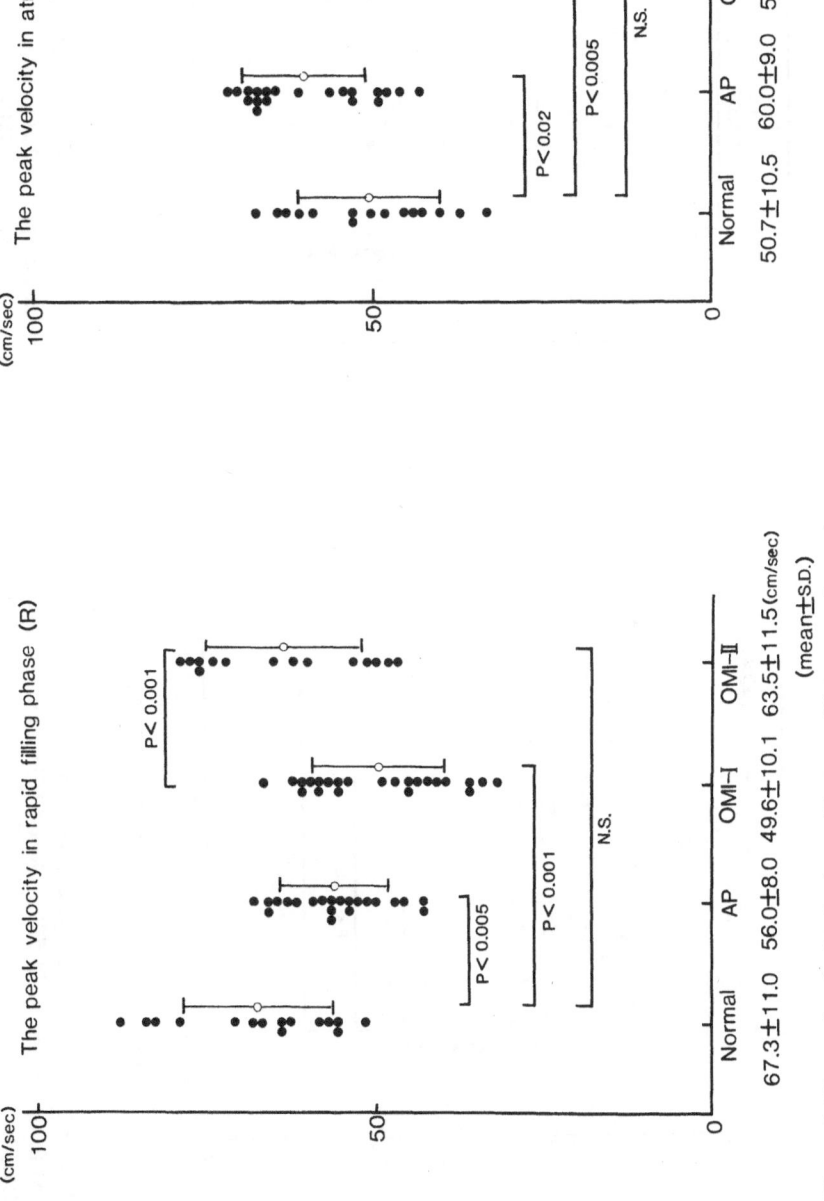

Figure 5. The peak velocity in the rapid phase (R) in normals, patients with effort angina pectoris (AP), patients with old myocardial infarction who have an LVEDP of less than 12 mm Hg (OMI-I) and have an LVEDP of higher than 12 mm Hg (OMI-II).

Figure 6. The peak velocity in the atrial contraction phase (A) in normals, AP, OMI-I and OMI-II.

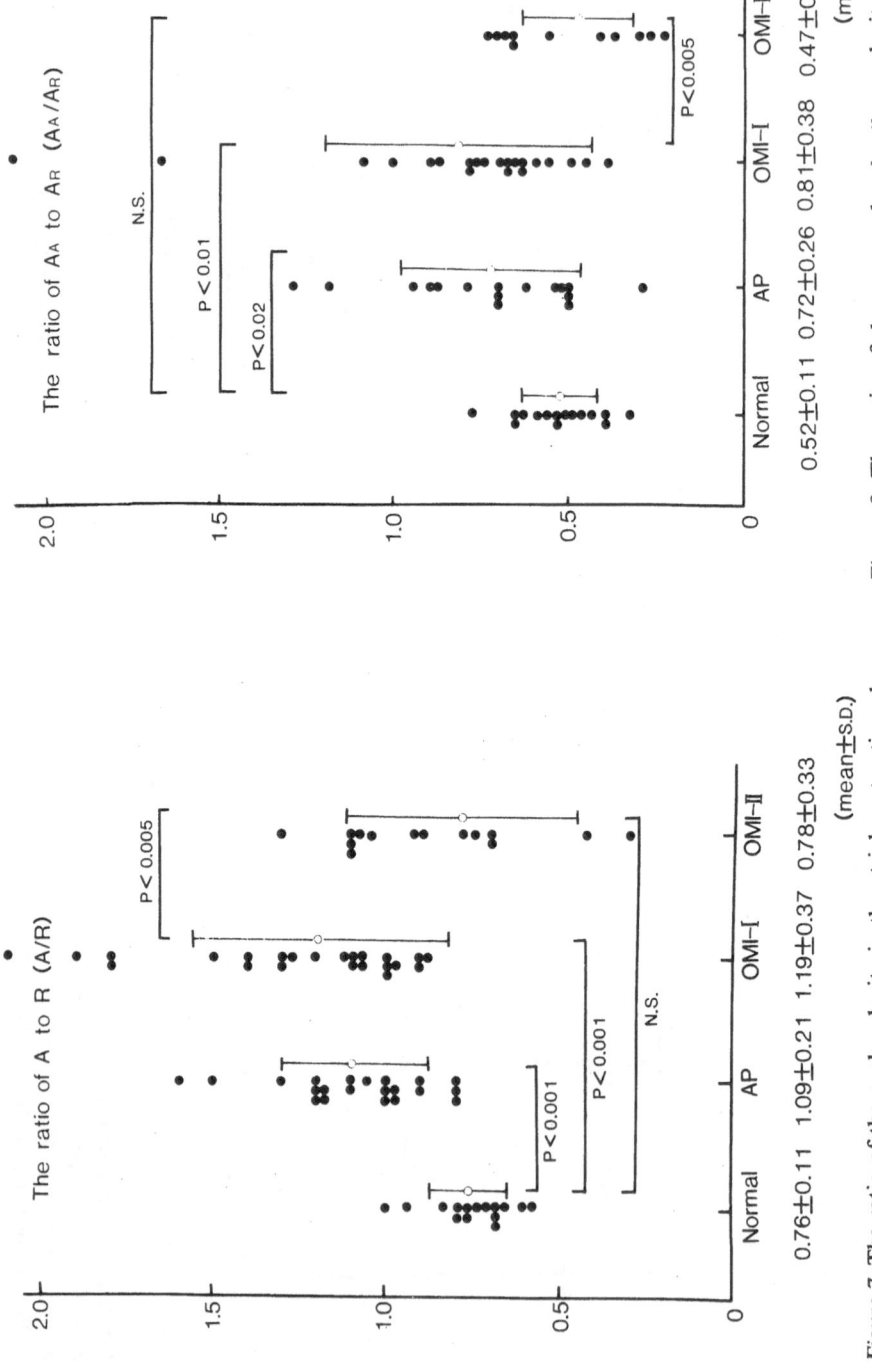

Figure 8. The ratio of the area under the flow velocity curve in the atrial contraction phase (A_A) to that in the rapid filling phase (A_R) in normals, AP, OMI-I and OMI-II.

Figure 7. The ratio of the peak velocity in the atrial contraction phase (A) to that in the rapid filling phase (R) in normals, AP, OMI-I and OMI-II.

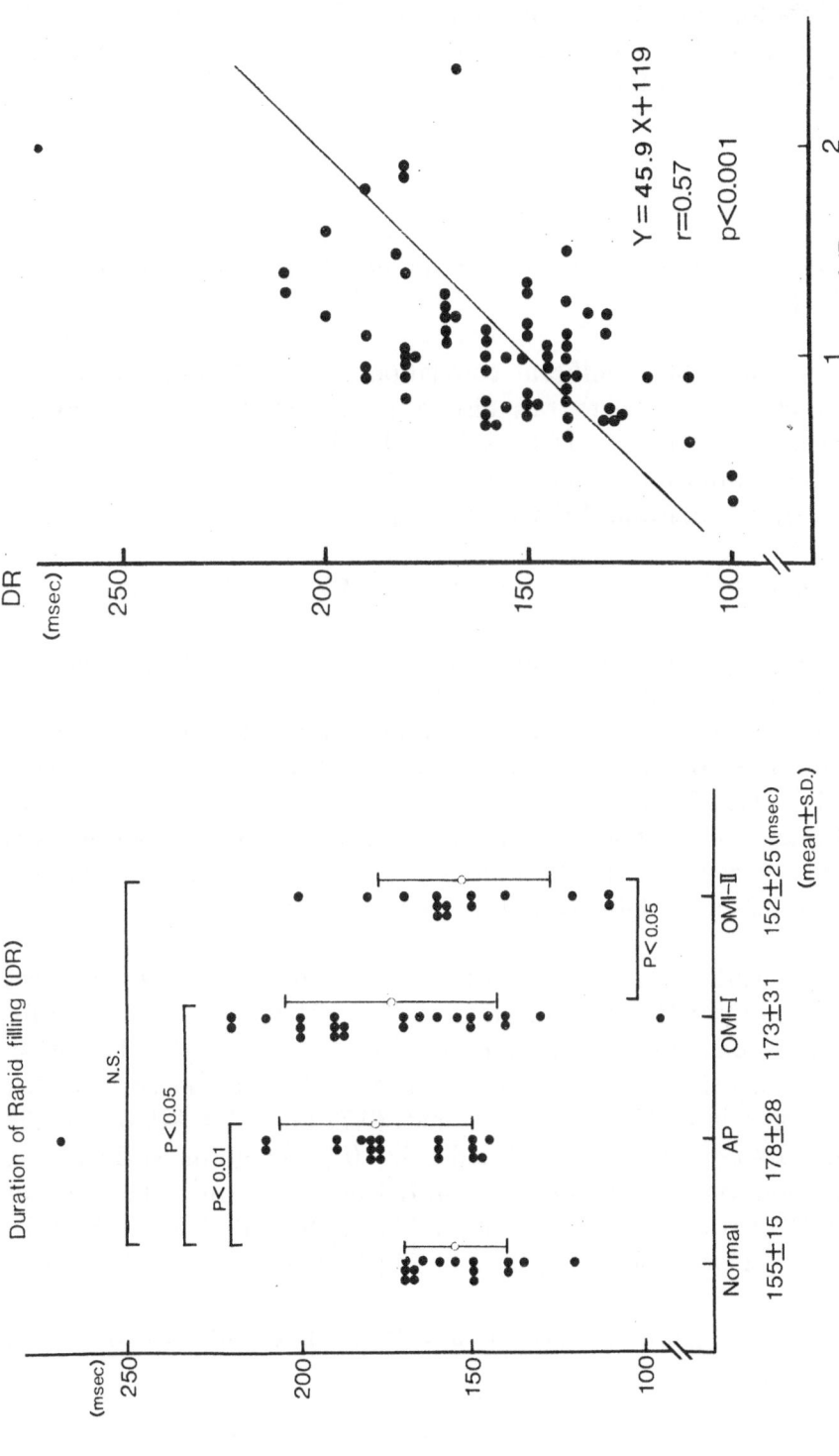

Figure 10. Relation between the duration of rapid filling (DR) and the ratio of the peak velocity A to the peak velocity R (A/R).

Figure 9. The width of rapid filling wave at the level of one-half of the peak velocity as the duration of rapid filling (DR) in normal, AP, OI-I and OI-II.

following parameters were obtained; (1) the ratio of LV volume changes in the atrial contraction phase to that in the rapid filling phase (V_A/V_R), (2) the ratio of the peak filling rate in the atrial contraction phase to that in the rapid filling phase (PFR_A/PFR_R).

RESULTS

The relations between the LV diastolic volume changes and transmitral flow velocity

There was a highly significant correlation between V_A/V_R and A_A/A_R (r = 0.88, p<0.001). There was also a significant correlation between PFR_A/PFR_R and A/R (r = 0.80, p<0.01) (Figure 3). These data indicated that the transmitral flow velocity measured by a pulse Doppler flowmeter well reflected the diastolic LV volume changes.

The transmitral flow velocity in AP. OMI-I, OMI-II and normals

Figure 4 shows the representative patterns of transmitral flow velocity. The peak velocity R was significantly smaller in AP or OMI-I than in normals, but was not smaller in OMI-II than in normals (The mean $\pm$SD was 56.0$\pm$8.0 cm/sec for AP, 49.6$\pm$10.1 cm/sec for OMI-I, 63.5$\pm$11.5 for OMI-II and 67.3$\pm$11.0 for normals) (Figure 5). The peak velocity A was significantly greater in AP or OMI-I than in normals, but was not greater in OMI-II than in normals (60.0$\pm$9.0 cm/sec for AP, 59.9$\pm$7.2 cm/sec for OMI-I, 50.5$\pm$12.0 cm/sec for OMI-II and 50.7$\pm$10.5 cm/sec for normals) (Figure 6).

A/R was significantly greater in AP or OMI-I than in normals, but was not greater in OMI-II than in normals (1.09$\pm$0.21 for AP, 1.19$\pm$0.37 for OMI-I, 0.78$\pm$0.33 for OMI-II and 0.76$\pm$0.11 for normals) (Figure 7). A_A/A_R was also significantly greater in AP or OMI-I than in normals, but was not greater in OMI-II than in normals (0.72$\pm$0.26 for AP, 0.81$\pm$0.38 for OMI-I, 0.47$\pm$0.16 for OMI-II and 0.52$\pm$0.11 for normals) (Figure 8). DR was significantly longer in AP or OMI-I than in normals, but was not longer in OMI-II than in normals (178$\pm$28 msec for AP, 173$\pm$31 msec for OMI-I, 152$\pm$25 msec for OMI-II and 155$\pm$15 msec for normals) (Figure 9).

There was a significant correlation between DR and A/R (r = 0.57, p<0.001) (Figure 10).

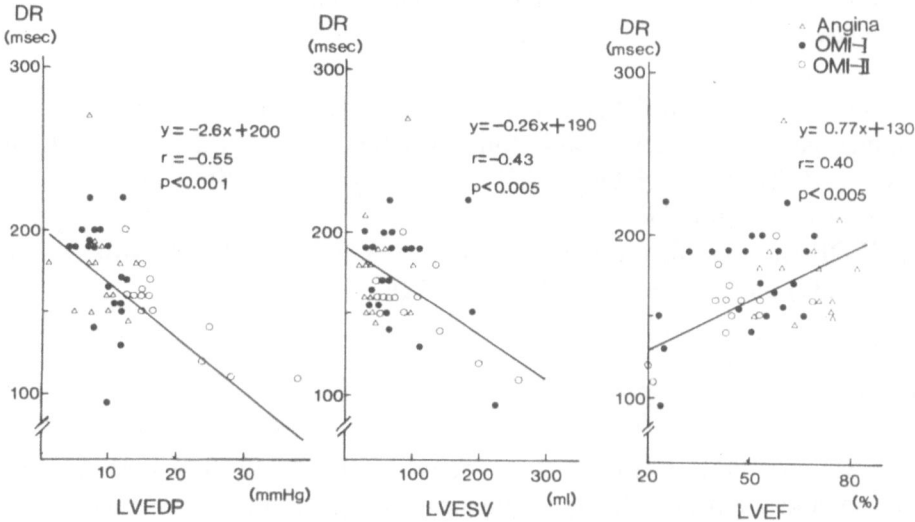

Figure 11. Correlation between the duration of rapid filling (DR) and left ventricular (LV) end-diastolic pressure (EDP) (left), between DR and LV end-systolic volume (ESV) (center) and between DR and LV ejection fraction (EF) (right).

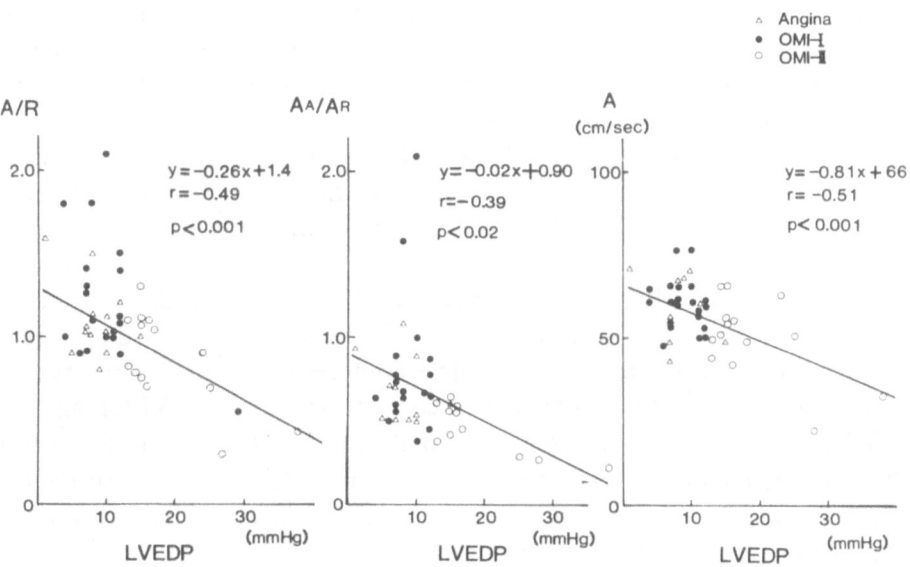

Figure 12. Correlations between the ratio of the peak velocity A to the peak velocity R (A/R) and left ventricular end-diastolic pressure (LVEDP) (left), between the ratio of the area A to the area R (A_A/A_R) and LVEDP (center) and between the peak velocity A and LVEDP (right).

The relations between the Doppler parameters and catheterization parameters

LVG score and stroke volume were not significantly correlated with Doppler parameters. LV end-systolic volume, ejection fraction and EDP were significantly correlated with DR (r = 0.43, r -w 0.40 and r = −0.55, respectively) (Figure 11).

LVEDP was significantly correlated with A/R (r = −0.49), with A_A/A_R (r = −0.39) and A (r = −0.51) (Figure 12).

DISCUSSION

In AP and OMI-I, the peak velocity in the rapid filling phase was reduced, and the peak velocity in the atrial contraction phase was increased. These results suggested the impairment of LV distensibility in early diastole and the compensatory augmentation of the atrial contraction in CAD, and well corresponded with the reports of Hammermister et al. who studied by a LV cineangiography [1] and Bonow et al. by a gated radionuclide angiograms [2].

In addition to these results, in AP and OMI-I, the prolongation of rapid filling phase, which was indicated by a significant prolongation of DR, was observed. This was thought to be related to the impairment of LV distensibility in early to mid diastole and to be the compensatory mechanism for the reduction of filling velocity, which was indicated by a significantly positive correlation between DR and A/R.

However, in OMI-II, there was no prolongation of DR or no augmentation of atrial contraction. There was a significantly inversed correlation between DR and LVEDP. There was also a significantly inversed correlation between DR and LVESV, and was a significantly positive correlation between DR and LVEF. In severe cases of OMI, LV distensibility could be highly disturbed, which caused the rapid increase of LV pressure in early diastole, so the rapid filling could have completed within a short period. There was also a significantly inversed correlation between LVEDP and any of A/R, A_A/A_R and A. This suggested that the LV filling due to atrial contraction was disturbed in the cases with a high LVEDP, because of the elevation of the LV pressure at the onset of atrial contraction and/or the disturbance of the atrial contraction itself.

As a cause of impaired LV filling, Kitabatake [3] and Florotti et al. [4] reported close relations between ventricular relaxation and early diastolic filling. In some patients with CAD, we measured LV pressure by a catheter-tipped micromanometer and found a well correlation between the time constant of isovolumic LV pressure decay and LV minimal pressure which was a major determinant of LV filling pressure in early diastole. Thus, impairment of LV relaxation was considered to a possible mechanism of depressed early diastolic filling in CAD.

In conclusion, the present study indicated that LV diastolic filling could be evaluated by measurement of transmitral flow velocity using a noninvasive pulse Doppler technique and also indicated that the rapid filling velocity was depressed with a prolongation of the rapid filling phase and the atrial contraction was compensatorily augmented in patients with CAD, but these findings were not recognized in severe cases of CAD with a high LVEDP.

REFERENCES

1. Hammermister KE, Warbasse JR: The rate of change of left ventricular volume in man. II. Diastolic events in health and disease. Circulation 49:739, 1974.
2. Bonow RO, Bacharach SL, Green MV, Kent KM, Rosing DR, Lipson LC, Leon MB, Epstein ST: Impaired left ventricular diastolic filling in patients with coronary artery disease: assessment with radionuclide angiography. Circulation 64:315, 1981.
3. Kitabatake A, Tanouchi J, Inouc M, Asano M, Morita T, Masuyama T, Ito H, Yasui K, Shimazu T, Hori M, Abe H: Relations between transmitral flow and ventricular relaxation: A study by pulsed Doppler flowmetry. Cardiac Doppler Dignosis, ed. Merrill P. Spencer. Martinus Nijhoff, p 111, 1983.
4. Floretti P, Brower RW, Meester GT, Serruys PW: Interaction of left ventricular relaxation and filling during early diastole in human subjects. Am J Cardiol 46:197, 1980.

14. Assessment of left ventricular end-diastolic pressure by Doppler velocity analysis across the mitral valve

KAINE IKWUEKE and ANDREW NICOLAIDES

INTRODUCTION

The use of doppler velocity analysis for the detection of abnormal jets within the cardiac chambers and the determination of direction of flow are now becoming firmly established [1–3]. It is currently used for the noninvasive determination of the gradient across the aortic valve, and there have been promising reports of the use of both transcutaneous aortovelography and trans-mitral Doppler velography for the noninvasive estimation of the cardiac output. There has recently been a growing interest in the use of Doppler velocity analysis for the determination of resting left ventricular end diastolic pressure as this is a sensitive measure of left ventricular function. Changes in the resting end diastolic pressure often preceed changes in other parameters of left ventricular function and provide an early marker of deterioration in left ventricular function. They also reflect early changes in response to treatment.

LEFT VENTRICULAR DIASTOLIC MECHANICS

At the end of left ventricular isometric relaxation, the mitral valve opens and the left ventricle fills passively as a result of the pressure difference between the left atrium and the left ventricle. There is an early rapid filling phase followed by a slow filling phase. Atrial systole then follows to complete left ventricular filling. The mitral valve then closes with the onset of ventricular systole. Both the passive filling phase and the atrial systole can be divided into acceleration and deceleration time intervals.

THE RATIONALE FOR THE ASSESSMENT OF LEFT VENTRICULAR END DIASTOLIC PRESSURE BY DOPPLER VELOCITY ANALYSIS

There have been several attempts at the noninvasive assessment of left ventricular function using various methods. Voigt [4] and Manolas [5], used the apex cardiographic tracings to evaluate left ventricular end diastolic pressure and found that an A/H ratio greater than 15% was highly predictive of raised end diastolic pressure. It is known that the velocity of filling of the left ventricle is a function of the distensibility of the left ventricle, the endsystolic volume, and the left atrial filling pressure. In the presence of a normal mitral valve the left atrial filling pressure equals the left ventricular end diastolic pressure. The advent of sophisticated duplex imaging systems, with pulsed Doppler capacity has enabled us to measure accurately, and from selected points, the velocity of filling of the left ventricle at the various phases of diastole. Further, the provision of simultaneous on line spectral analysis, has facilitated careful and accurate examination of the Doppler velocity pattern across the mitral valve and made it possible to determine the relationship between the left ventricular filling velocity pattern and the resting left ventricular end diastolic pressure.

DOPPLER VELOCITY RECORDING ACROSS THE MITRAL VALVE

Continuous wave doppler recording from normal mitral valves has been discussed else where in this book. The outline of the pulsed Doppler recording is similar except that since the sample volume is very small, the spectrum of velocities included in the spectral envelope is very limited. Thus it shows a sharp narrow spectral band with a wide clear window, Figure 1. The passive filling phase has a very rapid acceleration with an early peak. This is followed by gentle deceleration to the base line. Often the deceleration phase is interrupted by a secondary increase in the velocity of left ventricular filling. Atrial systole has a rapid acceleration with a late peak such that the spectral display is more symmetrical. In normal, young subjects the maximum doppler shift at atrial systole is usually less than at the passive filling phase.

TECHNICAL DETAILS

Good mitral valve recordings are obtained with the patients lying in the left lateral position and the transducer positioned over the apex to obtain adequate apical long axis or 4 chamber views. The doppler beam is posi-

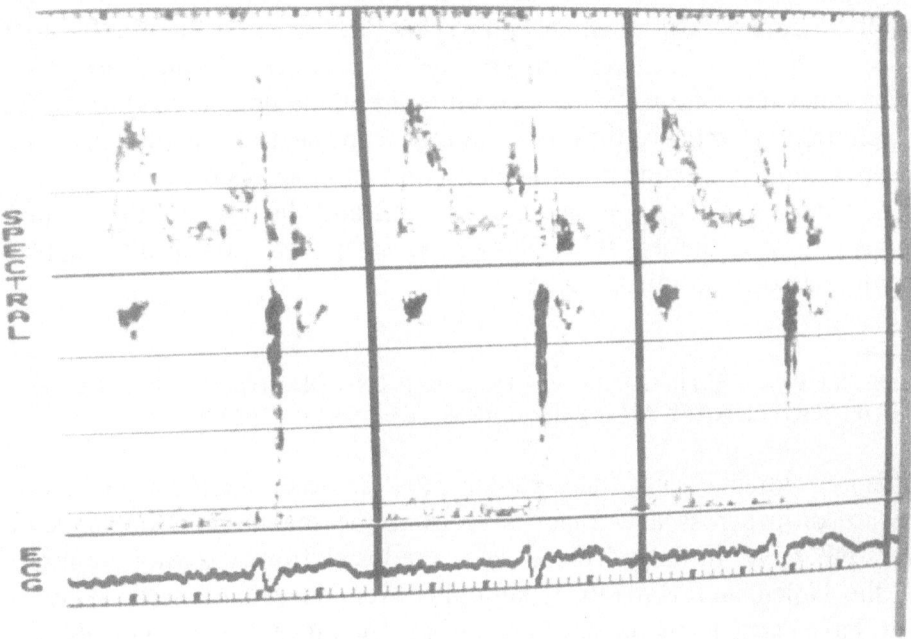

Figure 1. Spectral Display of Doppler recordings across the Mitral Valve.

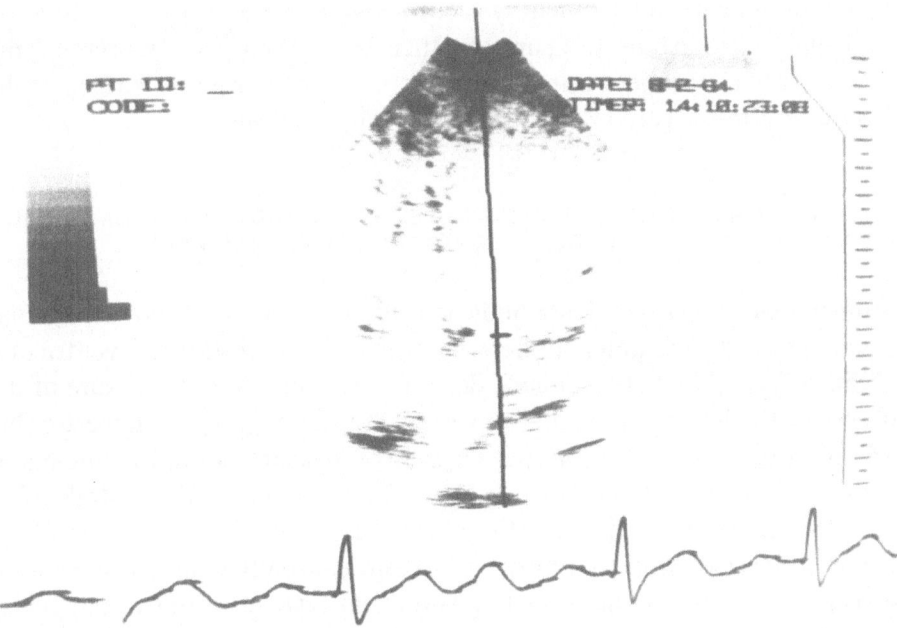

Figure 2. Apical four chamber view to show the direction of the Doppler beam and the position of the sample volume.

tioned along the axis from the apex to the middle of the mitral valve. The sample volume is positioned at a point along this axis, on the mitral valve orifice a little towards the left atrium, Figure 2. All the recordings are made during quiet respiration. When recordings are made during breath holding at expiration, to improve the quality of the recording, the patients often take a deep breath and expire incompletely, thus producing an increase in the thoracic diameter. The comined effect of this and the effect of diminished venous return on the left atrial filling produces a distortion of the Doppler recording across the mitral valve.

ASSESSMENT OF RESTING LEFT VENTRICULAR END DIASTOLIC PRESSURE BY DOPPLER VELOCITY ANALYSIS ACROSS THE AORTIC VALVE

It is now possible using the Bernoulli equation, to derive the instantanous pressure drop across a cardiac valve from the maximum Doppler shift across the valve. In large orifices where the losses from viscosity are neglible, the Holen and Hatle [6, 7] simplified version can be used. Popp et al. [8] have carried this further to determine the instantaneous pressure difference across the aortic valve at the end of ventricular diastole in patients with aortic regurgitation. This gives the difference between the aortic pressure and the left ventricular end diastolic pressure and since the aortic pressure can be roughly determined by cuff sphygmomanometry, the resting left ventricular end diastolic pressure can then be derived. This represents the first attempts at the determination of resting left ventricular end diastolic pressure non-invasively from Doppler velocity analysis.

ATTEMPTS AT ASSESSMENT OF RESTING LEFT VENTRICULAR END DIASTOLIC PRESSURE USING DOPPLER ANALYSIS ACROSS THE MITRAL VALVE

Whilst there are several methods for the assessment of left ventricular function by cardiac doppler studies, the assessment of resting left ventricular end diastolic pressure still remains desirable as it provides a measure of the stiffness of the left ventricle and in certain conditions notably hypertrophic cardiomyopathy (HCM), it provides a sesitive measure of improvement and response to treatment. Doppler velocity analysis across the mitral valve shows that in young patients with normal hearts, the passive filling phase has a rapid acceleration to a high peak, there is usually compete separation between the passive filling recording and atrial systole. In our initial study, we used the ratio of passive filling phase (PFP) to atrial systole (AS) as this appeared to be related to the resting EDP. The graph of the first 15 patients we studied is shown in Figure 3. The patients on the left limb of the graph

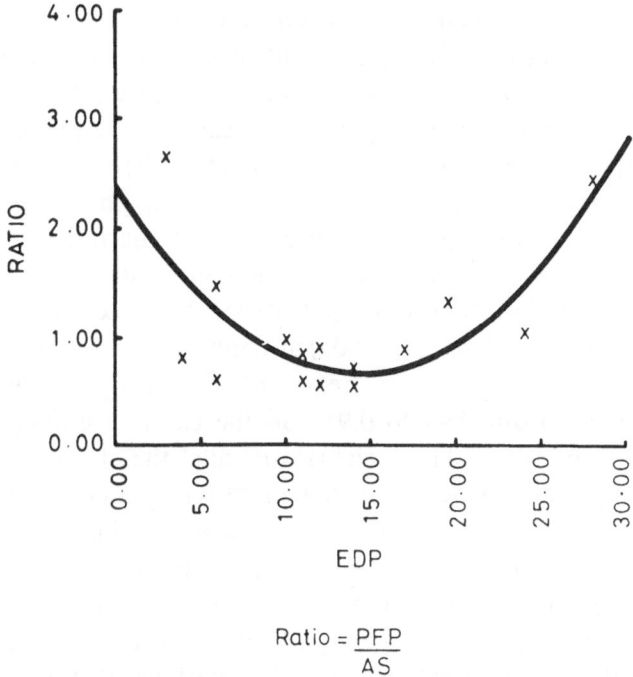

Ratio = $\dfrac{PFP}{AS}$

Figure 3. Doppler studies across the mitral valve. Plot of 'RATIO' against resting LVEDP in the first 15 patients studied. Ratio varied inversely with the resting LVEDP provided the resting LVEDP was less than 15 mm Hg.

were on the average younger than those on the right. This fits in with the expectation that younger patients have more compliant ventricles with easy distensibility which leads to high initial filling velocities. Gardin [9] has reported a progressive reduction in the velocity of the (PFP) with age. However as the resting EDP rises over 15 mm Hg in the group of patients with poor left ventricular function and reduced ejection fraction, there is a secondary rise in the velocity of the passive filling phase as shown in the right limb of the graph. The cause of this secondary rise is unclear but this may be due to a flabbly ventricle extremely compliant in the initial part of the passive filling phase but which quickly re-establishes the poor distensitility and poor compliance as the left ventricular filling progresses. The early rapid filling is consequently short lived and the entire duration of the PFP is shorter than in the patients with normal left ventricular function.

Takagi et al. [10] in Japan have studied a group of patients with ischaemic heart disease; with and without impaired left ventricular function and found that the ratio of the peak velocity in atrial systole to the peak velocity in the passive filling phase (A/R ratio) was greater (1.09 ± 0.21) for patients with angina pectoris than in normals (0.74 ± 0.11). The A/R ratio was also greater in patients with previous myocardial infarction than in normals provided their resting left ventricular end diastolic pressure was 13 mm Hg or less. This, generally, agrees with the graph shown in Figure 8 as the ratio of the passive filling phase to atrial systole begins to increase (or the ratio of atrial systole to passive filling phase begins to decrease) above the resting LVEDP of 15 mm Hg. Iwase et al. [11] have provided further indirect evidence of changes in the ratio of atrial systole to passive filling phase as a reflection of the changes in the resting left ventricular end diastolic pressure. They showed that the A/R ratio was higher in patients with hypertrophic cardio-myopathy at rest (0.99) than in normals (0.55). With exercise, it rose signif-icantly in this group to 1.20 (P<0.005) as compared with normals where the rise was insignificant (0.60). After treatment with diltiazem, the resting A/R ratio was reduced from 0.99 to 0.91 and the exercise induced increase in A/R ratio was abolished. These changes parallel the changes in the resting end diastolic pressure which is higher at rest in patients with HCM and increases significantly on exercise. Diltiazem is also known to abolish the exercise induced increase in left ventricular filling pressure as reflected by diastolic changes in the pulmonary artery pressure [12].

In our study at St Mary's Hospital [13] we measured the resting EDP with fluid filled catheters in 25 patients, and then performed transmitral doppler velocity analysis about 24 hours later, using the ATL Mark 500 duplex scanner.

We recorded:
Duration of passive filling phase (PFP).
Duration of atrial systole (AS)
Gradient of rising limb of the PFP
Gradient of rising limb of AS
Maximum Doppler shift at PFP
Maximum Doppler shift of AS.
Period from initial RQ deflection to the beginning of the passive filling phase (Figure 4).

Our aim was to evolve a relatively simple relationship for the derivation of the resting end diastolic pressure from the doppler velocity analysis across the mitral valve. The duration of the passive filling phase and dura-tion of atrial systole appeared to have an inverse relationship with the rest-ing end diastolic pressure. The increasing maximum velocity attained at atrial systole in patients with increased LVEDP suggests that atrial hyper-trophy occurs to compensate for the increased left ventricular filling pres-sure and the reduced duration of both phases in this group of patients points to a persistent increase in the resistance to left ventricular filling. The rela-tionship between the LVEDP and the Doppler readings was a complex one to which most of the readings contributed. We derived it from a multivar-iate analysis of regression based on a model

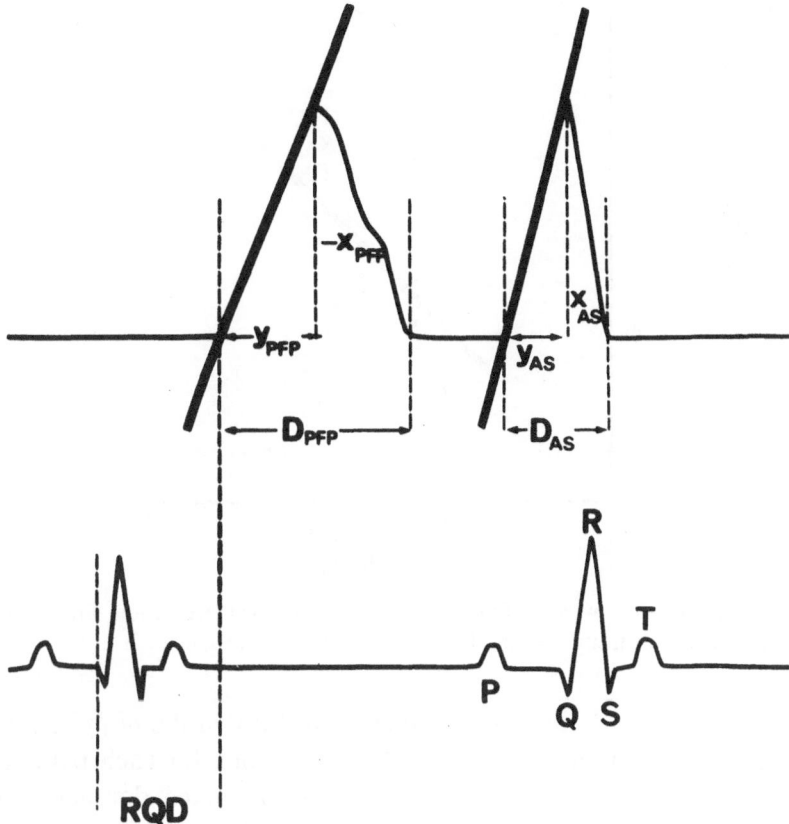

Figure 4. Doppler velocity analysis across the mitral valve. Spectral display.
D(PFP) = Duration of passive filling phase
D(AS) = Duration of atrial systole
X(PFP) = Maximum Doppler shift at passive filling phase
X(AS) = Maximum Doppler shift at Atria systole
X(PFP)/γ(PFP) = Gradient of rising limb of PFP
x(AS)γ(AS) = Gradient of rising limb of AS

$$Y = a \times 1 + b \times 2 + c \times 3 \ldots \ldots \ldots Oxn.$$

where Y was the dependent variable = resting LVEDP, ×1, ×2, ×3 .... were the Doppler measurements, and a, b, c ..... were constants to be detemined from the equation.

The relationship was given by:

Doppler Index = 20 − (0.02 × Duration of atrial systole)
+ (208.2 × Gradient of atrial systole)
− (4.747 × Maximum Doppler at AS)
+ (0.585 × Maximum Doppler shift at PFP)
− (0.0222 × Duration of PFP)
+ (304.27 × Gradient of PFP)

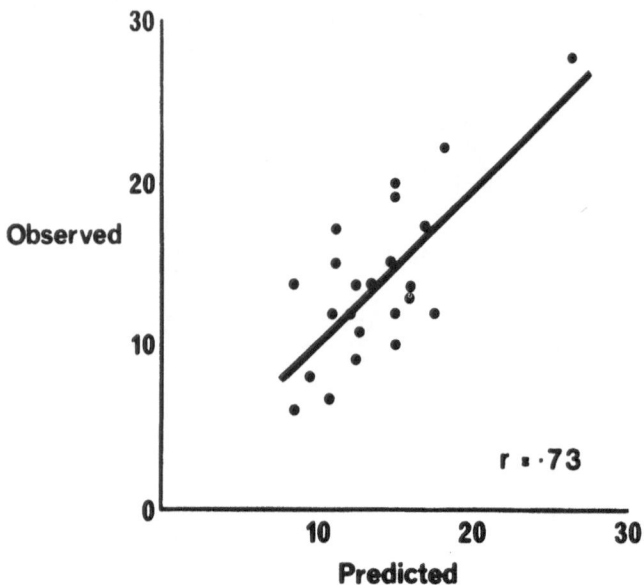

Figure 5. Observed values were LVEDP recorded at cardiac catheterisation. Predicted values were obtained from substitution of the Doppler readings into the equation.

Having derived the relationship, we then resubstituted the doppler readings in the equation to obtain a predicted Doppler index for each patient. The observed resting EDP was plotted against the predicted doppler index as shownin Figure 5. Good correlation was obtained between the two readings ($r = 0.73$, $P<0.05$). The mean ejection fraction in the group, determined from planimetry of the left ventriculograms was 56 ± 22 and the mean age was 53 ± 8.8 yrs. Eighteen of the 25 patients had significant coronary artery stenosis in one or more vessels.

DISCUSSION

The model was based on the assumption that the resting end diastolic pressure at rest would be equal both at cardiac catheterization and during subsequent 2D Echocardiograhic examination. However both the pulse rate

Table 1. The resting pulse rate and resting systolic blood pressures were lower during 2D echo than during cardiac catheterisation.

Cardiac catheterisation	2D Echo
Mean Sys BP 120.5 ± 22	112.3 ± 18
Mean Pulse rate 68.8 ± 9.5	60.6 ± 11.7

and the blood pressure were significantly lower during 2D echocardiographic examination (Table 1) so the expected EDP during 2D echocardiographic examination may have infact been lower. Nine doppler readings were taken during quiet respiration and the values entered were a mean of the nine readings. The variability within the Doppler readings was low (coefficient of variation = 3.8–8 %). Thus it would appear that the doppler readings are reliable and may provide a valuable tool for the non-invasive follow up of cardiac patients. Further work is however necessary to validate this relationship in a prospective study, and work is proceeding at St Mary's Hospital and various other centres in the United States and Japan to test this relationship.

Acknowledgements: We are grateful to Professors J. Egere and A. Ikeme for their help in preparing this chapter, to Mr John Ibrahim for his secretarial help and to all my colleagues at St Mary's Hospital without whose help this work would not have been possible.

REFERENCES

1. Stevenson JG, Kawabori I, Dooley T, Guntheroth WG: Diagnosis of ventricular septal defect by pulsed Doppler echocardiography; sensitivity, specificity and limitations. Circulation 58:2, 322–326, 1978.

2. Pearlman AS, Gentile R, Rubenstein SA, Dooley TK, Franklin DW: In: Echocrdiography. 3rd Symposium Erasmus University, Rotterdam. June 1979. Lancee CD (ed.). The Hague-Boston-London: Martinus Nijhoff 1979:255–260.

3. Ward JM, Baker DW, Rubenstein SA, Johnson SL: Detection of aortic insufficiency by pulsed Doppler echocardiography. Journal of Clinical Ultrasound, vol 5, No 1, 1976.

4. Voigt GC, Friesinger GC: The use of apexcardiography in assessment of left ventricular diastolic pressure. Circulation 41:1015–1024, 1970.

5. Manolas J, Rutishauser W, Wirz P, Arbenz U: Time relation between apex cardiogram and left ventricular events using simultaneous high-fidelity tracings in man. British Heart Journal 37:1263–1267, 1975.

6. Holen J, Aaslid R, Landmark K, Simonsen S: Determination of pressure gradient in mitral stenosis with a noninvasive ultrasound Doppler technique. Acta Med Scand 455–460, 1976.

7. Hatle L, Angelsen B: Doppler ultrasound in cardiology. Lea & Febiger, Philadelphia, 1982.

8. Yock PG, Popp RL: Noninvasive estimation of ventricular pressures by Doppler ultrasound in patients with tricuspid or aortic regurgitation. Circulation 68:Supp III, 230, 1983.

9. Gardin J: Effect of age on Doppler flow velocity measurements (personal communication).

10. Takagi S, Yokota M, Iwase M, Koide M, Ching CH: Evaluation of diastolic behavior of the left ventricle in patients with coronary artery disease by pulse Doppler combined with 2-D echocardiography. J of Card Ultrasonog 3:2, 199, Abstract, Summer, 1984, (Myron R Schoenfeld, ed.).

11. Iwase M, Yokota M, Takagi S, Koide M, Ching CH, Kawai N, Hayashi H and Sotobata I: Effects fo Diltiazem on left ventricular diastolic behavior in patients with hypertrophic

178

cardiomyopathy: Evaluation with exercise pulsed Doppler echocardiography. J of Card Ultrasonog 3:2, 199, Abstract, Summer, 1984, (Myron R Schoenfeld, ed.).

12. Nagao M, Yasue H, Omote S, Takizawa A, Hyon H, Nishida S, Horie M, Yamada K, Tanaka S: Diltiazem induced decrease of exercise-elevated pulmonary arterial diastolic pressure in hypertrophic cardiomyopathy patients. American Heart Journal 102(4):789–790, 1981.

13. Ikwueke JK, Vecht R, Nicolaides E, Sonecha T, Nicolaides AN; Noninvasive assessment of left ventricular end diastolic pressure by Doppler velocity analysis across the mitral valve. J of Card Ultrasonog 3:2, 199, Abstract, Summer, 1984 (Myron R Schoenfeld, ed.).

15. Doppler echocardiography in congestive cardiomyopathy and heart failure

JULIUS M. GARDIN and WALTER L. HENRY

INTRODUCTION

Doppler echocardiography has been shown to be a clinically useful non-invasive technique for evaluating beat-to-beat variations in stroke volume [1–4], and in characterizing the flow velocity patterns in the great arteries [5–9]. One important application of the Doppler technique is the evaluation of global ventricular function in patients with known or suspected heart disease. Unlike M-mode echocardiography, Doppler flow velocity patterns reflect the function of the entire ventricle and not just an 'ice pick' sample.

This report will summarize the Doppler findings in the ascending aorta and main pulmonary artery of patients with congestive cardiomyopathy and also the changes in various aortic flow velocity measurements in patients with congestive heart failure who receive vasodilator therapy.

PATIENT POPULATION

Our initial studies compared Doppler aortic and pulmonary flow velocity patterns in 12 patients known to have congestive cardiomyopathy, and 20 normal subjects [10]. There were 9 men and 3 women, age range 36 to 80 years. The patients with dilated cardiomyopathy had characteristic clinical findings and M-mode echocardiograms – including a left ventricular diastolic dimension greater than 25% above the normal value predicted on the basis of age and body surface area [11–12], a left-ventricular percentage fractional shortening less than 25% (normal range 28% to 44%) [12] and increased E-point septal separation [13]. Two-dimensional echocardiograms revealed a dilated, non-hypertrophic left ventricle with diffuse hypokinesis in all patients; four of the 12 had additional areas of mild dyskinesis. Four patients underwent coronary arteriography because of complaints of chest pain. Three of these patients were demonstrated to have greater than 50 % luminal narrowing in at least one coronary artery, but none had evidence of a discrete left ventricular aneurysm. The presumptive etiology of the cardio-myopathic in four patients. Most of the studies were performed at least 6 hours after the last dose of hydralazine, isosorbide dinitrate, or nitroglycerin ointment. Patients with atrial fibrillation were excluded from the study population.

Blood flow velocities were also recorded in the ascending aorta and main pulmonary artery of 20 normal subjects [9]. The normal group consisted of 12 men and eight women, age range 21 to 46 years. All had normal cardiovascular histories, physical examinations, and M-mode echocardiograms. None of our normal subjects was obese or a trained competitive athlete.

DOPPLER TECHNIQUE

Doppler echocardiographic studies were performed using an echocardiographic unit incorporating a spectrum analyzer-based, range-gated pulsed Doppler velocimeter interfaced with a mechanical sector scanner (Ultra Imager, Electronics for Medicine/Honeywell Corp., Denver, Colo.) [8–10]. Doppler frequency shifts were detected by a dual-channel spectrum analyzer, converted into the corresponding flow velocity using the Doppler equation, and displayed at 5 msec intervals on a strip chart record.

Ascending aortic flow velocity recordings were obtained using a 2.25 MHz right-angle M-mode echocardiographic transducer placed in the suprasternal notch position [9, 10]. Since the ascending aorta was not imaged, care was taken to record the maximum aortic blood flow velocity by mapping the ascending aorta at various sample depths from the transducer. Specifically, the distance from the transducer to the nearest boundary of the sample volume was varied at one cm intervals from a depth of 3 to 9 cm. At each sample volume depth, the transducer was angulated to obtain the peak flow velocity. By using the beats with the maximum peak flow velocity for analysis, we standardized our measurements for the effects of transducer angulation, respiration, pulsus alterans, etc.

Pulmonary flow velocity recordings were obtained using a 3.5 MHz sector scanner transducer to image the main pulmonary artery in the parasternal short-axis view. The Doppler sample volume was then electronically superimposed on the two-dimensional image of the proximal main pulmonary artery in a near-parallel orientation to the long axis of blood flow [9, 10]. As previsouly noted, if the angle of incidence of the ultrasound beam is within 20 % of the long axis of blood flow, the error introduced (underestimation)

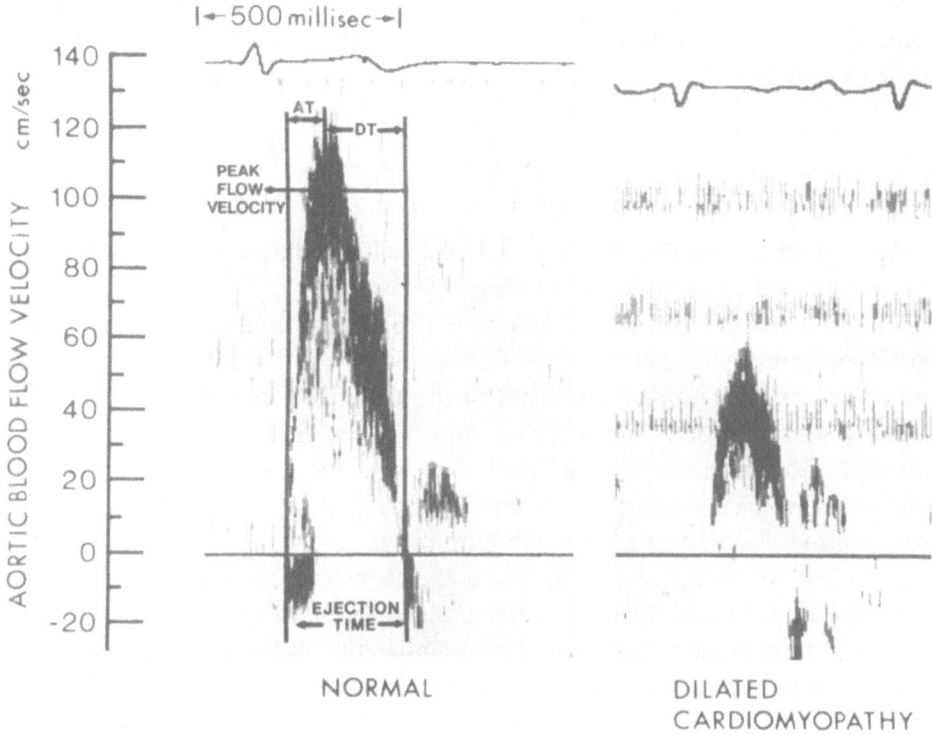

Figure 1. Doppler blood flow velocity recordings in the ascending aorta in a normal subject (left panel) and in a patient with dilated cardiomyopathy (right panel). Aortic blood flow velocity in cm/sec is displayed on the vertical axis and time on the horizontal axis. Normal Doppler aortic flow velocity recording is labelled to show how measurements were made of peak flow velocity, acceleration time (AT), deceleration time (DT), and ejection time. Note that aortic peak flow velocity, flow velocity integral, average acceleration time, and ejection time are greater in the normal subjects than in the cardiomyopathy patients. See text for details. (Reprinted from Gardin JM et al.: Evaluation of dilated cardiomyopathy by pulsed Doppler echocardiography. Am Heart J 106:1057-1065, 1983. Reproduced by permission.)

into the blood flow velocity measurement is less than 6% (cosine function in the Doppler equation) [9, 14]. Because the two-dimensional transducer was not available when four of the patients were studied, pulmonary flow velocity was recorded in only eight of the 12 cardiomyopathy patients.

By our convention, blood flowing in the normal direction within the circulatory system is indicated by a positive, or upward deflection of the recording. Therefore, in the ascending aorta, flow out of the heart and toward the suprasternal notch transducer was displayed as a positive deflection and flow away from the transducer was displayed as a negative deflection. In the main pulmonary, flow away from the transducer in the parasternal position was displayed as positive and flow towards the transducer was displayed as negative. The use of this convention facilitated a direct comparison between predominantly upright flow velocity records obtained from the ascending aorta and main pulmonary artery [9, 10].

BLOOD FLOW VELOCITY MEASUREMENTS

Figure 1 demonstrates the Doppler flow velocity parameters measured in the normal subjects and cardiomyopathy patients [9, 10]. These measurements were made from flow tracings recorded in both the ascending aorta and main pulmonary artery. Peak flow velocity was measured in cm/sec at the center of the Doppler spectrum at the time that maximum blood flow velocity was recorded. Acceleration time was measured in msec from the onset of ejection to the point of peak flow velocity. Average acceleration in cm/sec/sec was calculated by dividing the peak flow velocity by the acceleration time. Ejection time was measured in msec from the onset of systolic flow to the time at end-systole when the flow velocity curve crossed the zero-flow line. In each of the normal subjects and cardiomyopathy patients, the aortic flow velocity integral, or area under the aortic flow velocity curve in cm, was planimetered from the beat demonstrating the greatest peak flow velocity [10].

COMPARISON OF FLOW VELOCITY PARAMETERS

Aortic and pulmonary artery flow velocity data in the normal subjects and cardiomyopathy patients are displayed in Figures 2–4. Peak flow velocities in the aorta ranged from 35 to 62 cm/sec (mean 47 cm/sec) in the cardiomyopathy patients, and from 72 to 120 cm/sec (mean 92 cm/sec) in the normal subjects ($p < 0.001$). Furthermore, there was no overlap in the data points between the two groups. In the main pulmonary artery, peak flow velocities ranged from 38 to 78 cm/sec (mean 57 cm/sec) in cardiomyopathy patients and from 44 to 77 cm/sec (mean 62 cm/sec) in the normal subjects. This difference was not statistically significant and there was considerable overlap of the data in the two groups.

Data for average acceleration in the aorta and main pulmonary artery are plotted in Figure 3. In the aorta, average acceleration in the cardiomyopathy patients (range 389 to 921cm/sec/sec, mean 659) was significantly less ($p < 0.001$) than in the normal subjects (range 735 to 1318 cm/sec/sec, mean 955). However, there was modest overlap of the average acceleration data between the two groups. In the main pulmonary artery, average acceleration was significantly greater ($p < 0.05$) in the cardiomyopathy patients than in

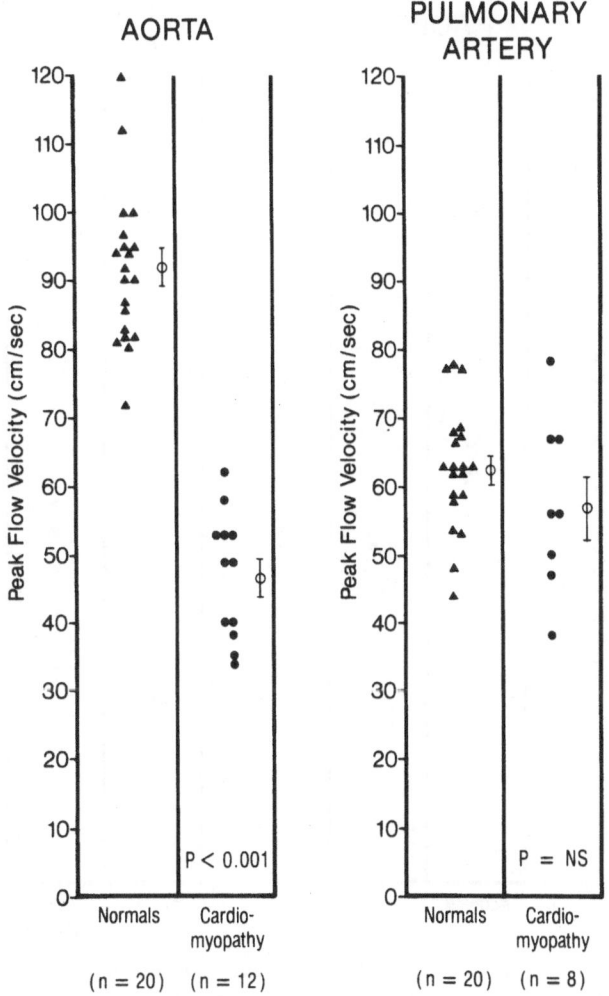

Figure 2. Peak flow velocity in the ascending aorta (left panel) and main pulmonary artery (right panel) are plotted for the 20 normal subjects and 12 cardiomyopathy patients. Pulmonary artery data are available in eight of the cardiomyopathy patients. The mean in each group is expressed by an open circle bisected by a horizontal line. The standard error of the mean is depicted on either side of the mean symbol. The p values reflect the comparison between the two groups in each panel. (Reprinted from Gardin et al.: Evaluation of dilated cardiomyopathy by pulsed Doppler echocardiography. Am Heart J 106:1057-1065, 1983. Reproduced by permission.)

the normal subjects. However, there was overlap in the data in the two groups, with average acceleration ranging from 392 to 800 cm/sec/sec (mean 594) in the cardiomyopathy patients, and from 270 to 515 cm/sec/sec (mean 396) in the normal subjects. The average acceleration in the pulmonary artery was greater in the cardiomyopathy patients because the mean acceleration time was decreased in the cardiomyopathy patients, while the peak flow velocity was similar to normals. Recent studies have demonstrated that

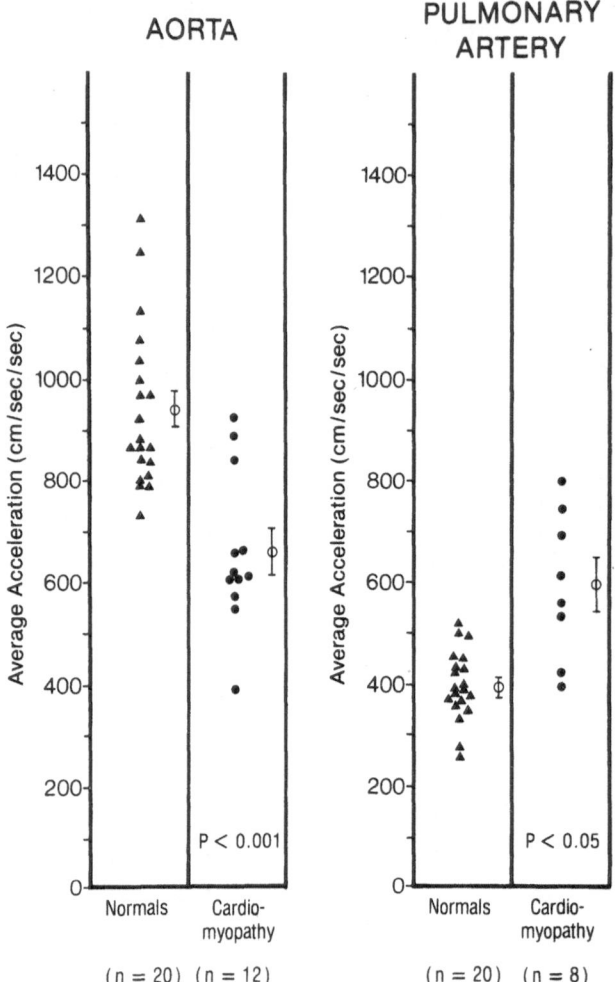

Figure 3. Average acceleration in normal subjects and cardiomyopathy patients are plotted for the ascending aorta (left panel) and the main pulmonary artery (right panel). Symbols are as in Figure 2. (From Gardin JM et al.: Evaluation of dilated cardiomyopathy by pulsed Doppler echocardiography. Am Heart J 106:1057-1065, 1983. Reproduced by permission.)

the acceleration time in the pulmonary artery is decreased in patients with elevated mean pulmonary artery pressure [15–17].

Data for ejection times measured in the ascending aorta and main pulmonary artery are plotted in Figure 4. In the aorta, ejection time ranged from 150 to 300 msec (mean 236 msec) and cardiomyopathy patients and from 265 to 325 msec (mean 294 msec) in normal subjets. Although there was moderate overlap in the data, there was a significant difference ($p < 0.005$) between the two groups. Although in the cardiomyopathy patients, the mean heart rate (79 beats per minute) was 16 beats per minute

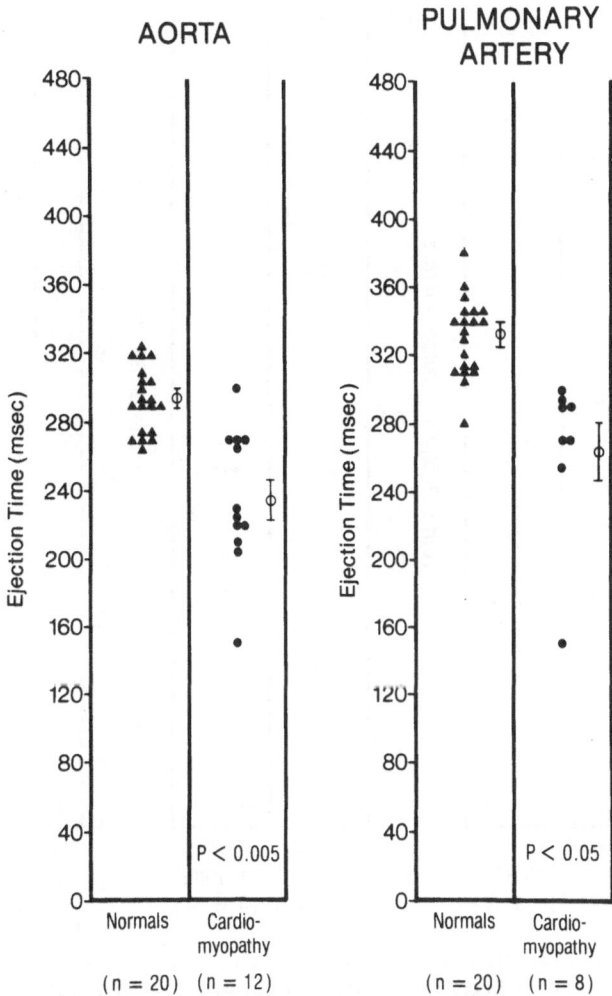

Figure 4. Ejection time measured in the ascending aorta (left panel) and main pulmonary artery (right panel) are plotted for normal subjects and cardiomyopathy patients. Symbols are as in Figure 2. (From Gardin et al.: Evaluation of dilated cardiomyopathy by pulsed Doppler echocardiography. Am Heart J 106:1057-1065, 1983. Reproduced by permission.)

greater than in the normal subjects, correction of the ejection times for heart rate utilizing the formula of Weissler et al. [18] still resulted in a statistically significant difference (p<0.05). In the main pulmonary artery, ejection time was also significantly shorter (p<0.05) in cardiomyopathy patients (range 150 to 380 msec, mean 331), with moderate overlap of data between the two groups. In both cardiomyopathy and normal groups, mean ejection time was longer in the pulmonary artery than in the ascending aorta.

In the normal subjects, mean aortic flow velocity integral determined by planimetry was 15.7 cm with a range of 12.6 to 22.5 cm, whereas in the

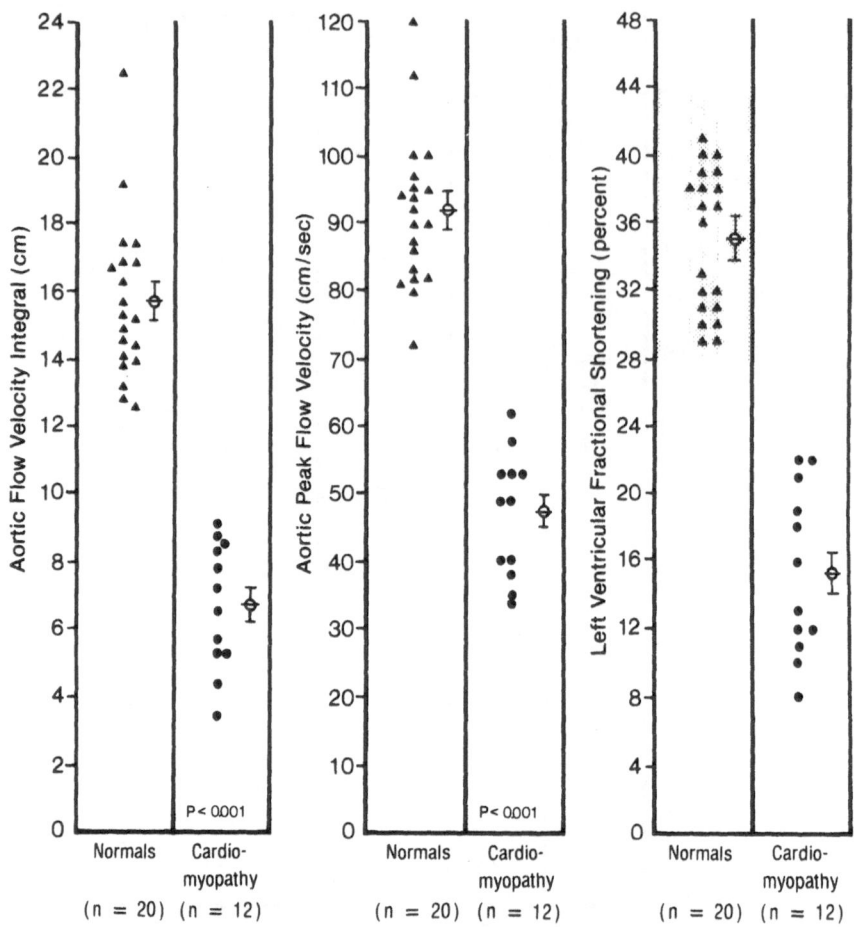

Figure 5. Aortic flow velocity integral (left panel), aortic peak flow velocity (middle panel), and left ventricular percentage fractional shortening from M-mode echocardiography (right panel) are compared in normal subjects and in patients with cardiomyopathy. Note that the data for all three measurments separate normal subjects from patients with cardiomyopathy to a similar degree. Shaded area represents normal range for left ventricular percentage fractional shortening. (From Gardin et al.: Evaluation of dilated cardiomyopathy by pulsed Doppler echocardiography. Am Heart J 106:1057-1065, 1983. Reproduced by permission.)

cardiomyopathy patients, mean flow velocity integral was 6.7 cm, with a range of 3.5 to 9.1 cm. Figure 5 displays a comparison of data for aortic flow velocity integral, peak aortic flow velocity, and left ventricular percentage fractional shortening in the normal and cardiomyopathy patients. The two groups were defined in such a manner that there was no overlap in data for left ventricular percent fractional shortening. There was an excellent correlation between aortic peak flow velocity and aortic flow velocity integral ($r = 0.98$) in the normal and cardiomyopathy groups.

AORTIC FLOW VELOCITY MEASUREMENTS IN CONGESTIVE HEART FAILURE
PATIENTS UNDERGOING VASODILATOR THERAPY

Vasodilators have been shown to be a useful adjunct in treatment of patients with various causes of congestive heart failure, including congestive cardiomyopathy. However, the individual variability in responses to vasodilator dosage has resulted in the common use of invasive hemodynamic monitoring to assess the efficacy of various doses. Because of the morbidity and increased cost associated with invasive monitoring, a simple and reliable noninvasive method for assessing the efficacy of vasodilator therapy would be extremely useful.

Consequently, we studied 13 patients (12 men and one woman, ages 34 to 79 years), who underwent treatment with vasodilators for congestive heart failure [19]. The etiology for the congestive heart failure was congestive cardiomyopathy in five and coronary artery disease in eight patients. The diagnosis was based on cardiac catheterization in seven of the patients and on clinical, electrocardiographic, echocardiographic and radioisotopic criteria in six patients. All patients were in sinus rhythm during the study. Eighteen drug interventions were performed in these 13 patients: intravenous nitroprusside in seven patients, oral hydralazine in six, oral isosorbide dinitrate in four, and a combination of oral hydralazine and nitroglycerin ointment in one patient. Invasive hemodynamic evaluation was performed using a Swan-Ganz thermodilution catheter (American Edwards Laboratories) inserted into the pulmonary artery. Cardiac output (CO) was determined by thermodilution as the mean of three consecutive determinations with less than 10% variation. The following additional calculations were made from the hemodynamic data: (1) mean arterial blood pressure (MBP) = $D+(S-D)/3$, where S = peak systolic BP and D = diastolic BP; (2) stroke volume (SV) = cardiac output/heart rate; and (3) systemic vascular resistance (SVR) = $80([MBP - \text{main right atrial pressure}]/CO)$.

Doppler aortic blood flow measurements

In this study peak aortic flow velocity (PFV), ejection time (ET) and aortic flow velocity integral were calculated. The flow velocity integral was calculated using the following formula [10, 19]:

$$FVI = 1.14(PFV \times 1/2\,ET) + 0.30.$$

This formula was obtained by comparing the planimetered area under the flow velocity curve during systole to a mathematical approximation in 34 patients with a wide range of flow velocity integrals. The mathematical approximation of the area under the flow velocity curve was based on mul-

188

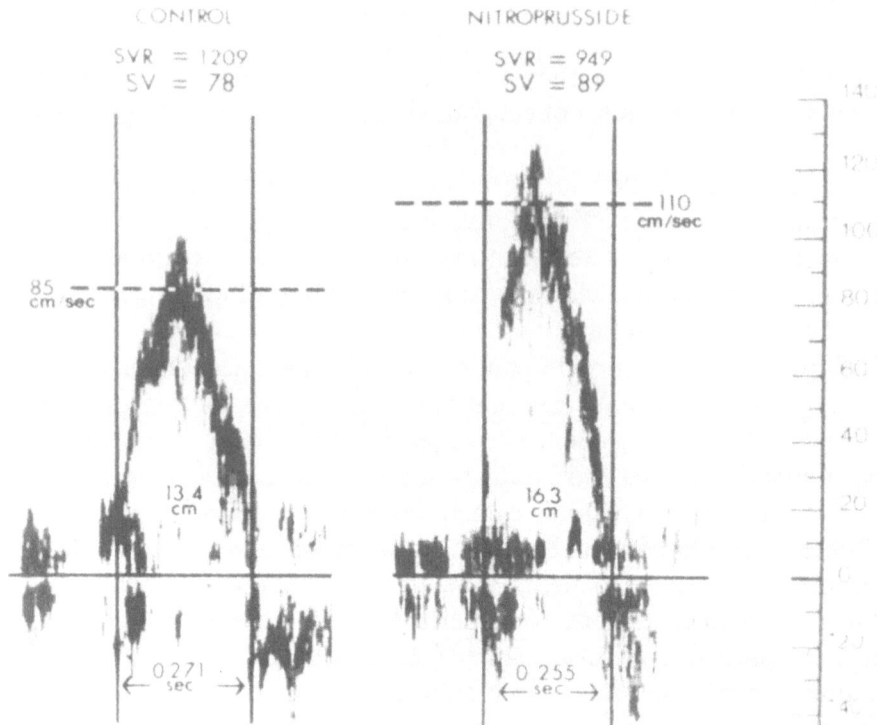

Figure 6. Ascending aortic blood flow velocity recordings performed in a patient with congestive heart failure during state (left panel) and after nitroprusside therapy (right panel). Note the increase in peak flow velocity (to 110 cm/sec from 85 cm/sec) and flow velocity integral (to 16.3 cm from 13.4 cm) after therapy. Systemic vascular resistance (SVR in dyn-sec-cm^{-5}) decreases, while stroke volume (SV in cc) increases with therapy. (From Elkayam U et al.: The use of Doppler flow velocity measurement to assess the hemodynamic response to vasodilators in patients with heart failure. Circulation 67:377-383, 1983. Reproduced by permission of the author and the American Heart Association, Inc.)

tiplying peak flow velocity times 1/2 the ejection time. The correlation coefficient between the estimated and the actually measured flow velocity integral was 0.97 [19].

Figure 6 demonstrates an aortic blood flow velocity recording before and during administration of intravenous nitroprusside. Note the increase in peak flow velocity and flow velocity integral which accompanied the decrease in systolic vascular resistance and increase in stroke volume measured invasively.

Peak flow velocity

Absolute values of Doppler peak flow velocity (PFV) and systemic vas-

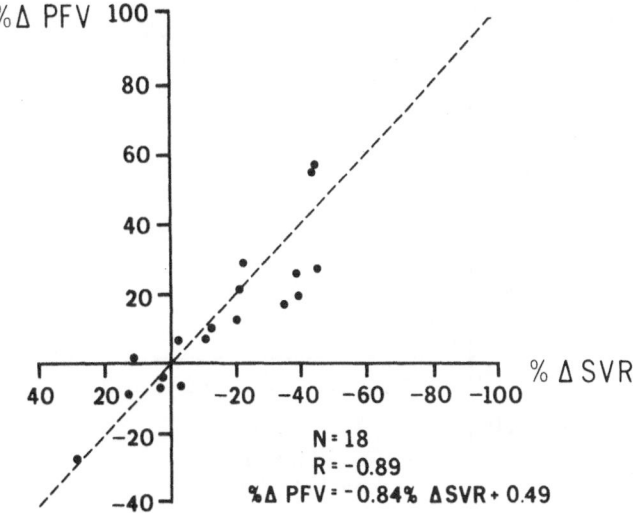

Figure 7. Relationship between percent change in systemic vascular resistance (percent Δ SVR) and change in aortic peak flow velocity (% Δ PFV) in patients with heart failure undergoing vasodilator therapy. See text for details. (From Elkayam U et al.: The use of Doppler flow velocity measurement to assess the hemodynamic response to vasodilators in patients with heart failure. Circulation 67:377-383, 1983. Reproduced by permission of the author and the American Heart Association, Inc.)

cular resistance (SVR) measured at control periods and during peak therapeutic effect during the 18 interventions were weakly correlated ($r = -0.38$). However, there was a good inverse correlation ($r = -0.89$) between *percent* change in both SVR and PFV during vasodilator therapy (Figure 7). The equation relating the two parameters was:

$$\% \Delta PFV = -0.84(\% \Delta SVR) + 0.49.$$

In nine of the 18 studies, percent change in SCR was in the range of 21 to 45%; in all nine studies, PFV changed 17 to 57%. In the other nine studies, in which a 2 to 20% change in SCR was noted, the change in PFV did not exceed 13%.

There was also a weak correlation between PFV and stroke volume (SV) ($r = 0.33$). However, a better correlation was demonstrated between the *percent* change in stroke volume and the *percent* change in peak flow velocity ($r = 0.75$).

Ejection time

The correlation between the absolute values and percent changes of ejection time and systemic vascular resistance revealed r values of 0.01 and −0.15, respectively. Correction of ejection time by heart rate improved these correlations with systemic vascular resistance only slightly.

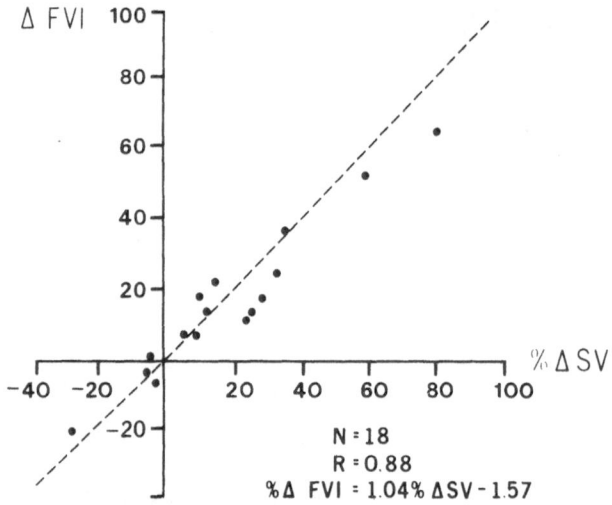

Figure 8. Relationship between percent change in stroke volume (% Δ SV) and percent change in flow velocity integral (% Δ FVI) in patients with heart failure undergoing vasodilator therapy. See text for details. (From Elkayam et al.: The use of Doppler flow velocity measurement to assess the hemodynamic response to vasodilators in patients with heart failure. Circulation 67:377-383, 1983. Reproduced by permission of the author and the American Heart Association, Inc.)

On the other hand, the correlation between ejection time and stroke volume was better: $r = 0.56$ for the absolute measurements and $r = 0.70$ for the *percent* changes. Correction of the ejection time by heart rate did not improve these correlations.

Flow velocity integral

Correlation between the absolute values of Doppler aortic flow velocity integral and systemic vascular resistance was -0.31 and between the percent change in these two parameters was $r = -0.65$. The relationship between the absolute values of flow velocity integral and stroke volume revealed an r value of 0.44; however, a very good correlation ($r = 0.88$) was found between the percent changes of these two measurements during therapy (Figure 8). The equation relating the two parameters was:

$$\% \Delta FVI = 1.04(\% \Delta SV) - 1.57.$$

DISCUSSION

Flow velocity measurements in congestive cardiomyopathy

Doppler blood flow measurements appear to be useful in differentiating normal subjects from patients with poor left ventricular function due to congestive cardiomyopathy. In our studies, both aortic peak flow velocity and flow velocity integral proved to be excellent discriminators between the normal and cardiomyopathy groups. That both aortic flow velocity integral and peak flow velocity were good discriminators of reduced left ventricular systolic function is not surprising. Several studies have suggested a relationship between aortic peak flow velocity and left ventricular stroke volume. Colocousis et al. [26] have demonstrated during experimental exsanguination and fluid infusion in dogs that Doppler aortic peak flow velocity is linearly related to stroke volume – except at higher cardiac outputs, where stroke volume is augmented by a prolongation of ejection time while peak velocity reaches a plateau. Spencer has shown in hypertensive patients that aortic PFV is increased after nadalol treatment [21]. This finding was felt to be secondary to a decrease in heart rate with a related increase in stroke volume. Furthermore, flow velocity integral (in cm), when multiplied by the cross-sectional area of the vessel (in cm^2), should theoretically give a non-invasive estimate of stroke volume (in cm^3).

Our observation that there was a relationship between average aortic flow acceleration and systolic left ventricular function reinforces preliminary findings of Chandraratna et al. [22] who found a positive correlation between maximum blood flow acceleration in the transverse aorta and left ventricular ejection fraction in patients with coronary artery disease [27]. However, we found that both aortic peak flow velocity and flow velocity integral appeared to better discriminate between the cardiomyopathy and normal groups than did average aortic flow acceleration. One explanation for this finding might be that small errors in measurement of acceleration time result in relatively larger errors in calculation of average acceleration [9].

The mean ejection time in both the ascending aorta and main pulmonary artery, whether uncorrected or corrected for heart rate, was significantly decreased in the cardiomyopathy patients relative to normal. This finding has been previously well documented in the presence of reduced left ventricular function and stroke volume. However, we found much more overlap in the two groups for ejection time measurements than for aortic peak flow velocity or flow velocity integral measurements [10]. The finding of decreased acceleration and increased average acceleration in the pulmonary artery of the cardiomyopathy patients differed from the aortic blood flow measurements in these patients. Although the data in this study do not directly explain the differences, it is possible that in light of recent studies demonstrating a decreased pulmonary artery acceleration time in patients with pulmonary hypertension, that the cardiomyopathy patients had elevated pulmonary artery pressures [15–17].

Review of our data indicates that ascending aortic flow velocity measurements can be used pulmonary artery flow measurements in identifying and following patients with dilated cardiomyopathy. Moreover, the ascending aortic flow measurements have the advantage that they can be obtained without the necessity of two-dimensional echocardiographic imaging. Therefore, as Light and others have also suggested, it is possible to evaluate and monitor these patients – e.g. in the intensive care unit setting – by obtaining data solely from the ascending aorta without imaging using the transducer in the suprasternal notch [1, 2, 5, 19].

Evaluation of vasodilators in congestive heart failure

Our studies in patients with congestive heart failure undergoing vasolidator therapy have demonstrated that the magnitude of the change in aortic peak blood flow velocity generally allows a separation between patients who do and do not have a clinically important effect of therapy on systemic vascular resistance [19]. The direction of change in SVR could be predicted in most cases by an opposite change in peak flow velocity. Two patients who did not follow this general rule demonstrated only small changes in both SVR and PFV. The discrepancy probably reflects the error inherent in the accuracy and reproducibility of both techniques and demonstrates the problem in trying to assess small hemodynamic changes by Doppler velocimetry. Although systemic vascular resistance decreased in most cases who responded to therapy, a paraxdoxical marked increase in resistance was observed in one case and could be identified by its association with a large decrease in aortic peak flow velocity.

Despite the close relationship between the percent changes in systemic vascular resistance and peak flow velocity, a poor correlation ($r = 0.38$) was found between the absolute values of these variables [19]. Aortic blood flow velocity, therefore, must be influenced by other factors in addition to vascular resistance. These factors may include the state of myocardial contractility, the size and shape of the aortic valve and aorta, etc. Furthermore, the absolute stroke volume did not seem to correlate strongly with the absolute peak flow velocity ($r = 0.33$); however, there was a better correlation between the change in these parameters ($r = 0.75$).

Our study also did not demonstrate a strong correlation between the absolute values of stroke volume and the area under the flow velocity curve ($r = 0.44$). The explanation is due, at least in part, to the fact that measurement of aortic diameter (and area) is required for the assessment of volumetric blood flow using the Doppler technique [3, 4]. Also, *changes* in stroke volume were not necessarily associated with *changes* in peak flow velocity or ejection time when evaluated separately. However, the effect on these two variables in combination, as reflected by changes in the area under the Doppler aortic flow velocity curve (FVI), was indicative of changes in stroke volume in most patients in our study. Careful analysis of the individual data showed a small decrease in thermodilution stroke volume with no change in FVI in one case, and a minimal increase in stroke volume associated with a small decrease in FVI in another case. Consequently, errors inherent in both Doppler and invasive techniques might limit the clinical usefulness of the Doppler technique in assessing small hemodynamic changes.

The correlation between changes in stroke volume and flow velocity integral obtained in our study is in agreement with data obtained in dogs by either manually positioning the Doppler transducer on the aortic arch [14] or by the suprasternal approach [20]. Our results are an extension of these experimental studies and demonstrate the clinical application of the technique for the noninvasive evaluation of acute hemodynamic changes in patients with congestive heart failure. Further studies are warranted to evaluate the potential application of this technique in the long term assessment of vasodilator therapy in patients with congestive heart failure.

REFERENCES

1. Buchtal A, Hanson GC, Peisach AR: Transcutaneous aortovelography. Potentially useful technique in management of critically ill patients. Br Heart J 38:451, 1976.
2. Sequeira RF, Light LH, Cross G, Raftery EB: Transcutaneous aortovelography: A quantitative evaluation. Br Heart J 38:443, 1976.
3. Magnin PA, Stewart JA, Myers S, von Ramm O, Kisslo JA: Combined Doppler and phased-array echocardiographic estimation of cardiac output. Circulation 63:388–392, 1981.
4. Huntsman LL, Stewart DK, Barnes SR, Franklin SB, Colocousis JS, Hessel EA: Noninvasive Doppler determination of cardiac output in man. Clinical validation. Circulation 67:593–601, 1983.
5. Light LH: Non injurious ultrasonic technique for observing flow in the human aorta. Nature 224:1119, 1969.
6. Huntsman LL, Gams E, Johson CC, Fairbanks E: Transcutanesous determination of aortic blood flow velocities in man. Am Heart J 89:605, 1975.
7. Angelsen BAJ, Brubakk AO: Transcutaneous measurement of blood flow velocity in the human aorta. Cardiovasc Res 10:368, 1976.
8. Griffith JM, Henry WL: An ultrasound system for cardiac imaging and Doppler blood flow measurement in man. Circulation 56:925, 1978.
9. Gardin JM, Burn C, Childs W, Henry WL: Evaluation of blood flow velocity in the ascending aorta and main pulmonary artery of normal subjects by Doppler echocardiography. Am Heart J 107:310–319, 1984.
10. Gardin JM, Iseri LT, Elkayam U, Tobis J, Childs W, Burn CS, Henry WL: Evaluation of dilated cardiomyopathy by pulsed Doppler echocardiography. Am Heart J 106:1057–1065, 1983.

194

11. Fisher DC, Sahn DJ, Friedman MJ et al.! The mitral valve orifice method for noninvasive two-dimensional echo Doppler determinations of cardiac output. Circulation 67:872–877, 1983.
12. Henry WL, Gardin JM, Ware JH: Echocardiographic measurements in normal subjects from infancy to old age. Circulation 62:1054, 1980.
13. Massie BM, Schiller NB, Ratshin RA, Parmley WW: Mitral-septal separation: A new echocardiographic index of left ventricular function. Am J Cardiol 39:1008, 1977.
14. Steingart RM, Meller J, Barovick J, Patterson R, Herman MV, Teichholz LE: Pulsed Doppler echocardiographic measurements of beat-to-beat changes in stroke volume in dogs. Circulation 62:542, 1980.
15. Kitabatake A, Inoue M, Asao M: Noninvasive evaluation of pulmonary hypertension by pulsed Doppler technique. Circulation 68:302–309, 1983.
16. Kosturakis D, Goldberg SJ, Allen HD, Loeber C: Doppler echocardiographic prediction of pulmonary arterial hypertension in congenital heart disease. Am J Cardiol 53:1110–1115, 1984.
17. Mahan G, Dabestani A, Gardin J et al.: Estimation of pulmonary artery pressure by pulsed Doppler echocardiography (Abstract). Circulation 68(III):III–367, 1983.
18. Weissler Am, Harris WS, Schoenfeld CD: Systolic time intervals in heart failure in man. Circulation 37:149, 1968.
19. Elkayam J, Gardin JM, Berkley R, Hughes CA, Henry WL: The use of Doppler blood flow measurement to assess the hemodynamic response to vasodilators in patients with heart failure. Circulation 67:377–383, 1983.
20. Colocousis JS, Huntsman LL, Curreri PW: Estimation of stroke volume changes by ultrasound Doppler. Circulation 56:914, 1977.
21. Spence JD: Alteration of blood velocity: A 'new' property of antihypertensive drugs. Proceedings of the Seventh Meeting of the International Society of Hypertension, 1980, p. 125.
22. Chandraratna PAN, Silveira B, Aronow WS: Assessment of left ventricular function by determination of maximum acceleration of blood flow in the aorta using continuous Doppler ultrasound (Abstract). Am J Cardiol 45:398, 1980.

16. Effects of diltiazem on left ventricular diastolic behavior in patients with hypertrophic cardiomyopathy: Evaluation with exercise pulse Doppler echocardiography

MASATSUGU IWASE, MITSUHIRO YOKOTA, SHIGEHITO TAKAGI, MASABUMI

KOIDE, HU XIAO JING, NAOKI KAWAI, HIROSHI HAYASHI, IWAO SOTOBATA

INTRODUCTION

Recently, some authors have reported the effectiveness of the slow calcium channel-blocking agents, such as verapamil [1], nefedipine [2], and diltiazem [3] for the treatment of hypertrophic cardiomyopathy (HCM). However, few data [4, 5] are available on the hemodynamic effects of these drugs on left ventricular (LV) diastolic behavior during exercise. To estimate the effect of diltiazem on the LV diastolic abnormality in patients (pts) with HCM, transmitral flow velocity during diastole was studied before and after dynamic leg exercise using a pulse Doppler combined with 2-D echocardiograph.

METHODS

The subjects consisted of 23 healthy males (25 to 41 yrs; with mean age of 33 yrs) and 12 pts with HCM (28 to 69 yrs; with mean age of 51 yrs). All subjects showed normal sinus rhythm.

The pulse Doppler systems (ATL Mark V, ATL 500 and Aloka SSd-720+UGR-23) with a 3 MHz transducer were used, combined with a 2-D echocardiograph with mechanical sector scanning. The 2-D echocardiograms in the apical long axis views were monitored with the subjects in the supine position, breathing normally, and the sampling site was positioned at the center of the mitral ring. True transmitral flow velocity was calculated from the shifted frequency using the Doppler equation. The pattern of transmitral flow velocity in diastole consisted of two components. The first component corresponded to the rapid filling phase in early diastole, and the second one to the atrial contraction phase in late diastole.

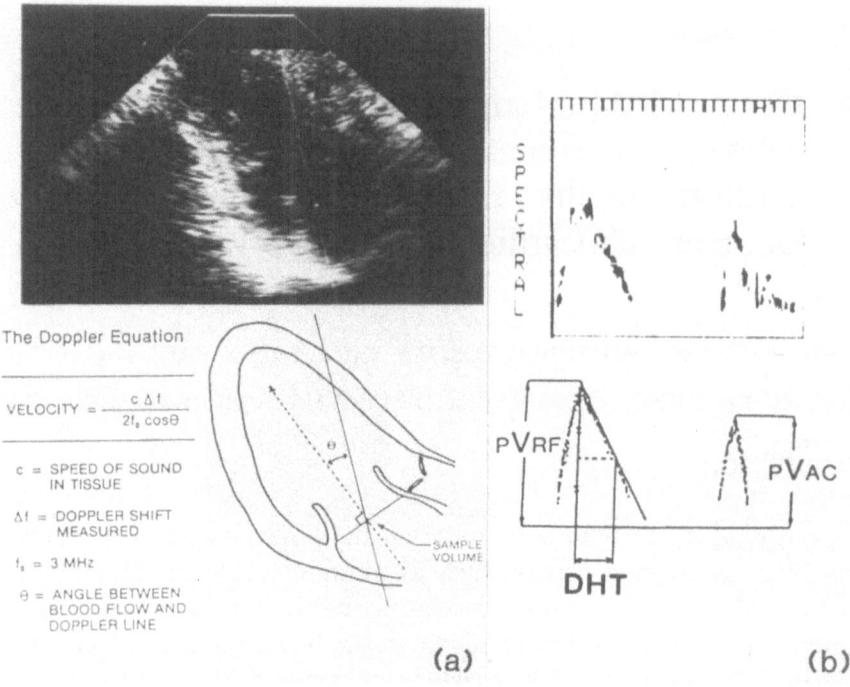

Figure 1. (a) Measurement of corrected transmitral flow velocity. Monitoring the apical long axis view with the 2-D echocardiogram, the sampling site was positioned at the center of the mitral ring. The Doppler shift measured was corrected by the Doppler equation to the velocity, by the angle (θ) between the Doppler line and the true diastolic blood flow direction, from the mitral orifice to the LV apex. (b) The measurement of 4 parameters from the transmitral flow velocity pattern.

Peak velocity in the rapid filling phase (P^{V}RF; cm/sec), deceleration half time of rapid filling velocity (DHT; msec), peak velocity in the atrial contraction phase (P^{V}AC; cm/sec) and the ratio of P^{V}AC over P^{V}RF (A/R) were measured to estimate the LV diastolic behavior (Figure 1). The P^{V}RF and DHT are considered to represent LV distensibility, and A/R to represent the contribution of left atrial (LA) contraction to LV filling.

The multistage exercise testing was carried out using a bicycle ergometer with subjects in the supine position. The initial load was 25 watt for pts with HCM and 50 watt for healthy subjects; the load was increased by 25 watt every 3 minutes. The exercise end point was the target heart rate (HR) of 120 beats/min. The HCM pts were directed to perform the exercise of the same intensity after oral administration of diltiazem (90–180 mg/day) for one week or longer.

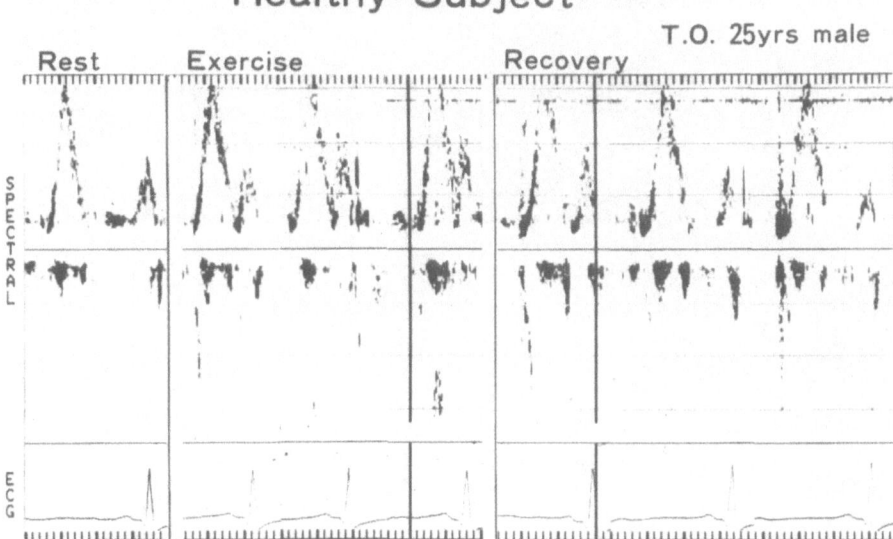

Healthy Subject

T.O. 25yrs male

Rest   Exercise   Recovery

S P E C T R A L

E C G

1min   3min   6min   1min   3min   5min

Figure 2. Case 1. 25-year-old healthy male. HR, P^VRF, and P^VAC increased during exercise, but DHT shortened and A/R did not change. Rapid filling and LA contraction flow tracings did not fuse together throughout the exercise testing. During the recovery phase, these parameters returned gradually except for A/R. A/R did not change before, during, or after exercise.

RESULTS

Case presentation

In a 25-year-old healthy male, HR, P^VRF, and P^VAC increased during exercise, but DHT shortened and A/R did not change. The rapid filling and LA contraction flow tracings did not fuse together. During the recovery phase, HR, P^VRF, P^AC and DHT returned gradually to their resting levels. A/R did not change throughout the exercise testing (Figure 2). In a 51-year-old HCM male at rest before diltiazem administration, transmitral flow velocity patterns showed slightly depressed P^VRF, slightly prolonged DHT, and slightly increased P^VAC and A/R compared to these of normal subject. During exercise, P^VRF increased very little, DHT prolonged, and P^VAC and A/R increased markedly. During the fifth minute of exercise, at HR of 86 bpm, rapid filling and atrial contraction flow tracings could not be detected separately, and almost all of the transmitral flow tracings were dominated by the LA contraction flow. After exercise, these two components separated again. P^VRF increased very little, DHT prolonged while

198

Hypertrophic Cardiomyopathy

I.M. 51yrs male

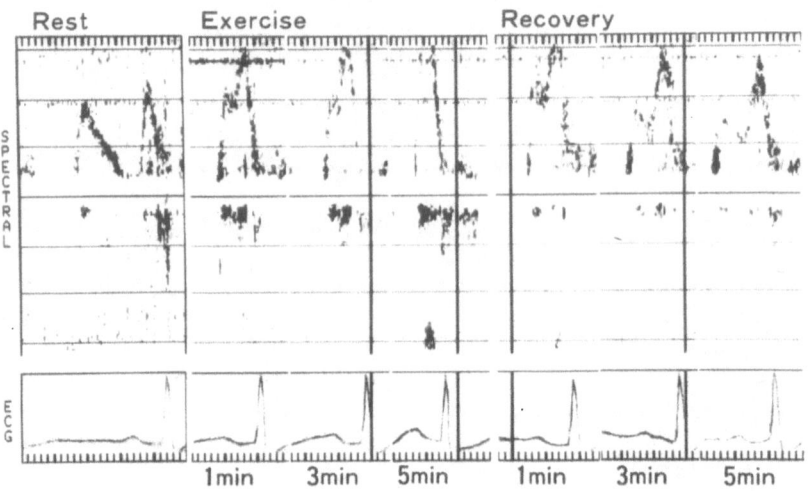

Before Diltiazem

Figure 3. Case 2. 51-year-old male with HCM before diltiazem administration. At rest all 4 parameters were abnormal. During exercise, P^VRF increased very little, DHT prolonged, and P^VAC and A/R increased markedly. After the first 5 minutes of exercise, rapid filling and the LA contraction flow pattern were not detectable separately, and almost all of the transmitral flow pattern consisted of the LA contraction flow pattern. After exercise, these two components separated again, P^VRF decreased and DHT prolonged, while P^VAC and A/R markedly increased. In this case, the patient needed longer than the five minutes of monitoring to regain the pre-exercise levels.

P^VAC and A/R increased markedly. These markedly increased P^VAC and A/R would represent the left atrial compensatory mechanism for the poor LV distensibility in HCM pts during and after dynamic exercise (Figure 3). After diltiazem administration (180 mg/day) of one week in this HCM patient, the transmitral flow velocity patterns at rest showed increased P^VRF, shortened DHT, increased P^VAC and unchanged A/R. During exercise, P^VRF increased and DHT did not prolong as compared with the levels before diltiazem administration. During the fifth minute of exercise, at HR of 82 bpm, rapid filling and atrial contraction flow tracings did not fuse together. After one minute of exercise, P^VRF and P^VAC increased, DHT shortened and A/R did not change. These increased P^VRF and reduced DHT levels would represent the improved LV distensibility as a result of diltiazem therapy during and after dynamic exercise. The small increase in P^VAC and unchanged A/R would demonstrate that improved LV distensi-

Hypertrophic Cardiomyopathy

I.M. 51yrs male

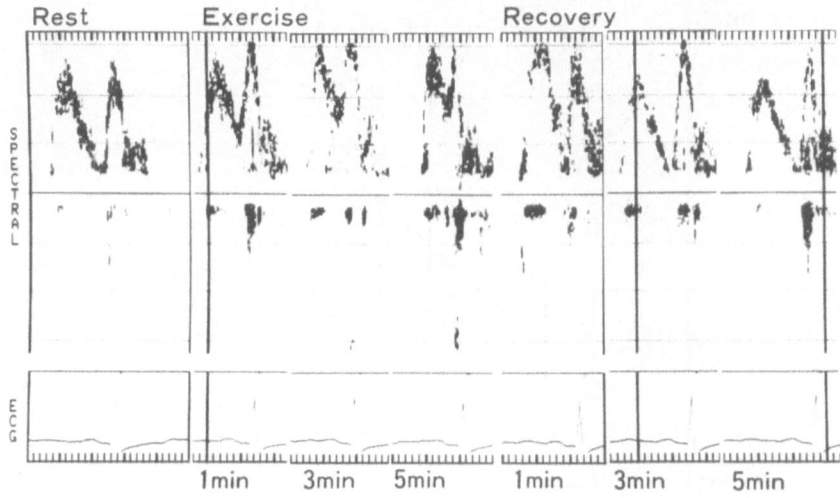

After Diltiazem

Figure 4. Case 2. 51-year-old male with HCM after diltiazem. At rest P^{V}RF increased and DHT shortened. During exercise P^{V}RF increased and DGT did not prolonged as compared with the levels before diltiazem administration. After the first 5 minutes of exercise, rapid filling and atrial contraction flow tracings did not fuse together. After one minute of exercise, P^{V}RF and P^{V}AC increased and DHT shortened. A/R did not change significantly throughout the exercise testing.

bility by diltiazem does not necessitate the compensatory mechanism of the LA (Figure 4).

In order to analyze the two components of the transmitral flow velocity patterns, the data at rest and after the first minute of recovery were statistically analyzed. HR increased significantly from the resting state to the first minute of recovery in all three groups, but no significant differences were observed among the three groups at rest and after first minute of recovery (Figure 5). The P^{V}RF increased significantly from 81 to 94 cm/sec in healthy subjects ($p < 0.001$). For the HCM pts, P^{V}RF increased significantly from 50 to 55 cm/sec ($p < 0.05$). After diltiazem administration, P^{V}RF increased significantly from 56 to 65 cm/sec ($p < 0.001$). The increase of P^{V}RF after diltiazem was larger after one minute of recovery than that in the resting state. The DHT decreased significantly from 84 to 76 msec in healthy subjects ($p < 0.001$). For the HCM pts, DHT increased from 125 to 141 msec. After diltiazem, DHT decreased from 113 to 105 msec, but neither change was

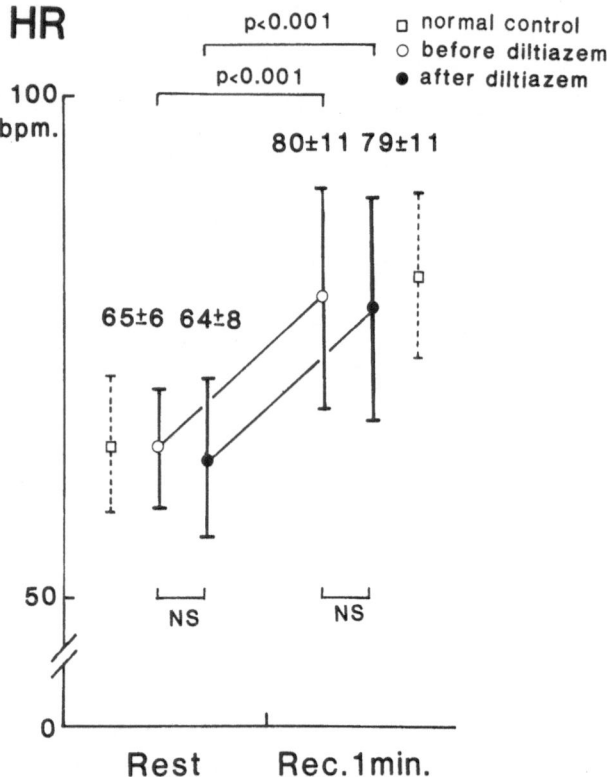

Figure 5. HR response to exercise. After the first minute of recovery HR increased significantly in all three groups, but no significant differences were observed before and after diltiazem administration.

significant. With diltiazem the significant difference in DHT levels appeared after one minute of recovery in HCM pts (p<0.05) (Figure 6). The P^VAC increased significantly from 44 to 56 cm/sec in healthy subjects (p<0.001). For HCM pts, P^VAC increased significantly from 47 to 62 cm/sec (p<0.001), after diltiazem, P^VAC increased significantly from 48 to 58 cm/sec (p<0.01). Increase of P^VAC after diltiazem was smaller than that before diltiazem. A/R increased insignificantly from 0.55 to 0.60 in healthy subjects, but increased significantly from 0.99 to 1.20 in HCM pts (p<0.005). After diltiazem, A/R increased insignificantly from 0.91 to 0.93 in HCM pts (Figure 7).

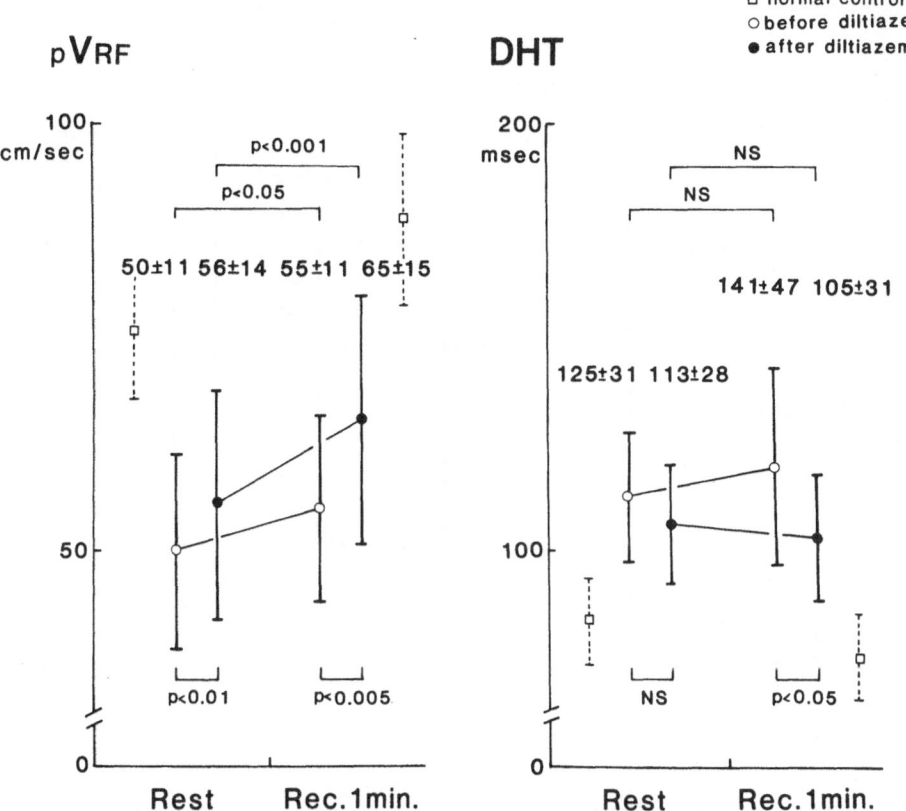

Figure 6. P^VRF and DHT responses to exercise. After the first minute of recovery P^VRF increased significantly in healthy subjects and HCM pts before diltiazem administration. The increase of P^VRF after diltiazem was larger after one minute of recovery than that in the resting state. DHT decreased significantly in healthy subject but increased in HCM pts after one minute of recovery. With diltiazem, the significant difference in DHT levels appeared after one minute of recovery in HCM pts.

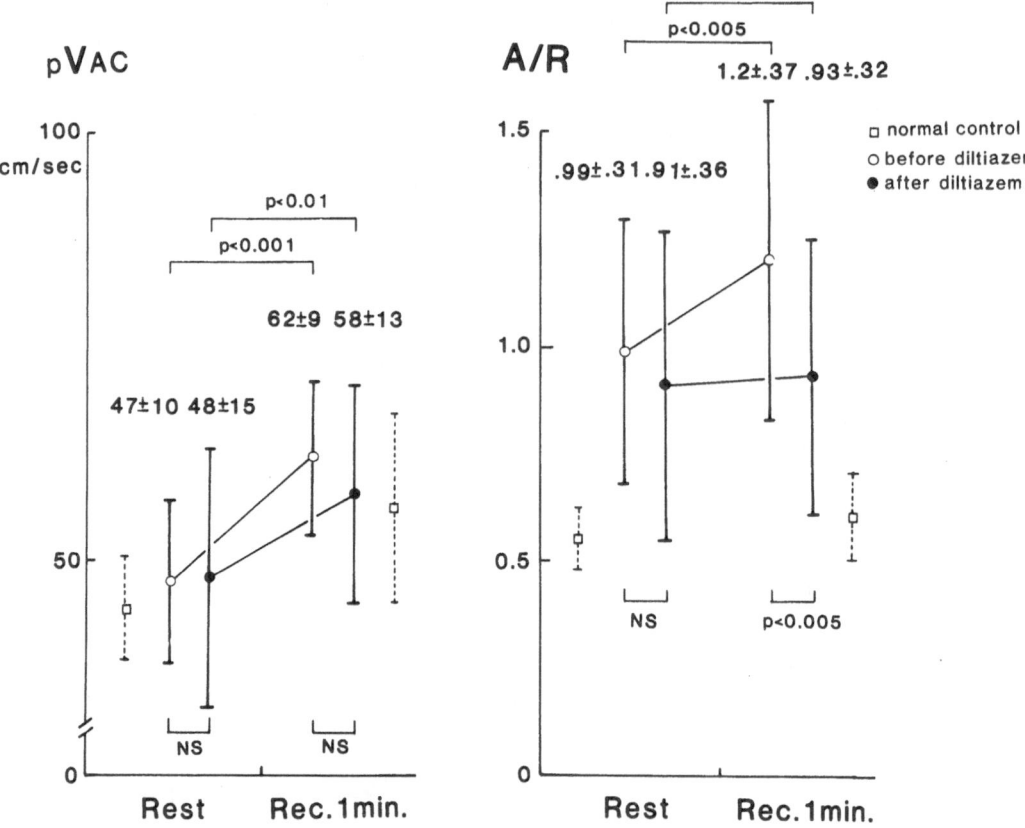

Figure 7. P^{V}AC and A/R responses to exercise. The P^{V}AC increased significantly after one minute of recovery in all three groups. However, increase of P^{V}AC after diltiazem was smaller than that before diltiazem. A/R increased insignificantly in healthy subjects, but significantly in HCM pts. After diltiazem, A/R increased insignificantly in HCM pts.

DISCUSSION

The healthy subjects demonstrated a markedly increased rapid filling of the LV after mild dynamic exercise, while HCM pts showed only a minimal increase in rapid filling of the LV. The increase in flow velocity during LA contraction phase during and after exercise was almost parallel to the increase in rapid filling velocity of the LV in healthy subjects; but much more marked in HCM. These responses to exercise may possibly be the mechanism which compensates for the poor LV distensibility in HCM pts. After diltiazem administration in HCM pts, the increase in rapid filling velocity of the LV was more marked after one minute of recovery than at rest, and the increase in flow velocity during LA contraction phase was less marked after one minute of recovery. These results suggest that diltiazem could improve the abnormal LV diastolic behavior in HCM pts not only at rest but also after mild dynamic exercise. Hanrath et al. [5] reported that chronic verapamil therapy in pts with HCM had a beneficial effect on LV hemodynamics at rest and during exercise, using invasive measurement of PA pressure and cardiac output.

The exact mode of action of slow calcium channel-blocking agent in improving the abnormal LV diastolic behavior in HCM pts is still unclear and several possible mechanisms are suspected. One of the most supported mechanisms is to improve the subendocardial ischemia by coronary arterial dilatation. However, these abnormal LV diastolic behaviors in HCM pts differed from those in coronary artery disease pts [6], but resembled to those of pts with secondary hypertrophied LV [7]. The increased Ca influx in hypertrophied myocardium might be the main factor to induce the abnormal LV diastolic behavior. Therefore Ca channel-blocking agent, diltiazem, decrease the Ca influx in these myocardium and could improve the abnormal LV diastolic behavior in HCM pts. Until recently, non-invasive estimation of LV diastolic behavior after exercise was difficult, however, exercise pulse Doppler echocardiography can repeatedly and easily be used to estimate not only abnormal LV distensibility in HCM pts [8] but also the efficacy of the drugs on LV distensibility.

REFERENCES

1. Bonow RO, Rosing DR, Bacharach SL, Green MV, Kent KM, Lipson LC, Maron BJ, Leon MB, Epstein SE: Effects of verapamil on left ventricular systolic function and diastolic filling in patients with hypertrophic cardiomyopathy. Circulation 64:787, 1981.
2. Lorell BH, Paulus WJ, Grossman W, Wynne J, Cohn PF: Modification of abnormal left ventricular diastolic properties by nifedipine in patients with hypertrophic cardiomyopathy. Circulation 65:499, 1982.
3. Suwa M, Hirota Y, Kawamura K: Improvement in left ventricular diastolic function during intravenous and oral diltiazem therapy in patients with hypertrophic cardiomyopathy: An echocardiographic study. Am J Cardiol 54:1047, 1984.
4. Nagao M, Yasue H, Omoto S, Takizawa A, Hyon H, Nishida S, Horie M, Yamada K, Tanaka S: Diltiazem-induced decrease of exercise elevated pulmonary arterial diastolic pressure in hypertrophic cardiomyopathy patients. Am Heart J 102:789, 1981.
5. Hanrath P, Schluter M, Sonntag F, Diemert J, Bleifeld W: Influence of verapamil therapy on left ventricular performance at rest and during exercise in hypertrophic cardiomyopathy. Am J Cardiol 52:544, 1983.
6. Carroll JD, Hess OM, Hirzel HO, Krayenbuehl HP: Exercise-induced Ischemia: The influence of altered relaxation on early diastolic pressures. Circulation 67:521, 1983.
7. Eichhorn P, Grimm J, Koch R, Hess O, Carroll J, Krayenbuehl HP: Left ventricular relaxation in patients with left ventricular hypertrophy secondary to aortic valve disease. Circulation 65:1395, 1982.
8. Iwase M, Yokota M, Takagi S, Koide M, Kawai N, Yoshida R, Hayashi H, Sotobata I: Analysis of diastolic behavior of the left ventricle on dynamic exercise by pulse Doppler combined with 2-D echocardiograph. In: Cardiac Doppler Diagnosis, Spencer MP (ed.), Martinus Nijhoff, Publishers, Boston, p 121–130, 1983.

17. The disturbance of left ventricular inflow by prolapsing and non-prolapsing left atrial myxoma: Estimation with pulse Doppler echocardiography

MASATSUGU IWASE, MITSUHIRO YOKOTA, SHIGEHITO TAKAGI, MASABUMI KOIDE, HU XIAO JING, NAOKI KAWAI, HIROSHI HAYASHI, IWAO SOTOBATA and MINORU TANAKA

Diagnosis of left atrial myxoma [1] is relatively easily carried out by echocardiography [2], in particular by two-dimentional (2-D) echocardiography [3], which is a useful method for diagnosis of not only the presence of myxoma but also the characteristics of myxoma. Characteristics of the myxoma would include its size, the site of attachment and it is prolapsing or not. However, the hemodynamic alteration of left ventricular (LV) filling where a myxoma is present cannot be fully assessed by echocardiography alone [4], and hemodynamics have been studied by cardiac catheterization technique [5, 6], although there are some dangers especially in patients with embolization episodes. The purpose of the present study is to estimate the severity of the LV inflow disturbance by left atrial (LA) myxoma using the pulse Doppler method.

MATERIALS AND METHODS

Subjects consisted of 5 patients with LA myxoma diagnosed by 2-D echocardiography. Catheterization by Swan-Ganz catheter was performed on all 5 patients to measure pulmonary arterial pressure and cardiac output before and after surgical removal of the myxoma. The transmitral flow velocity was recorded by monitoring the apical long axis view, using pulse Doppler combined with a 2-D echocardiograph (Toshiba SSH-11A+SDS10A and Aloka SSD-880).

206

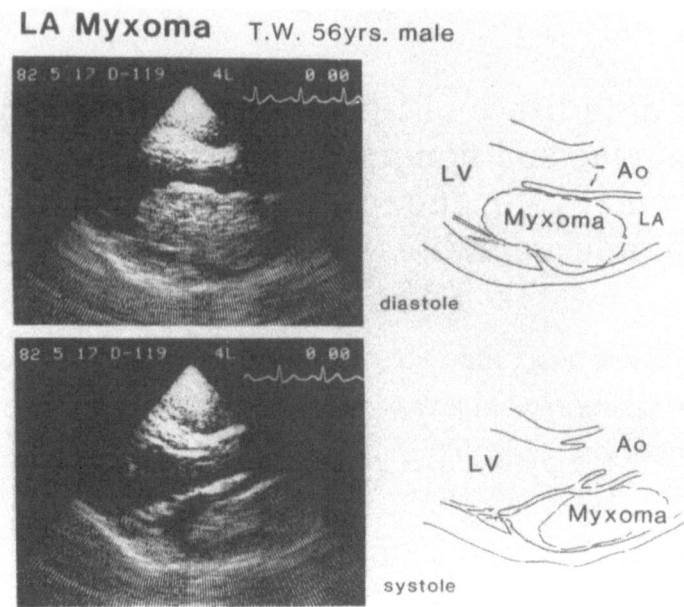

Figure 1. 2-D echocardiograms in case 2. A large myxoma prolapses into the mitral annulus and is coactated by the mitral annulus which suggests the complete obstruction of the mitral orifice in mid diastole.

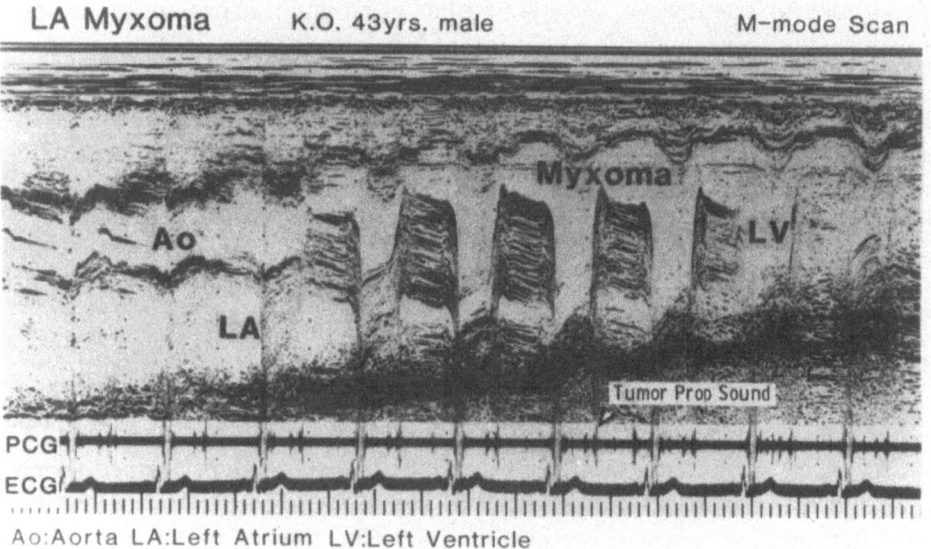

Figure 2. M-mode scan in case 2. The myxoma echoes are visible behind the anterior leaflet of the mitral valve during diastole and the diastolic slope of the mitral valve is reduced as in mitral stenosis.

LA Myxoma

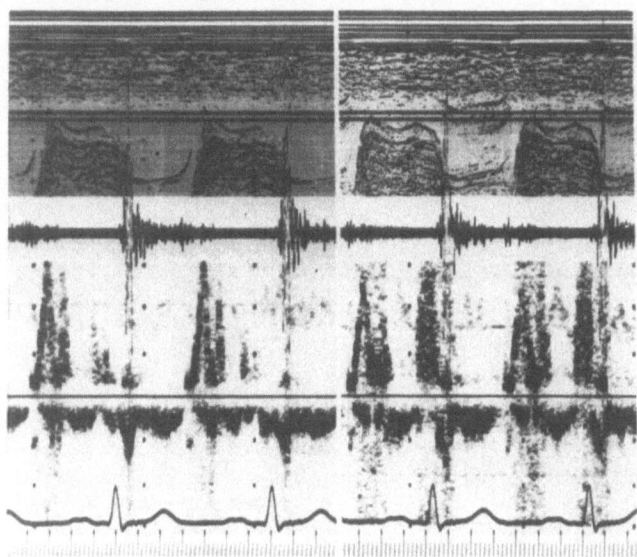

Figure 3. Pulse Doppler echocardiograms in case 2. A high LV inflow with short duration is observed jut before the prolapse of the myxoma into the mitral annulus, and after prolapsing, LV inflow disappeared almost completely. During the LA contraction phase, the LV inflow can be seen at some of the sampling points.

LA Myxoma 60yrs. female

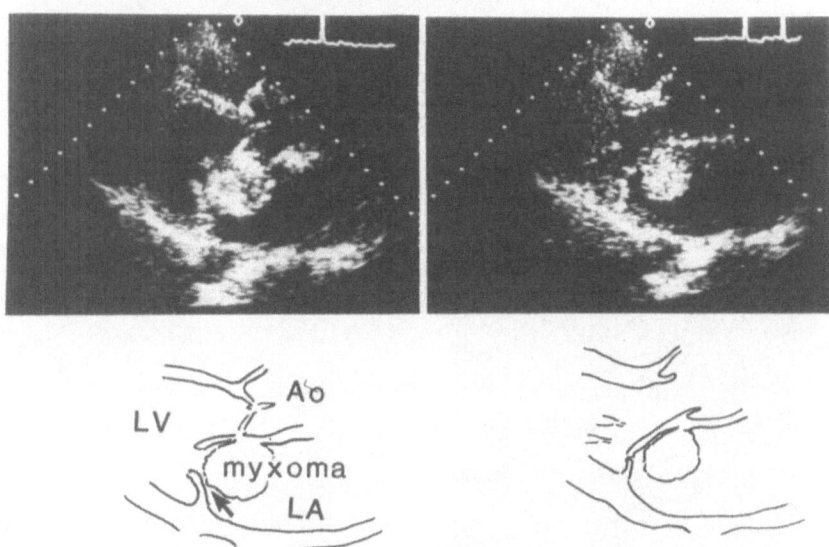

Figure 4. 2-D echocardiograms in case 3. A middle-sized myxoma prolapses into the mitral annulus but a small space is visible behind the myxoma and the posterior leaflet of mitral valve (arrow) since the myxoma is relatively smaller than the mitral orifice.

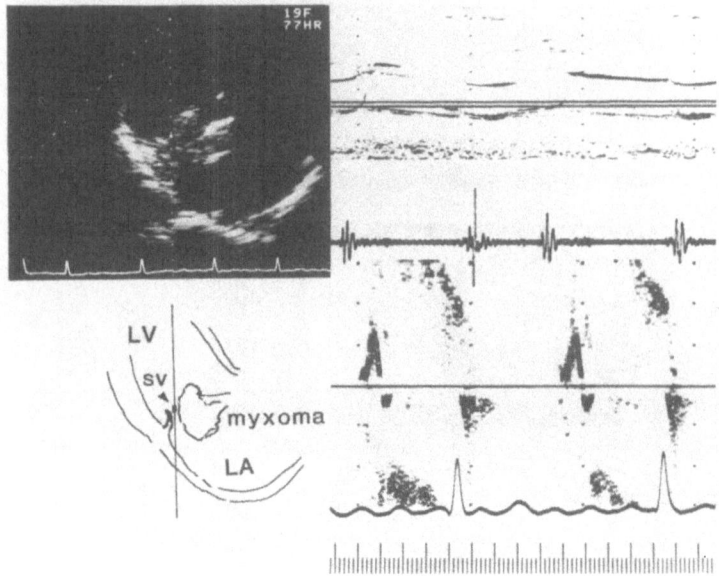

LA Myxoma 60yrs. female

Figure 5. Pulse Doppler echocardiograms in case 3. The LV inflow with short duration is observed just before the prolapse of myxoma into the mitral annulus, and after prolapsing, the LV inflow shows prolonged deceleration of the rapid filling velocity like mitral stenosis.

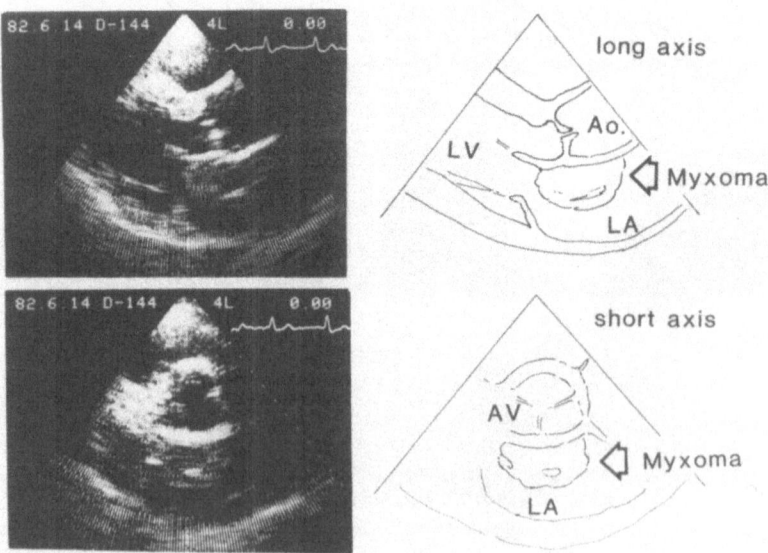

LA Myxoma M.H. 73yrs. male

Figure 6. 2-D echocardiograms in case 4. A moderate-sized myxoma is shown on the anterior side of the LA without a stalk and with no movement during the entire cardiac cycle.

LA Myxoma M.H. 73yrs male   M-mode Scan

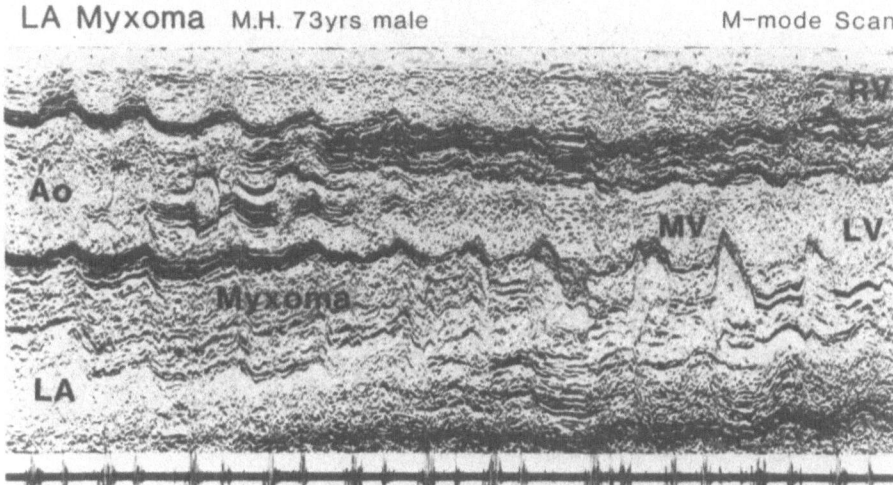

Figure 7. M-mode scan in case 4. The myxoma echoes are visible behind the posterior aortic wall throughout the cardiac cycle but not visible behind the anterior leaflet of the mitral valve during diastole. The movements of the mitral valve leaflets is almost normal.

RESULTS

Case 1, a 43-yr-old male and case 2, a 56-yr-old male had complaints of general fatigue and dyspnea after the slightest exertion, very similar to a case of mitral stenosis. These two patients had almost the same echocardiographic and pulse Doppler findings. 2-D and M-mode echocardiograms showed a large and mobile LA myxoma which prolapsed into the mitral annulus and almost completely blocks the mitral orifice in diastole (Figure 1 and 2). On the pulse Doppler echocardiograms, a high LV inflow with short duration was observed just before prolapsing of the myxoma into the mitral annulus and LV inflow disappeared almost completely after prolapsing. During the LA contraction phase, the LV inflow could be seen at some of the sampling points. Catheterization data showed that mean pulmonary arterial (PA) pressure was 25 mm Hg in case 1 and 23 mm Hg in case 2, and suggested that the LV inflow was hemodynamically disturbed in two cases. The weight of the myxoma in case 1 was 33 g and that in case 2 was 73 g.

Case 3, a 60-yr-old female had complaint of slowly progressive general fatigue and weight loss from 60 kg to 44 kg during 2 years. 2-D echocardiograms of this case showed a middle sized and mobile LA myxoma which

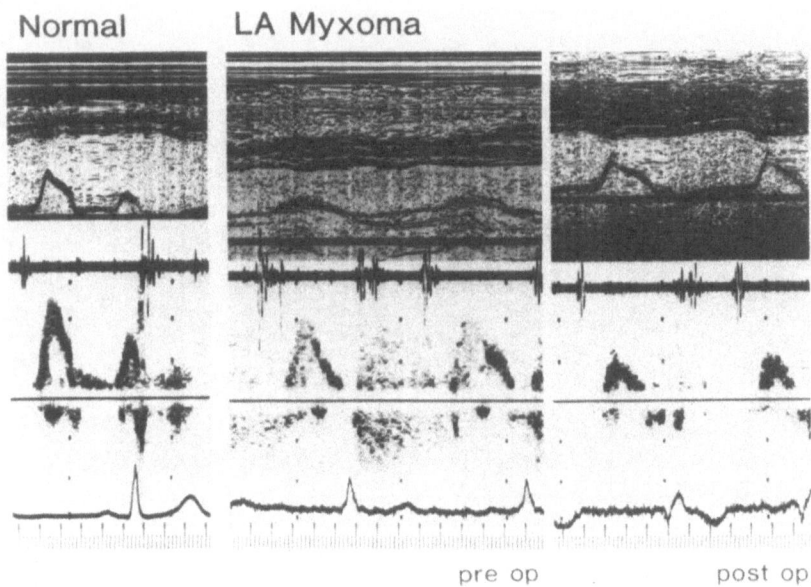

Normal   LA Myxoma

pre op   post op

Figure 8. Pulse Doppler echocardiograms in case 4. The LV flow is almost the same as that of the normal apart from the lack of LA contraction flow caused by atrial fibrilation. The mitral regurgitant signals are seen before operation, but disappeared after the simple removal of myxoma.

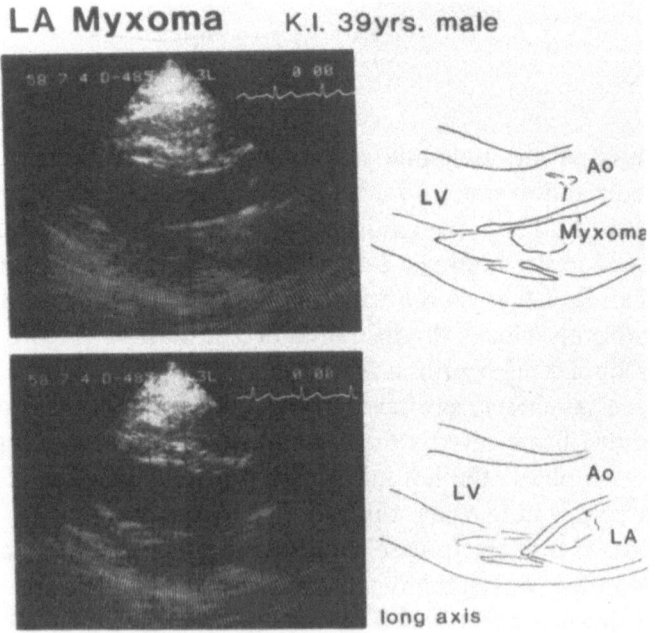

LA Myxoma   K.I. 39yrs. male

long axis

Figure 9. 2-D echocardiograms in case 5. A small and pedunculated myxoma is seen behind the anterior mitral leaflet, but the mitral orifice is only partially occluded because of the small size.

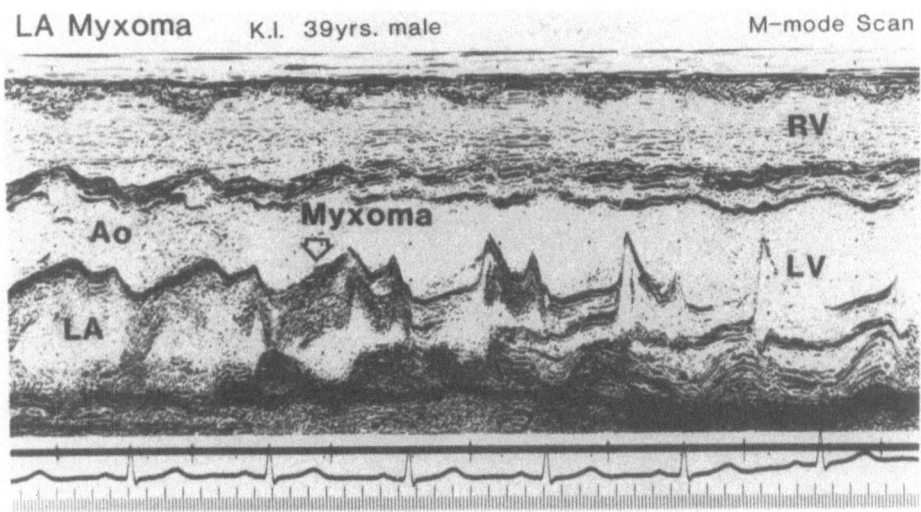

Figure 10. M-mode scan in case 5. The myxoma echoes are visible behind the anterior mitral leaflet, but its diastolic slope is almost normal which suggests no LV inflow disturbance.

prolapsed into the mitral annulus but does not completely obstruct its orifice in diastole (Figure 4). On the pulse Doppler echocardiograms, the LV inflow with short duration was observed just before prolapsing like case 1 and 2, but the LV inflow showed prolonged deceleration of the rapid filling velocity after prolapsing (Figure 5). The mean PA pressure in this case was 20 mm Hg, and the weight of the myxoma was 15 g.

Case 4, a 73-yr-old male had multiple embolization episodes for the previous three years, but no physical abnormality such as general fatigue or dyspnea. 2-D and M-mode echocardiograms of this case showed a moderate-size myxoma attached widely to the anterior wall of the LA without a stalk and movement to the mitral orifice (Figures 6 and 7).

On the pulse Doppler echocardiograms in this case, the pattern of LV inflow is almost the same as that of the normal apart from the lack of LA contraction flow caused by atrial fibrilation, and the mitral regurgitant signals. However, these mitral regurgitant signals disappeared after the simple removal of the myxoma (Figure 8). The mean PA pressure in this case was 12 mm Hg, and the weight of the myxoma was 35 g.

Case 5, a 39-yr-old male suddenly lost the sight of his right eye and thereafter had an attack of hemiparalysis from which he recovered almost completely. The diagnosis of LA myxoma was carried out by echocardiography two months after this first episode. This patient had no physical complaints such as general fatigue or dyspnea on exertion. 2-D and M-mode echocardiograms of this case showed a small and pedunculated myxoma

LA Myxoma

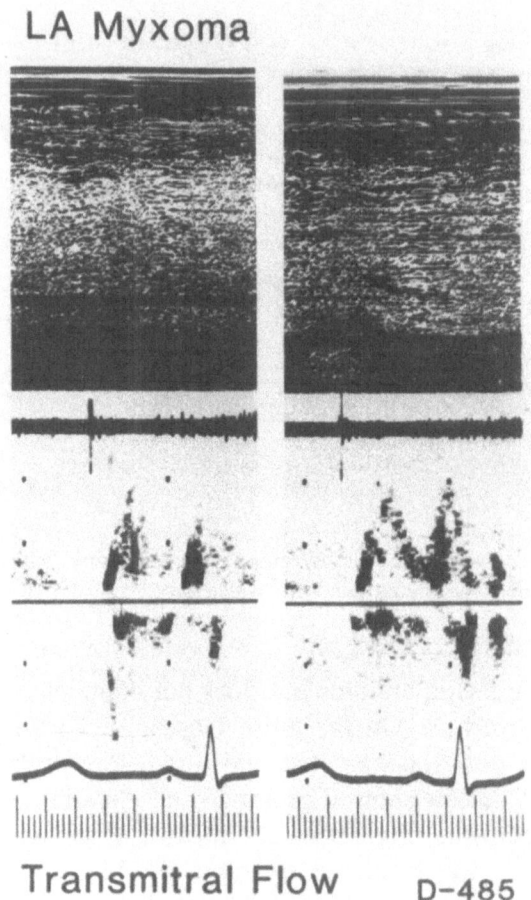

Transmitral Flow   D-485

Figure 11. Pulse Doppler echocardiograms in case 5. Disturbed LV inflow like case 1 and 2 is seen at the sampling site of the posteromedial commisura, where the myxoma prolapses, but LV inflow recorded at the other sampling points is almost normal.

behind the anterior mitral leaflet, but the mitral orifice is only partially occluded because of the small size of the myxoma (Figures 9, 10).

On the pulse Doppler echocardiograms, LV inflow was interrupted as if there was a large and prolapsing myxoma at the sampling site of the postero-medial commisura, where the myxoma prolapsed, but LV inflow recorded at the other sampling points was almost normal (Figure 11). The mean PA pressure was 15 mm Hg and the weight of the myxoma was only 3 g.

DISCUSSION

Concerning the hemodynamic features of prolapsing and nonprolapsing LA myxoma, Ruey J. Sung et al. [6] investigated the two types using simultaneous recordings of left ventricular and left atrial or pulmonary arterial wedge pressures and cineangiocardiograms. In their type I, prolapsing LA myxomas moved from LA to LV and prominent C and V waves accompanied by a rapidly descent was shown in the pulmonary wedge or left atrial pressure pulse. This rapidly descent seems to correspond to the early diastolic high LV inflow velocity with a short duration observed in pulse Doppler methods.

In their type II, nonprolapsing LA myxomas remained in LA during entire cardiac cycle and impeded flow across the mitral valve. In this type, the y descent was slow and the large pressure differences between LA and LV persisted during diastole as if there was mitral stenosis. To impede the LV inflow throughout diastole like mitral stenosis, the nonprolapsing LA myxoma would have to be larger than the prolapsing LA myxoma or prolapsing LA myxoma would not have to be so large to obstruct the mitral orifice completely. However, the LV inflow was almost normal in our cases 4 and 5. Therefore, hemodynamically normal pressure patterns would be presented in some cases of LA myxoma.

In the course of the evaluation of five patients with LA myxoma, it was noted that the movement and the size of myxoma was related to hemodynamic characteristics of LV inflow and three types of LV inflow patterns would be conceivable in LA myxoma. Type A: high LV inflow of short duration in early diastole and almost no LV inflow in mid to late diastole after prolapsing of myxoma. Type B: continuous LV inflow interruption throughout diastole as in mitral stenosis. Type C: no disturbance of LV inflow. Type A pattern was shown in large and prolapsing myxomas (cases 1 and 2) and considered to coincide with type 1 suggested by Sung et al. Type B pattern was demonstrated in a prolapsing and moderate-sized myxoma (case 3) or possibly in a non-prolapsing and very large myxoma. This type seemed to be consistent with type II by Sung et al. Type C pattern was shown in a nonprolapsing and moderate-sized myxoma (case 4), or in a prolapsing and small myxoma (case 5).

To clinically evaluate the LV inflow disturbances caused by LA myxoma, a pulse Doppler combined with 2-D echocardiography is a useful non-invasive technique in clinical practice.

REFERENCES

1. Zitnik RS, Giuliani ER, Rochester M: Clinical recognition of atrial myxoma. Am Heart J 80:689, 1970.
2. Wolfe SB, Popp RL, Feigenbaum H: Diagnosis of atrial tumors by ultrasound. Circulation 39:615, 1969.
3. Lappe DL, Bulkley BH, Weiss JL: Two-dimensional echocardiographic diagnosis of left atrial myxoma. Chest 74:55, 1978.
4. Gershlick AH, Leech G, Mills PG, Leatham A: The loud first heart sound in left atrial myxoma. Br Heart J 52:403, 1984.
5. Pitt A, Pitt B, Schaefer J, Criley JM: Myxoma of the left atrium: Hemodynamic and phonocardiographic consequences of sudden tumor movement. Circulation 36:408, 1967.
6. Sung RJ, Ghahramani AR, Mallon SM, Richter SE, Sommer LS, Gottlieb S, Myerburg RJ: Hemodynamic features of prolapsing and nonprolapsing left atrial myxoma. Circulation 51:342, 1975.

18. Evaluating the fetal circulation by combined pulsed Doppler and 2-D echocardiography

HIDEYO SHIMADA, MICHIKO TAKAHASHI, HIROSHI YANAGISAWA,

SHIZUO KATAGIRI, and HIDEO KOBAYASHI

INTRODUCTION

Recent advances of 2D echocardiography and Doppler method have enabled us to record the states of fetal heart and to analyse fetal cardiac anatomy and physiology.

The present study explains the techniques to record fetal Doppler flow patterns with 2D echocardiography and their clinical applications based on our experiences.

METHODS

Three-hundred and twenty-five fetuses of healthy mothers varying 30 to 38 weeks gestation were performed 2D echocardiography in the past 4 years in our laboratory. Twenty-three cases from which clear apical four-chamber view tracings could be obtained went to pulsed Doppler study. Apical four chamber view tracings of the fetus, adequate to get Doppler flow patterns of the cardiac chambers, could be recorded only when the fetus was located in the right cephalic presentation (Figure 1).

The sampling volume for Doppler flow patterns of the left ventricle was set in the center of the mitral orifice just below the mitral valve, and of the right ventricle in the center of the tricuspid orifice just below the tricuspid valve (Figure 2).

Doppler flow patterns of the pulmonary artery and of the aorta could not be obtained, mainly because of technical difficulties.

A Toshiba SSH-11A real-time, phased-array ultrasonic sector scanner with a hand-controlled 2.4 MHz transducer was used to perform 2D and M-mode echocardiography. The pulsed Doppler examinations were performed with a Doppler flow meter Toshiba SDS-10A with the echocardiographic systems.

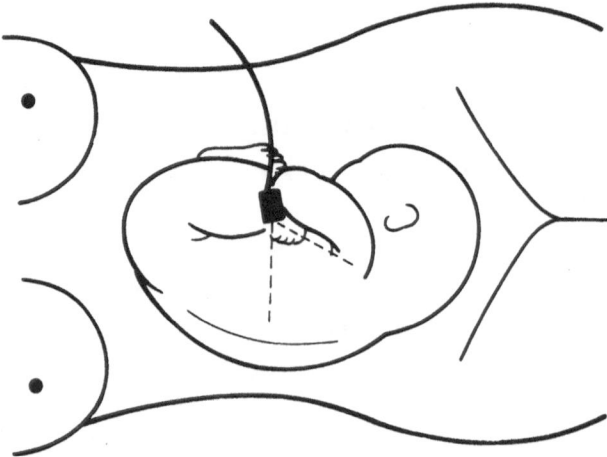

Figure 1. The transducer position. The fetus is located in the right cephalic presentation. Transducer is set on maternal naval region.

The flow velocity was calculated by using the formula as follows:

$$v = \frac{f_2 \cdot C}{2 f_0 \cos \theta}$$

C : speed of sound in tissue
v : maximum velocity
f_2 : frequency shift
f_0 : Transducer frequency
θ : angle between ultrasound beam and blood flow

RESULTS

(1) Doppler flow pattern of the mitral orifice showed twin-peaked toward flow in diastole. The first one occurred in the rapid filling phase of the left ventricle, and the other one occured coincident with the left atrial contraction phase. The atrial contraction wave showed much faster velocity than that of the rapid filling waves (Figure 2).

(2) Doppler flow pattern of the tricuspid orifice was essentially the same as that of the mitral orifice. But the faster flow velocity than that of the mitral orifice was observed both in rapid filling wave and atrial contraction wave (Figure 2).

(3) The maximum mitral flow velocity was 52.1 ± 9.9 cm/sec (mean $\pm$ SD). The maximum tricuspid flow velocity was 56.1 ± 8.7 cm/sec (Figure 3).

— Doppler Spectrum —

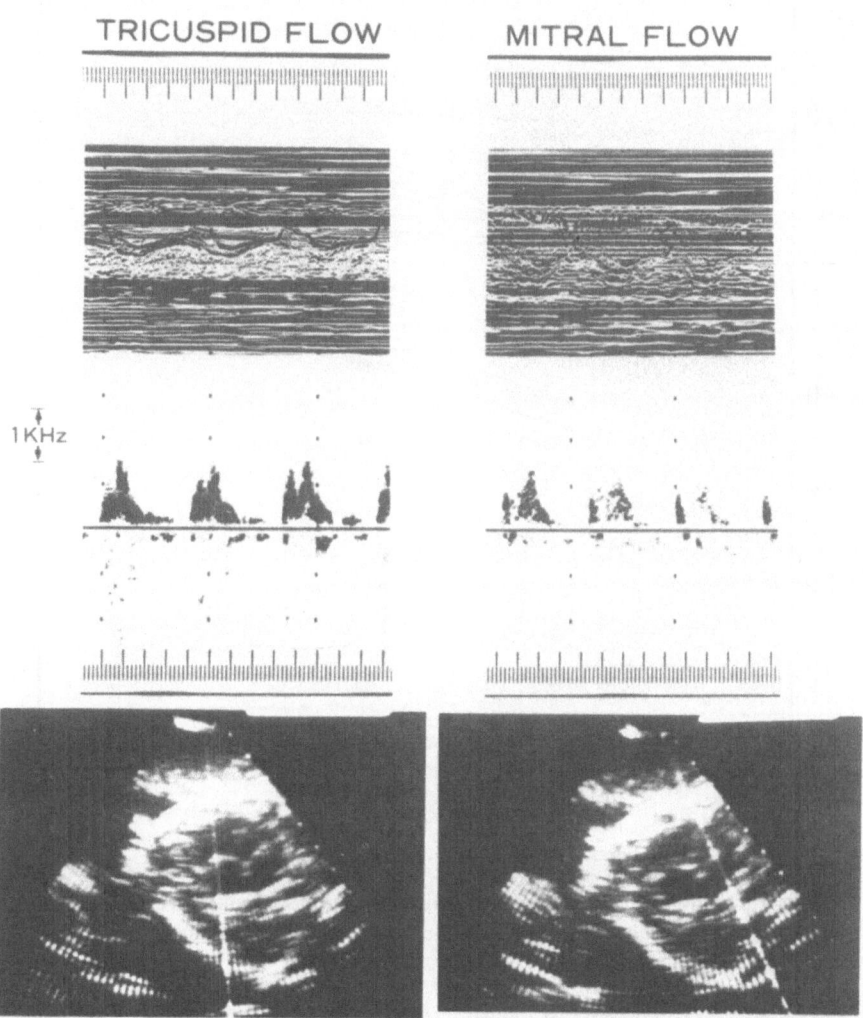

Figure 2. The site of the sampling volume and the Doppler flow patterns of the mitral and of the tricuspid valves. The sampling volume of the left ventricle was set in the center of the mitral orifice just below the mitral valve and that of the right ventricle was set in the center of the tricuspid orifice just below the tricuspid valve as shown on the 2D echocardiograms (bottom). Both flow patterns through the mitral and tricuspid valves showed twin peaded patterns (top).

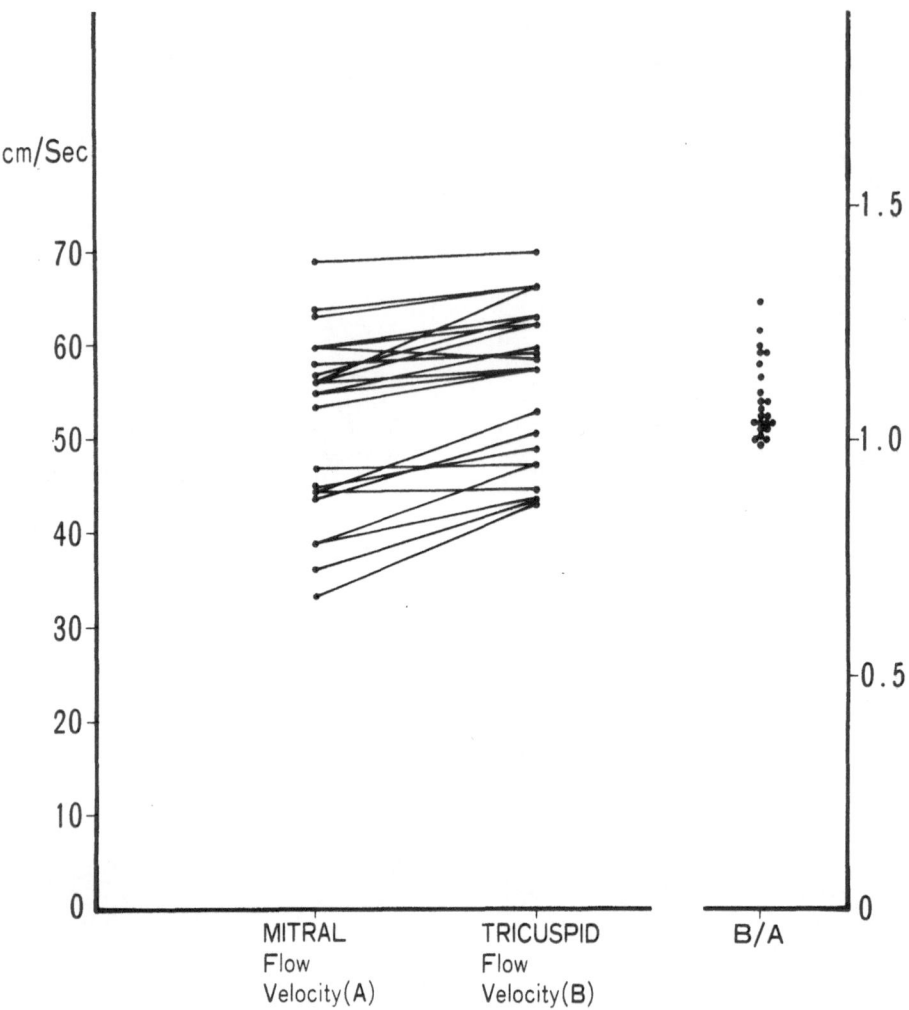

Figure 3. The maximum flow velocity of the mitral and tricuspid valve. The maximum mitral flow velocity was 52.1 ± 9.9 cm/sec. The maximum tricuspid flow velocity to mitral flow velocity was 1.09 ± 0.09.

(4) The ratio of tricuspid flow velocity to mitral flow velocity was 1.09 ± 0.09 (Figure 3).

DISCUSSION

Only a few studies have been reported in the field of the fetal Doppler echocardiography [1].

At the fetal stage, since lungs do not work, pulmonary circulation cannot be detected. Therefore, the blood stream through Foramen ovale supplies the mitral flow, and the blood stream through Ductus arteriosus is supplied by the tricuspid flow.

Then, if the flow volume through the mitral and tricuspid valve could be detected, it is possible to estimate blood flow volume through Foramen ovale and Ductus arteriosus.

We have calculated the mitral flow velocity and tricuspid flow velocity by using the pulsed Doppler method. The flow velocity is not equal to the flow volume. But, if the size of the mitral valve orifice and that of tricuspid valve orifice could be measured, the mitral and tricuspid flow volume could be estimated from the mitral flow velocity and from the tricuspid flow velocity, respectively.

Unfortunately, it was impossible to calculate the size of the mitral valve orifice and the tricuspid valve orifice in the fetus. As, widely accepted, the excursion of the mitral and tricuspid valves reflects the size of the mitral and tricuspid valve functional orifice, then the amplitude of the both valves might be used as the size of the functional orifice of the valves.

The mitral valve excursion and the tricuspid excursion of the fetus was almost equally based on our studies [2], so the mitral valve orifice and the tricuspid valve orifice were thought to be almost equally functional.

Therefore, the mitral flow velocity and the tricuspid flow velocity, calculated from the Doppler method, might substitute the flow volume of the mitral valve and the tricuspid valve.

As already mentioned, the ratio of the tricuspid flow velocity to the mitral flow velocity was 1.09 (mean). It means when the left ventricle ejects 1, the right ventricle ejects 1.09.

There have been no report about the fetal cardiac circulations in the human heart. The only report by Rudolph and Heyman [3] based on animal experiments, was described that the left ventricle ejected only 1/3 of the total cardiac output. But our data suggested at least more than 1/3 of the total cardiac output was ejected from the left ventricle before birth.

CONCLUSION

The fetal Doppler method with 2D echocardiography is to be thought very useful to evaluate cardiac hemodynamics before birth.

REFERENCES

1. Maulik D, Nanda NC, Saini VD: Fetal Doppler Echocardiography: Method and Characterization of Normal and Abnormal Hemodynamics. Am J Cardiol 53:572, 1984.

2. Takahashi M, Shimada H, Yanagisawa H, Katagiri S, Kobayashi H: Trial to Evaluate Fetal Hemodynamics by Pulsed Doppler Echocardiography. J Cardiography, in press, 1984.
3. Rudolph AM, Heyman MA: Circulatory Changes during Growth in the Fetal Lamb. Cir Res 26:289, 1970.

19. Application of multigate pulsed Doppler systems in congenital heart disease

O. DANIËLS, S. DE KNECHT, J.C.W. HOPMAN, A.P.G. HOEKS and R.S. RENEMAN

INTRODUCTION

Single gate pulsed Doppler systems enable the transcutaneous investigation of the hemodynamic behavior at a rather well determined site. The spatial resolution of pulsed Doppler systems in both axial and lateral direction with respect to the ultrasound beam provides a means to emphasize specific phenomena without interference caused by Doppler signals originating from outside the sample volume. However, a single gate system obscures the three-dimensional nature of blood flow in the cavities of the heart. A multigate pulsed Doppler system allows the assessment of the hemodynamic behaviour in a number of sample volumes simultaneously. Preferable a large number of sample volumes of small dimensions hould be employed to maintain detail in the velocity distribution along the ultrasound beam. To provide feedback about the position of the ultrasound beam with respect to the structures investigated a multigate pulsed Doppler system should be connected to a two-dimensional imaging system. Operating alternately the echo- and the Doppler system allows verification of the position of the ultrasound beam intermittently.

SYSTEM DESCRIPTION

The multigae pulsed Doppler system used in this study operates at an emission frequency of 5 MHz, Hoeks [1]. Because of the limited range of penetration due to the frequency-dependent attenuation of ultrasound by the medium, in its present form the system is restricted to pediatric cardiology. The selection of 5 MHz for the emission frequency allows the connection of the system to a commercially available echo device (ATL, Mark V), the echo- and the Doppler system sharing the same probe. When either of both systems is in operation the other is switched off to avoid interference. Selection of systems is facilitated by a foot switch.

The pulse repetition frequency of the Doppler system is set at 16 kHz (allowing a range of 48 mm) while the duration of emission can be selected (0.8 or 1.2 usec). A short duration of emission enhances the axial resolution of the Doppler system, while a longer duration of emission improves the signal-to-noise ratio of the Doppler signal. Even for the long ultrasound burst the size of the sample volume is considerably less than 2 mm^3; the sample volume being defined as the region where 90 % of the energy of the received Doppler signal is originating from Hoeks et al. [1].

The time-dependent gain can be adjusted for range intervals of 5 mm independent of the gain setting of the echo system. To suppress high-amplitude low-frequency Doppler signals originating from tissue interfaces a cascade of two high-pass digital filters of the first order is incorporated in the system. The cut-off frequency of these filters can be selected at either 250 Hz or 500 Hz. The higher cutt-off frequency is especially convenient when the ultrasound beam intersects with fast moving tissue interfaces like cardiac walls and/or valve leaflets. The digital filter can accomodate 64 quadrature Doppler signals originating from 64 sample volumes distributed at 0.6 mm intervals along the ultrasound beam.

The position of the first sample volume with respect to the transducer can be varied with 6 mm increments, allowing shifting of the position of the sample volumes along the ultrasound beam. Any sample volume can be selected for aural evaluation. The quadrature Doppler signals of this volume are made available for spectral analysis.

To retrieve the average Doppler frequency in each of the sample volumes the instantaneous phase of the filtered quadrature Doppler signal is computed in each processing cycle following emission. The time-average of the change in phase in subsequent processing cycles is derived by using a digital filter of the first order, with a cut-off frequency of either 18 Hz or 36 Hz. A correction procedure acting on the instantaneous change of phase is incorporated to reduce the effect of noise on the detected average frequency (Hoeks et al.) [3]. The resulting instantaneous velocity distribution is displayed on a video screen where the horizontal axis represents depth and the vertical deflection indicates the local average velocity. The sample volume selected for aural evaluation is identified by a marker.

To appreciate the time-dependent nature of the velocity distribution observed along the ultrasound beam the instantaneous velocity profiles are stored in a memory at a rate of 60 Hz. The velocity distribution as function of time is made available on a second display in scroll mode. The memory can accommodate a maximum of 256 velocity profiles equivalent to a time span of over 4 seconds. The number of velocity profiles per second and the total number on display can be adjusted to enhance detail. The spacing between two subsequent velocity profiles on display equals a calibrated value in Doppler shift frequency independent of the total number of velocity profiles displayed. In all cases the whole range of 64 sample gates (38.4 mm) is visualized. A bottom trace provides a reference signal e.g. the ECG. The total content of the memory can be dumped in a computer for off-line evaluation.

METHOD OF INVESTIGATION

As stated before the multigate pulsed Doppler system is connected to a two-dimensional duplex scanner (ATL Mark V). This is necessary because

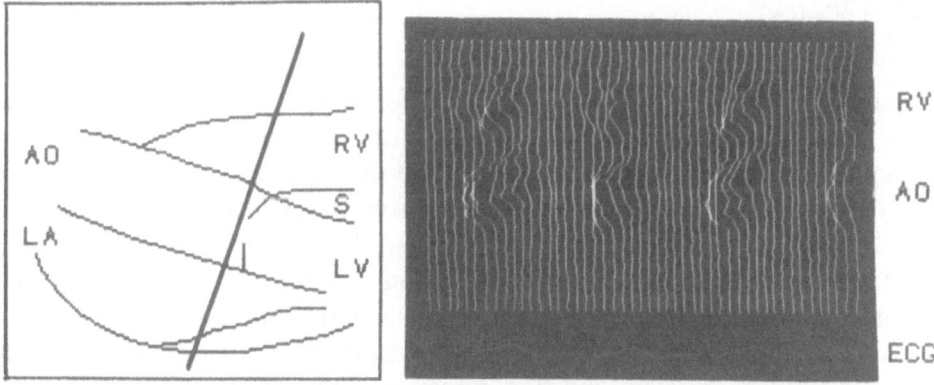

Figure 1. Flow profiles, obtained along the M-line as indicated, in a parasternal long axis view of the aorta and left ventricle. The flow in the right ventricular outflow tract (RV) and ascending aorta (AO) can be recognized. (LA = left atrium; LV = left ventricle; S = septum).

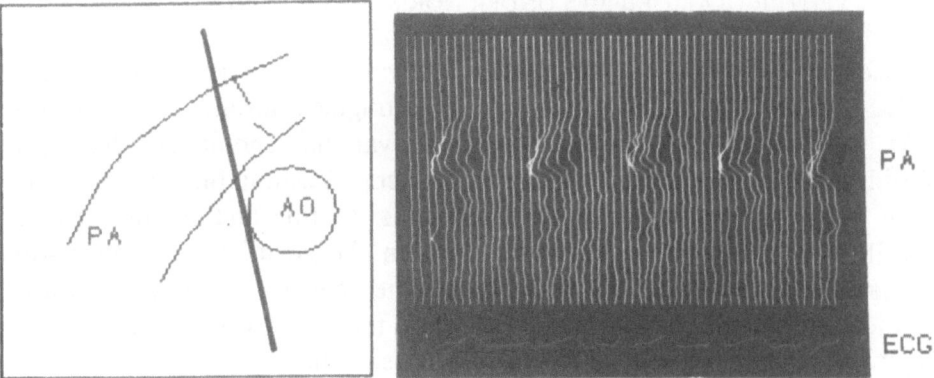

Figure 2. Flow profiles, obtained along the M-line as indicated, in a parasternal long axis view of the main pulmonary artery (PA).

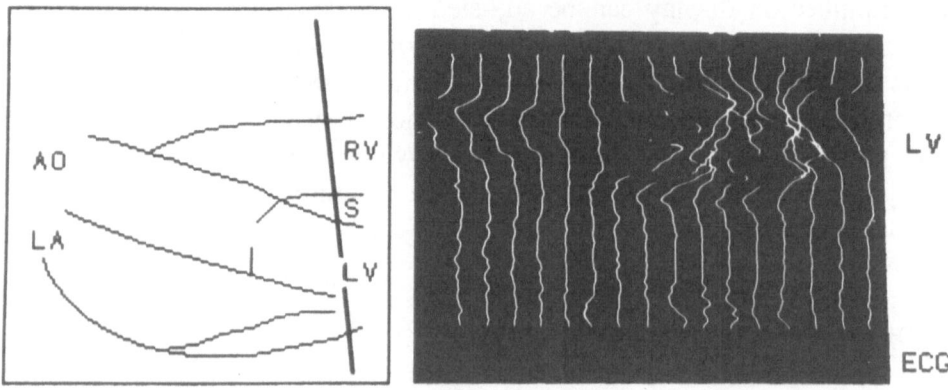

Figure 3. Flow profiles, obtained along the M-line as indicated, in a parasternal long axis left ventricular view. By the introduction of a time delay the 64 sample gates are positioned over the left ventricle (LV).

one ought to know where the Doppler information is originating from in such a complex structure as the heart. With this set-up it is possible to visualize the heart and great vessels by two-dimensional echocardiography. On the screen the M-line can be placed across the structure of interest and the depth of the site of investigation can be assessed. In the multigate pulsed Doppler system the delay between emission and the first sampling gate is adjusted so that the site to be examined falls within the 64 sampling gates. In contrast to single gate pulsed Doppler systems an obtuse angle is chosen between ultrasound beam and flow direction. This results in a profile with little or no aliasing under normal conditions.

VELOCITY PROFILES AS RECORDED IN GREAT ARTERIES AND
ATRIO–VENTRICULAR ORIFICES UNDER NORMAL CIRCUMSTANCES

Information about the shape of velocity profiles in great arteries and valve orifices is important to be able to distinguish normal from disturbed flow patterns as for example induced by valvular anomalies, Hoeks [4]. Besides, it provides insight into the error made in estimating cardiac output with single gate pulsed Doppler techniques. In this method the velocity profile is assumed to be flat (plug flow) in the great arteries and artrio-ventricular orifices. In Figures 1, 2 and 3 the velocity profiles as measured in the aorta, the main pulmonary artery and the mitral valve orifice, respectively, of a child without heart disease are shown.

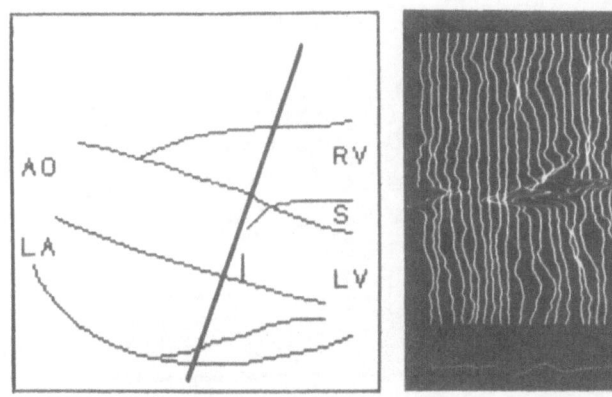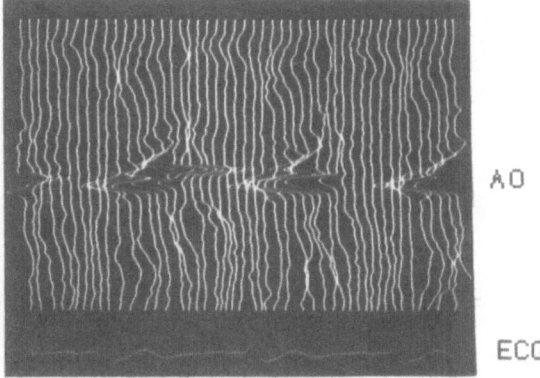

Figure 4. Flow profiles, obtained along the M-line as indicated, in a parasternal long axis view of the aorta and left ventricle in case of an aortic valve stenosis as decribed in case 1. Note the abnormal high velocity in the ascending aorta accentuated by aliasing.

ESTIMATION OF THE SEVERITY OF VALVULAR STENOSIS

In case of a valvular stenosis the orifice of the valve is narrowed. In this constricted opening and just downstream to it the blood flow velocity is faster than normal and a jetstream may exist in the more severe cases. The location and the width of these jetstreams can be determined with the multigate pulsed Doppler system by assessing the number of gates in which high velocities, generally accentuated by aliasing, are present (Figure 4). The diameter of the jetstream as measured just downstream to the valve should correspond with the hemodynamic orifice. So with the multigate pulsed Doppler system the severity of a valvular stenosis can be estimated independent of cardiac output measurements (de Knecht et al. [5, 6]).

CASE HISTORIES

Case 1. A 2.5 month old boy visited our clinic because of feeding problems. On admission he had a bodyweight of 5.4 kg. A grade 3/6 low frequency murmur was heard on the 1-2 right intercostal space. The ECG showed a left ventricle strain pattern. On the chest X-ray a cardiomegaly and signs of pulmonary venous congestion where seen. By echo-Doppler cardiography severe aortic valve stenosis and mitral regurgitation were diagnosed. With multigate pulsed Doppler echocardiography a disturbed flow pattern was seen in the ascending aorta. The measured diameter of the jet was 3.5-4 mm (Figure 4).

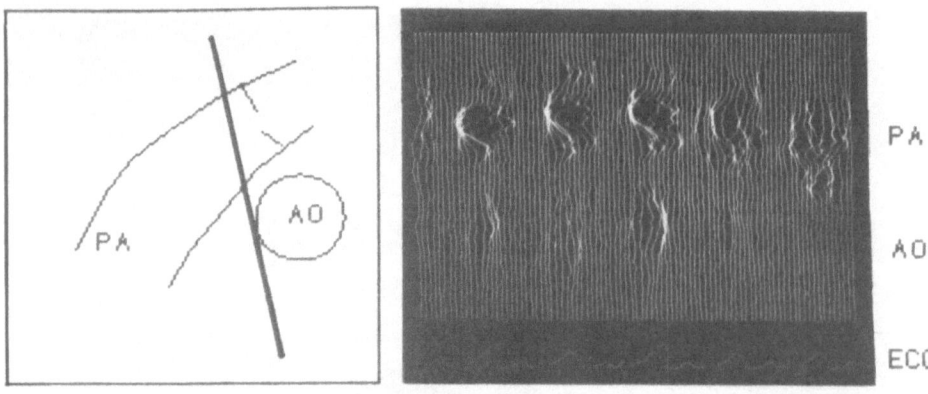

Figure 5. Flow profiles, obtained along the M-line as indicated, in a parasternal long axis view of the main pulmonary artery in case of a pulmonary valve stenosis as described in case 2. Note the region with high velocities in the late systole.

At heart catheterization a left ventricular aorta gradient of 75 mm Hg was found. On a left ventricular angiography just downstream the narrowed aortic valve a jet with a diameter of 3.6 mm was visualised. At heart operation the surgeon found a bicuspid valve with an opening of 3 mm in diameter.

Case 2. A boy of 3 years old with a bodyweight of 15 kg was known in our clinic for several years. At the age of 5 days a valvulotomy (Brock) was performed because of severe pulmonary valve stenosis with cyanosis. On physical examination he was again cyanotic and had a grade 2–3/6 low frequency systolic murmur in the second left intercostal space. The ECG showed a P-pulmonale and right ventricular hypertrophy. By echo-Doppler cardiography a right ventricular hypertrophy with pulmonary valve stenosis and tricuspid regurgitation was found. With multigate pulsed Doppler an ostium flow diameter of 5 mm was measured for the pulmonary valve (Figure 5).

During heart catheterization a right ventricular-pulmonary artery gradient of 115 mm Hg was measured. The valve ostium was calculated to be 0.13 cm^2 (according to the formula of Gorlin). This yields an ostium diameter of 4 mm assuming a round valve stenosis. On right ventricular cineangiography a jet diameter of 5.0 mm was found. Three weeks later at heart surgery a 5 mm probe could just pass the stenotic pulmonary valve ostium.

Case 3. A 9 days old neonate with a bodyweight of 2.8 kg was referred to our clinic because of severe heart failure. On physical examination a galop rhythm was heared, but no heart murmur. The femoral pulses were weak and the brachial pulses were well palpable. Echo-Doppler cardiography

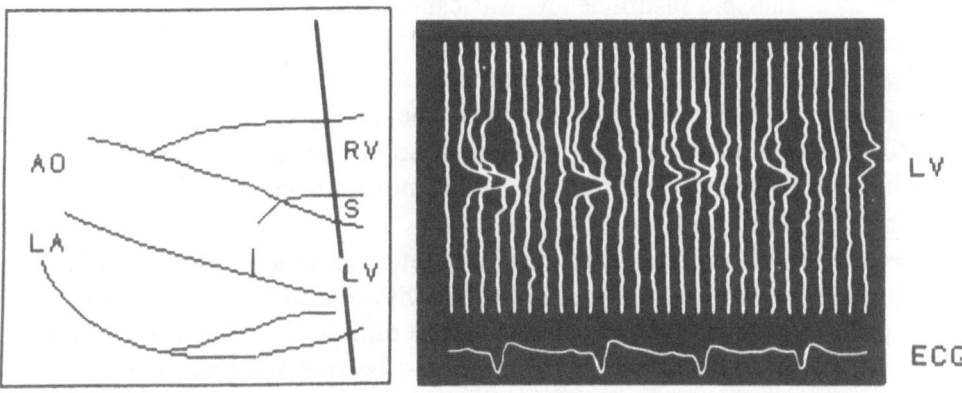

Figure 6. Flow profiles, obtained along the M-line as indicated, in a parasternal long axis left ventricular view in case of a hypoplastic mitral valve. By the introduction of a time delay the 64 sample gates are positioned over the left ventricle. A small region of high velocity in early diastole (4 mm) is interpreted as mitral valve orifice flow.

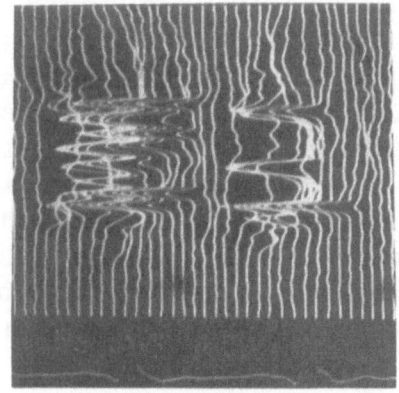

Figure 7. Flow profiles, obtained from a parasternal view, of a Ionescu Shiley bioprothesis nr. 17 in tricuspid position as described in case 4. There is a clear high velocity region, accentuated by aliasing, caused by the relative stenotic valve.

showed a preductal aortic coarctation with a hypoplastic arch, patent ductus arteriosus with right to left shunt, mitral valve hypoplasia with a maximal separation of the valve leaflets of 5 mm (M-mode), severe subvalvular aortic stenosis and tricuspid regurgitation. A VSD was not seen. With multigate pulsed Doppler a mitral valve ostium flow of 4 mm was measured (Figure 6).

At autopsy a 4 mm probe could pass the dysplastic mitral valve. There was a small VSD in the left ventricular outflow tract which drained to the right atrium. The systolic turbulence, as found in the right atrium and interpreted as a tricuspid insufficiency, was caused by this VSD. The other malformations as described above were confirmed.

Case 4. An 8 year old girl was operated for her ASD, VSD and infundibular and valvular pulmonary stenosis. She also got a Ionescu Shiley low profile nr. 17 bioprothesis for her hypoplastic tricuspid valve. The internal diameter of this valve was 13.4 cm. It was not possible to implant a greater prothesis in this child.

Because of anatomically circumstances one is generally not able to investigate the flow across the tricuspid valve with a sufficient obtuse angle. In this particular case, however, this could be done and a flow ostium of the prosthetic tricuspid valve of 12.3 mm could be assessed (Figure 7).

CONCLUSION

At the moment the multigate pulsed Doppler system is under investigation in our clinic for determination of the severity of aortic and pulmonary valvular stenosis in infants and children. At the present state of the art, this method is accurate in diagnosing the more severe cases. When a moderate stenosis is present, there seems to be a difference between the flow diameter, as determined with multigate pulsed Doppler and cine-angiography, and the orifice as measured at surgery: the surgeon finds a larger ostium.

So the question arises whether there is a difference between the anatomical orifice (as measured at operation) and the functional orifice (as estimated from jet measurements). This problem is subjected to further investigation. Multigate pulsed Doppler may be an asset in quantifying valvular stenoses and regurgitations and the size and number of ventricular septal defects.

REFERENCES

1. Hoeks APG: On the development of a multigate pulsed Doppler system with serial data-processing. Thesis, University of Limburg, Maastricht, the Netherlands, 1982.
2. Hoeks APG: Doppler measurement in heart chambers and ascending aorta: comparing single and multichannel systems. In: Cardiac Doppler Diagnosis, Spencer MP (ed.), Publ Martinus Nijhoff, The Hague, pp 43–50, 1983.
3. Hoeks APG, Ruissen CJ, Hick P, Reneman RS: Methods to evaluate the sample volume of pulsed Doppler systems. Ultrasound Med Biol, Vol 10:427–434, 1984a.
4. Hoeks APG, Peeters HPM, Ruissen CJ, Reneman RS: A novel frequency estimator for sampled Doppler signals. IEEE Trans Biomed Eng, Vol BME-31, nr 21, 212–220, 1984a.
5. de Knecht S, Daniëls O, Reneman RS: Non-invasive assessment of pulmonary valve stenosis with a multigate pulsed Doppler system. Br Heart J, Vol 50:592–593, 1983.
6. de Knecht S, Hopman JCW, Daniëls O, Reneman RS, Hoeks APG: Multigate pulsed Doppler assessment of jet stream in infants and children with pulmonary or aortic valve stenosis. In: Angio Archiv, Publ Demeter, Munich W-Germany, in press.

20. Assessment of systemic to pulmonary artery anastomoses by pulsed Doppler echocardiography

SAMUEL B. RITTER

Infants and children with cyanotic congenital heart disease characterized by diminished pulmonary blood flow often require a surgical systemic to pulmonary artery anastomosis. Clinical evaluation of cyanosis in these patients is often difficult. Differentiating systemic-to-pulmonary artery shunt patency from patent ductus arteriosus and from collateral aortic to pulmonary artery blood flow are just two examples. Also, cyanosis may be due to progressive pulmonary vascular disease in the face of large systemic to pulmonary artery runoff. Neonatal shunt candidates often having a patent ductus arteriosus is yet another group in whom the importance of non-invasive determination of shunt status is best exemplified: a continuous murmur undifferentiated from the surgical shunt may be present concurrently. Finally, in the post-operative period a ductus-like shunt murmur may not be audible for the first several days or may be masked by other murmurs. Assessment of shunt patency has traditionally been by cardiac catheterization and cineangiography, invasive and often risky procedures. Another method used for detection and measurement of shunts is radionuclide angiography: this method requires injection of a radioisotope and often has less than optimal resolution when performed at the bedside in the infant. In many children with cyanotic heart disease there is shunting as well at sites proximal to the area under investigation. Reliable, safe, non-invasive assessment and differentiation of these systemic-to-pulmonary artery shunts is therefore advantageous. Range-gated pulsed Doppler echocardiography offers such an alternative.

Systemic to pulmonary artery communications may occur naturally as in patent ductus arteriosus and descending aorta to pulmonary artery collateral vessels, or are surgically created: the Blalock Taussig (subclavian artery to pulmonary artery) shunt, the Waterston (ascending aorta to right pulmonary artery) shunt, and the Potts (descending aorta to left pulmonary artery) anastomosis are the more common ones encountered (Figure 1).

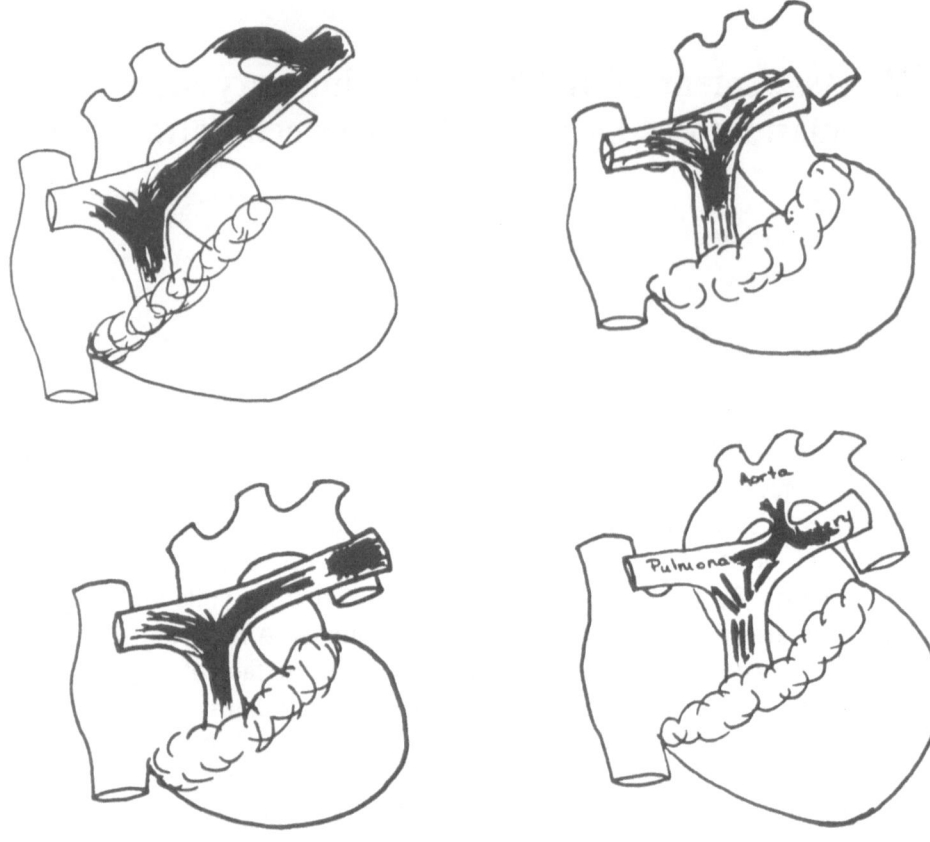

Figure 1. Systemic to Pulmonary Artery Anastomoses-Upper Left: Blalock-Taussig Shunt; Upper Right-Waterston Shunt; Lower Left; Pott's Anastomosis; Lower Right: Patent Ductus Arteriosus.

A small group of patients who had undergone systemic artery to pulmonary artery shunts were studied by Allen et al. [1]. Visualization and Doppler study of the right pulmonary artery were accomplished from the suprasternal notch position. The results of that study suggested that range-gated pulsed Doppler echocardiography is effective in confirming the patency of surgical systemic to pulmonary artery shunts even in cases where ausculatory evidence was absent. Continuous turbulent flow in the right pulmonary artery, normally laminar, identified shunt patency. However, this is not specific for the Blalock Taussig shunt function since this turbulent flow pattern could also arise from patent ductus arteriosus. Stevenson et al. [2] evaluated 35 infants and children with Blalock Taussig shunts from the suprasternal or high parasternal approach examining flow characteristics of the right pulmonary artery and in the Blalock Taussig shunts themselves.

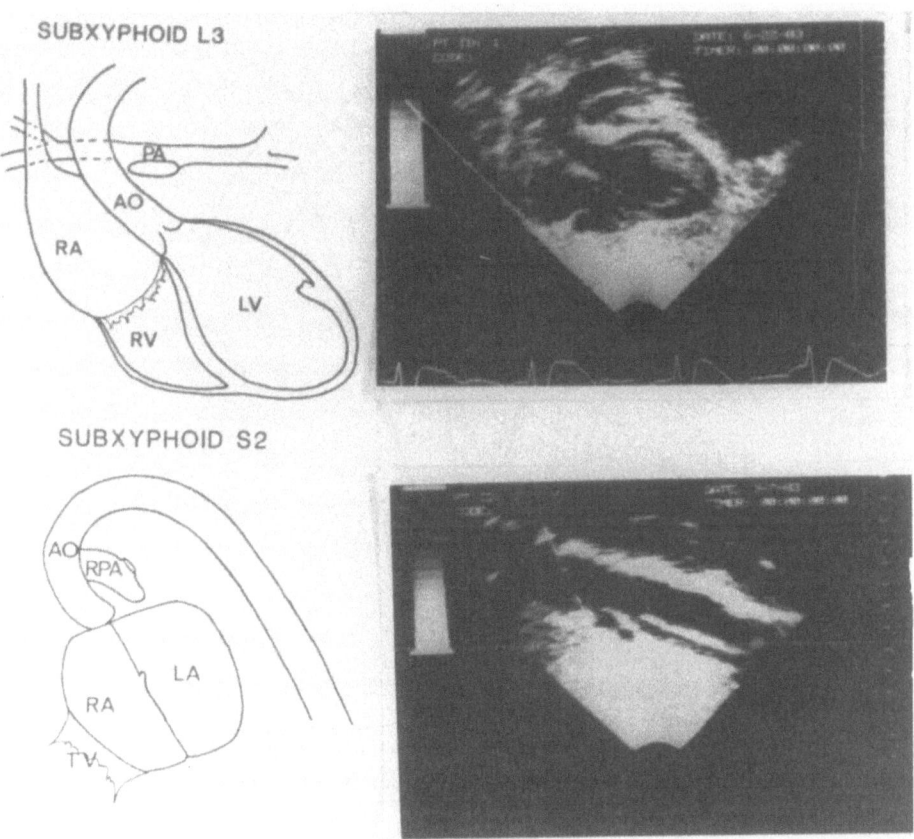

Figure 2. Upper Left: Subxiphoid Long Axis View of the Ascending Aorta, Upper Right: Two Dimensional Echocardiogram Subxiphoid Long Axis of Ascending Aorta. Lower Left: Subxiphoid Transverse View, Lower Right: Two Dimensional Echocardiogram Subxiphoid Transverse of Descending Aorta.

Although the study was successful in determining shunt status and differentiating patent ductus by Doppler, there were a number of difficulties and pitfalls: small vessel size, present in many of these patients, may produce difficulty in vessel imaging and flow sampling. Also, considerable detailed anatomic knowledge is often required by the examiner in such patients. Finally, locating the shunt is often problematic. Adequate imaging of the aortic arch from the suprasternal notch or high parasternal view in infants may often be difficult as well.

In our patients all imaging was performed using a commercially available Advanced Technology Laboratories Mark 600 Duplex system with a 459 pulsed Doppler flow analyzer and a 3.0 or 5.0 MHz transducer. This pro-

232

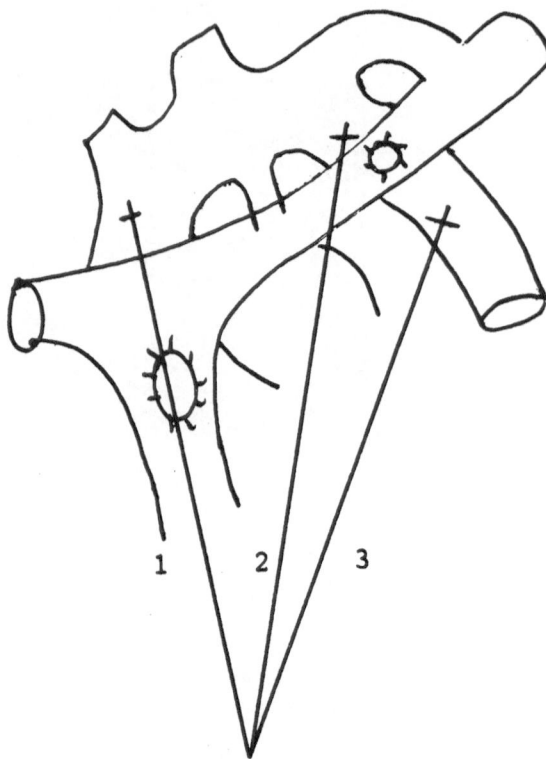

Figure 3. Subxiphoid Positioning of the Doppler Volume: Position 1 Corresponds to the Ascending Aorta, Position 2 to the Aortic Arch, Position 3 to the Descending Aorta.

vided real time two dimensional echocardiogram and bidirectional range-gated pulsed Doppler simultaneously. The Doppler sample volume represented by a small transvere line on a straight line cursor is superimposed on the 2-D image. Flow was therefore able to be characterized in any selected teardrop-shaped region approximately 2×4 mm on the 2-D image. The Doppler mode provided a graphic display of Doppler shifts processed by a microprocessor-based fast Fourier transform analyzer.

The vertical axis provided a calibrated KHz scale for Doppler shift above (flow towards the transducer) and below (flow away from the transducer) the zero reference line [3].

Subxiphoid two dimensional echocardiography was performed with the patients in the supine position. The transducer was placed in the subxiphoid area with the plane of the echobeam parallel to the horizontal plane of the trunk, perpendicular to the coronal plane. Cranial or anterior angulation of the transducer from this position with clockwise or leftward rotation displays all four cardiac chambers: additional cranial angulation toward the left mid-clavicle produces the standard longitudinal projection approximat-

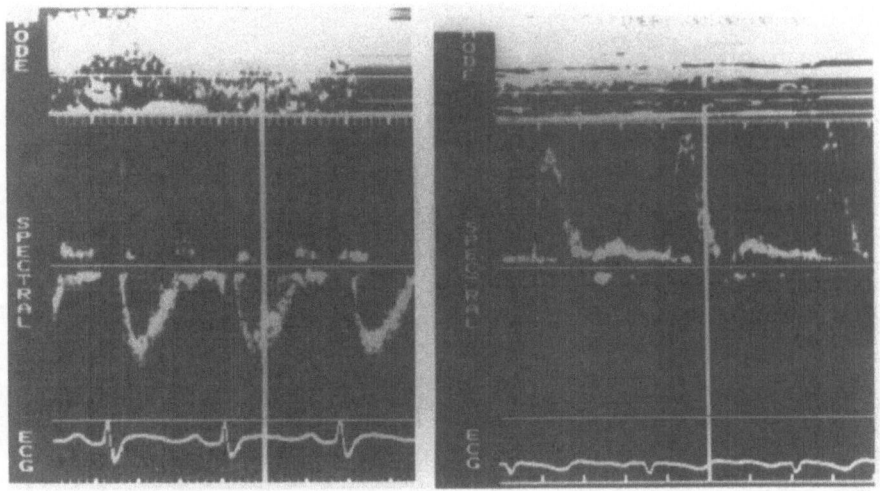

Figure 4. Normal Doppler Spectral Wave Form in Position 1 (left) and in Positions 2 and 3 (right): there is no net diastolic flow.

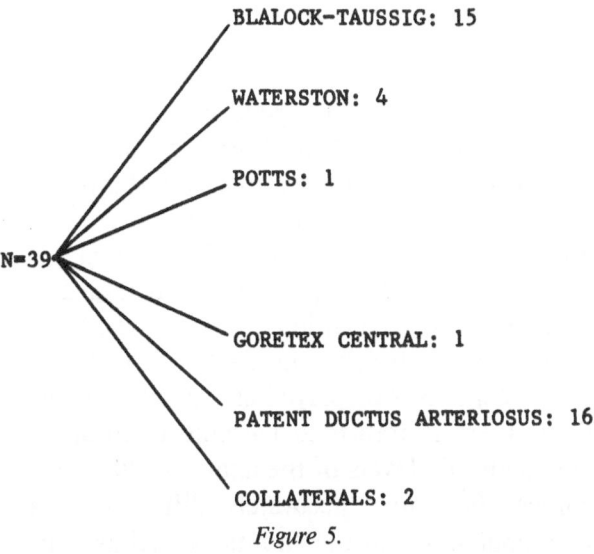

Figure 5.

ing a right anterior oblique cineangiogram and displays the left ventricle, left ventricular outflow tract and ascending aorta. Clockwise rotation (90°) of the transducer about its long axis produces a transverse or cross sectional view of the heart. Angling the transducer toward the left displays the ascending and descending aorta: this transverse projection simulates a lateral cineangiogram (Figure 2) [4, 5].

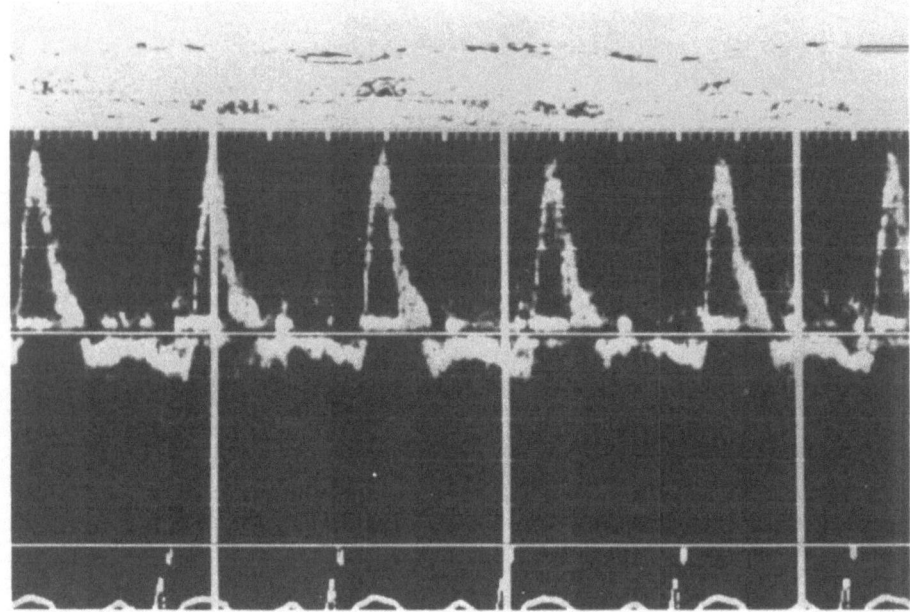

Figure 6. Doppler Flow in the Descending Aorta (positions 2 and 3) with a Blalock-Taussig Shunt: There is Diastolic Reversal of Flow Demonstrated.

From ths subxiphoid position, the gated pulsed Doppler sample volume was positioned in the aorta in each of three positions demonstrated in Figure 3: position 1 corresponds to the ascending aorta, position 2 at the level of the junction of the aortic arch and descending aorta, and position 3 in the descending aorta above the diaphragm. The normal graphic display of Doppler frequency shifts in these positions is demonstrated in Figure 4: ascending aortic blood flow in position 1 is displayed as a negative systolic Doppler shift with return to baseline in diastole: the descending aortic flow pattern in positions 2 and 3 is displayed as a positive Doppler shift with no net diastolic flow: there is return to baseline in diastole. Because of the differences in the anatomic levels of the anastomoses in each type of shunt, range-gated Doppler flow may accurately differentiate and discriminate between the functional status of the shunts as well as between the types of shunts. The common thread in all the shunts mentioned above is that they share the same diastolic flow property: reversal of flow in the aorta in diastole up to the level of the communication between the aorta and the pulmonary circuit but not proximal to that level is common in all these anastomoses.

39 patients with various systemic to pulmonary artery communications either alone or in combination, were evaluated (Figure 5).

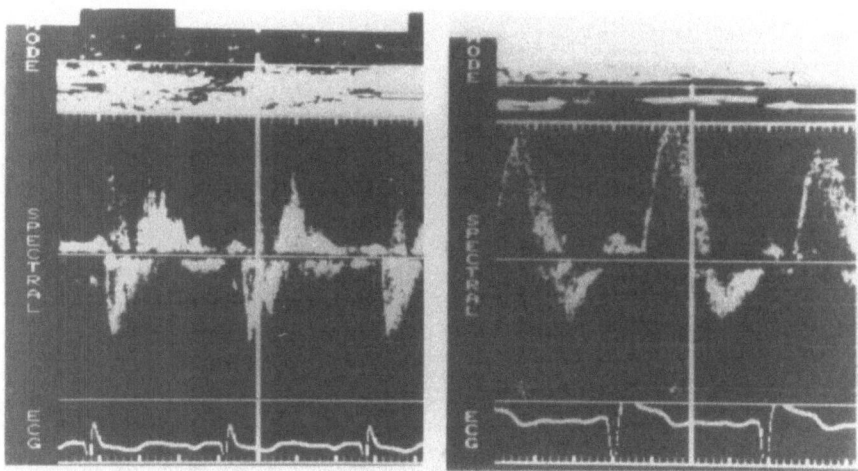

Figure 7. Waterston Shunt: left: ascending aorta with diastolic flow reversal. Right: descending aorta with smaller but present reversal of flow in diastole.

Of the 15 patients with Blalock Taussig anastomoses, all 15 demonstrated normal Doppler flow patterns with the sample volume placed in the ascending aorta (position 1): normal systolic aortic flow with return to baseline during diastole. In 14 of these patients with the sample volume in positions 2 and 3 in the descending aorta, there was diastolic flow reversal noted (Figure 6). In one of these patients, return to baseline in diastole of the Doppler waveform with no negative deflection, no flow reversal, was recorded. Angiographic data confirmed this last patient to be the only one in the group with a non-functioning shunt. Differentiation of the right and left Blalock-Taussig shunt is possible as well. With the sample volume in position 1, normal ascending aortic flow pattern would be found in either case. In the aortic arch between positions 2 and 3 diastolic flow reversal would signify systemic to pulmonary artery runoff proximally, a right Blalock-Taussig shunt; in left sided Blalock-Taussig anastomoses diastolic Doppler flow in this position would be normal; Doppler flow in position # 3 again would reveal diastolic flow reversal, present in Blalock-Taussig shunts on either side.

Four patients had an ascending aorta to right pulmonary artery communication, a Waterston shunt. Here the subxiphoid systolic Doppler flow pattern in the ascending aorta reveals a negative systolic deflection: there is reversal of flow in diastole (positive deflection). Descending aorta blood flow in all four revealed positive systolic deflection with a smaller reversal of flow in diastole (Figure 7).

One older patient had a Pott's anastomosis between the descending aorta and the left pulmonary artery: this type of shunt is no longer commonly

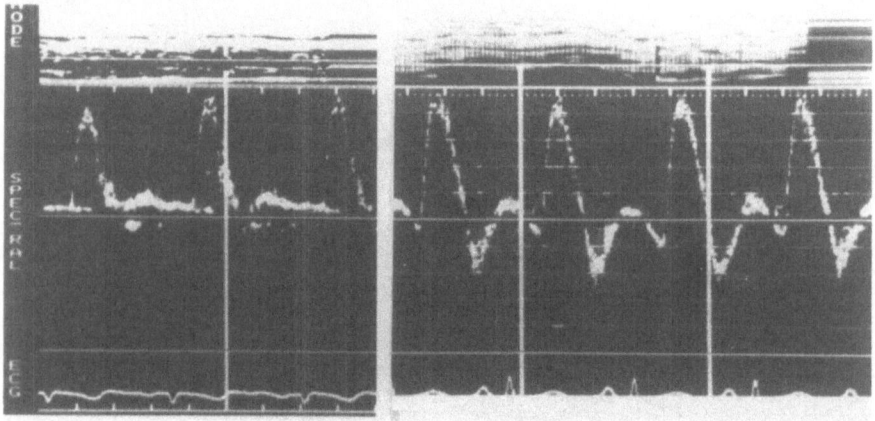

Figure 8. Pott's Anastomosis: Left: Doppler flow in position 2 is normal whereas in position 3 there is diastolic flow reversal indicating the level of the shunt in the descending aorta (right).

employed. Subxiphoid imaging in position 1 in the ascending aorta demonstrated normal spectral wave form pattern with return to baseline in diastole: this normal flow pattern is also seen in position 2 which is proximal to the level of the anastomosis. However, in the distal descending aorta, the typical wave from pattern of systemic to pulmonary artery diastolic runoff is noted: a positive Doppler shift in systole with reveral of flow in diastole (Figure 8).

11 patients had clinical findings consistent with a patent ductus arteriosus: all had typical continuous murmurs at the left intraclavicular area. All had classic Doppler flow study patterns consistent with patency of the ductus. In position 1 in the ascending aorta all 11 revealed normal Doppler wave form patterns. However, in positions 2 and 3, there was diastolic reversal of flow signifying a systemic to pulmonary artery runoff in diastole (Figure 9). 4 patients in the group had no clinical evidence at the time of examination of a patent ductus arteriosus. Pulsed Doppler evaluation however, suggested patency of the ductus in all four. One was a newborn infant with physical stigmata of Trisomy 21, Down's Syndrome. Because of the high association of congenital heart defects (endocardial cushion defects) with this chromosomal abnormality a two dimensional/pulsed Doppler echocardiographic study was performed during the first day of life. The physical examination revealed an acyanotic infant with no murmurs. The two dimensional echocardiogram revealed endocardial cushion defect of the atrioventricular canal type. Gated pulsed Doppler examination demonstrated normal ascending aortic blood flow with return to baseline in dias-

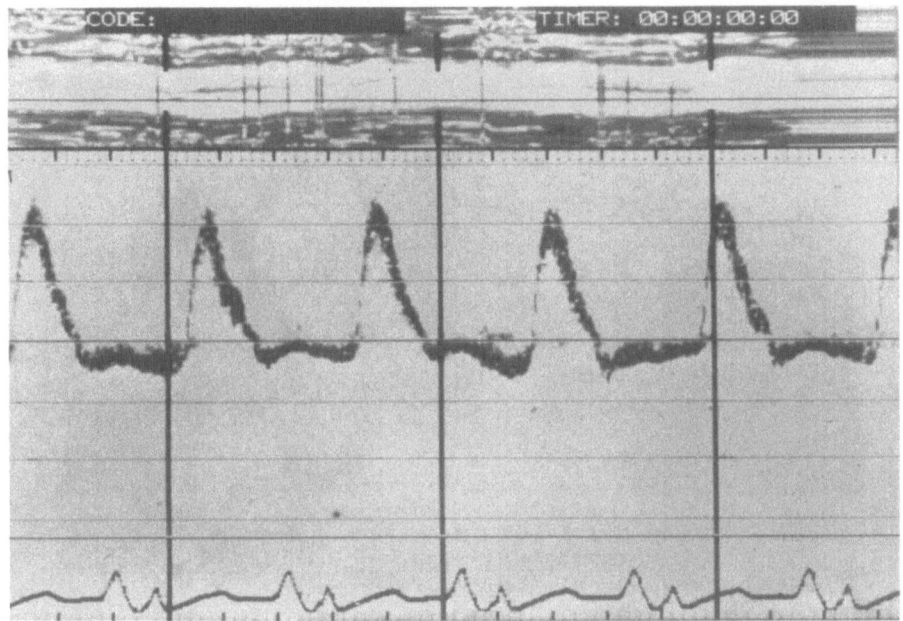

Figure 9. Descending Aorta Doppler Flow in Patent Ductus Arteriosus demonstrating diastolic flow reversal.

tole: in the descending aorta there was reversal of diastolic flow consistent with a patent ductus arteriosus. The patient had no clinical auscultatory evidence of this lesion.

A second patient, 3 ½ months old with a ventricular septal defect and pulmonary hypertension was evaluated. There was no evidence on physical examination of systemic to pulmonary artery runoff. Range-gated pulsed Doppler flow study in the ascending and descending aorta revealed normal spectral wave form patterns in room air. In 100% inspired oxygen the ascending aortic blood flow pattern remained normal while that in the descending aorta demonstrated diastolic flow reversal consistent with left to right shunting via a patent ductus arteriosus (Figure 10). The above findings were confirmed in these two patients as well as in one of the remaining two by cardiac catheterization and angiography. One newborn with transposition of the great vessels showed initial Doppler evidence of a closing patent ductus arteriosus: the infant responded clinically to prostaglandin E_1 infusion: Doppler flow evidence of reopening of the ductus arteriosus was confirmed.

Two patients with complex cyanotic congenital heart disease demonstrated the advantages of gated pulsed Doppler echocardiography in patients with complex heart disease and multiple shunts. The first was a 12 year old

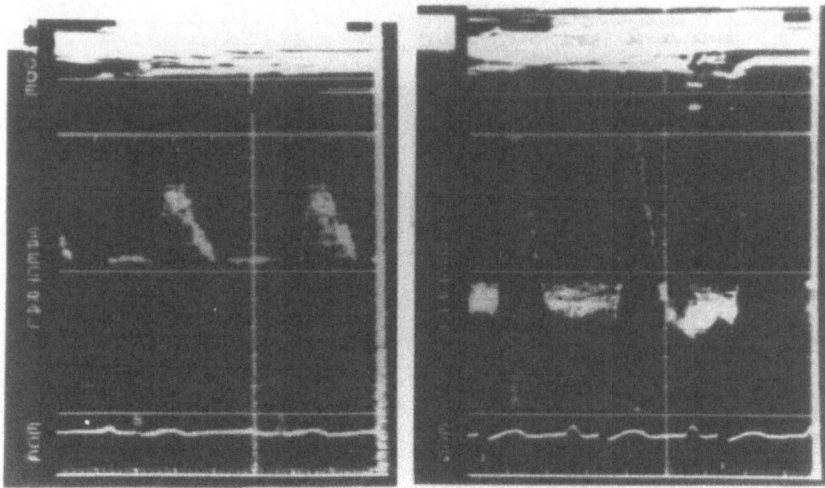

Figure 10. Left: Descending Aortic Flow in a 3½ month old infant with VSD and Pulmonary Hypertension: There is no diastole flow reversal noted. This implies no left to right shunt at the ductal level. Right: In 100% FiO2 there is marked reversal of flow in diastole signifying large left to right shunt at the level of the ductus.

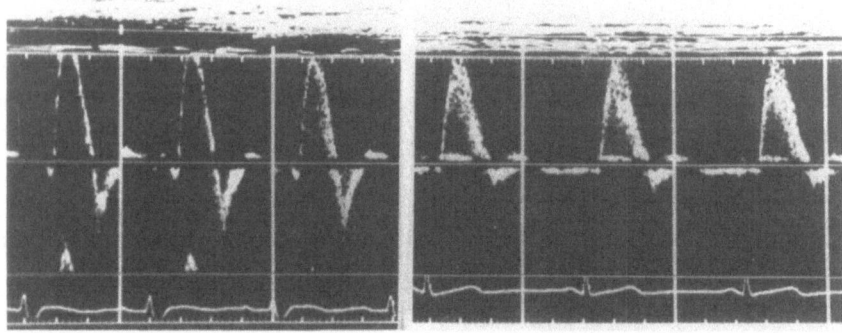

Figure 11. Left: Pre-operatively there is large diastolic flow reversal in the descending aorta suggesting large systemic to pulmonary artery flow at this level. Right: Post-operatively after surgical ligation of left sided aortic collateral vessels there remains diastolic flow reversal albeit diminished.

young man with pulmonary atresia and bilateral continuous murmurs over the entire chest suggesting large descending aorta-to-pulmonary collateral blood flow. Ascending aortic blood flow patterns were normal. The Doppler flow pattern in positions 2 and 3 in the descending aorta demonstrated large diastolic flow reversals suggesting collateral blood flow. The patient underwent surgical correction for pulmonary atresia: large collateral vessels were

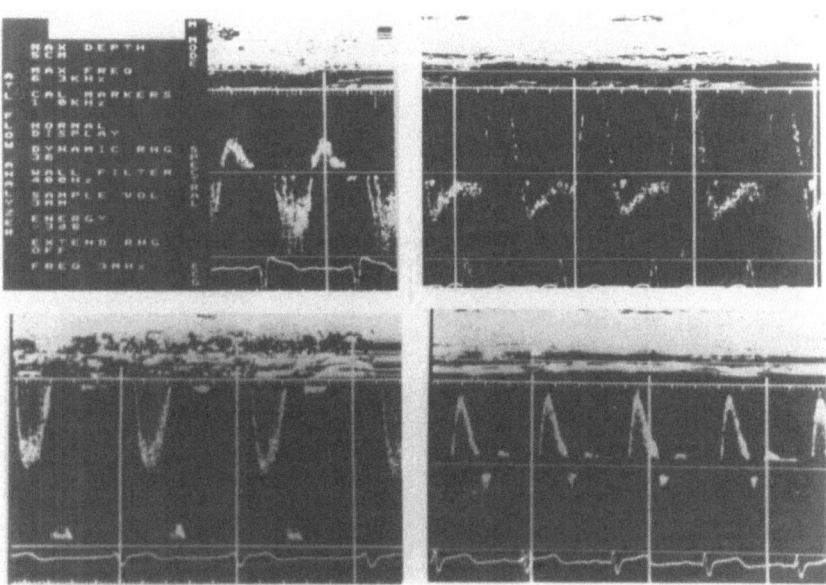

Figure 12. Doppler flow study in a child with pulmonary atresia, Waterston Shunt, and aortic-to-pulmonary artery collateral vessels. Upper Left: Pre-operatively, ascending aortic blood flow shows diastolic reversal of flow signifying patency of Waterston shunt. Upper Right: Large diastolic flow reversal of collateral aortic blood flow is noted in the descending aorta. Lower Left: Post-operatively, normal ascending aortic blood flow after takedown of the Waterston Shunt. Lower Right: Descending aortic blood flow post-operatively is normalized after collateral vessels are ligated.

also ligated at the time of surgery. Postoperatively, Doppler flow studies in the descending aorta showed persistent albeit diminished diastolic flow reversal suggesting persistent collateral flow which was confirmed at follow-up catheterization (Figure 11).

A second patient with severe Tetralogy of Fallot and pulmonary atresia had a Waterston shunt. Physical examination revealed loud continuous murmurs over both sides of the chest thereby making differentiation between shunt patency and collateral flow virtually impossible. Doppler flow in the ascending aorta showed diastolic flow reversal consistent with a patent ascending aorta-to-right pulmonary artery of Waterston shunt. The descending aortic diastolic flow pattern showed an even larger reversal of flow consistent with a second shunt at this level, collateral blood flow. These were both confirmed at the time of cardiac catheterization (Figure 12). After corrective open heart surgery which included ligation of the collateral vessels and takedown of the Waterston shunt, repeat Doppler study demonstrated no reversal of flow in diastole in the descending aorta signifying no remaining collateral blood flow: the ascending aortic blood flow

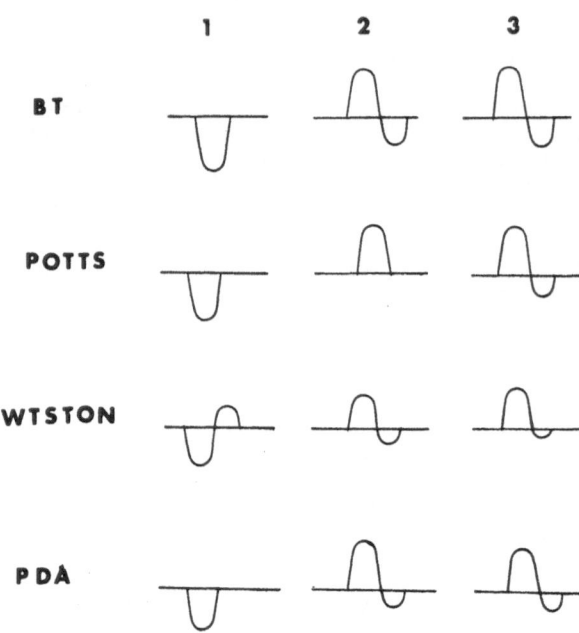

Figure 13. Summary of Pulsed Doppler spectral wave forms in systemic to pulmonary artery anastomoses (see text).

pattern returned to normal as well. That in patients with multiple systemic to pulmonary artery shunts, it is clinically difficult to distinguish patency of one versus the other anastomosis, is demonstrated in this last patient: range-gated Doppler flow study clearly demonstrated a proximal systemic to pulmonary artery runoff as well as distal shunt patency. This is most important especially in the newborn period where there may be the concurrent presence of patent ductus arteriosus in conjuntion with surgical systemic to pulmonary artery anastomoses.

The Doppler spectral wave form patterns in the various types of shunts are summarized in the final figure (Figure 13). In the Blalock-Taussig shunt ascending aortic blood flow patterns are normal: in right sided anastomoses of this type, in positions 2 and 3 in proximal and distal descending aorta, there is diastolic flow reversal while in left sided anastomoses flow is normal in position 2, but shows diastolic flow reversal in position 3 in the descending aorta. In the Pott's anastomosis, only descending aortic blood flow in position 3 shows diastolic flow reversal. In the proximally placed Waterston shunt, there is marked diastolic flow reversal in the ascending aorta in position 1 with somewhat diminished but present reversal of flow in both positions 2 and 3 in the descending aorta. In patent ductus arteriosus, ascending aortic blood flow patterns are normal with abnormalities seen in both the proximal and distal aortic positions, 2 and 3.

We correctly identified the type of shunt in all instances. In each instance, patency or closure was also correctly defined. The co-existence of multiple shunts as well as persistence of shunting post-operatively were also identified.

Range-gated pulsed Doppler echocardiography is an effective and sensitive noninvasive method of evaluation systemic of pulmonary artery shunt patency and of differentiating between the types of shunts. This is of particular importance when multiple shunts may coexist.

REFERENCES

1. Allen QD, Sah, DJ, Lange Lothar SJ: Noninvasive Assessment of Surgical Systemic to Pulmonary Artery Shunts by Range Gated Pulsed Doppler Echocardiography. The Journal of Pediatrics, March 1979, pages 395–402, volume 94 # 3.
2. Stevenson JG, Kawabori I, Bailey WW: Noninvasive Evaluation of Blalock-Taussig Shunts: Determination of Patency and Differentiation from Patent Ductus Arteriosus by Doppler Echocardiography. American Heart Journal, November 1983, pages 1121–1132, volume 106 # 5 part 1.
3. Stevenson JG: Pulsed Doppler Characterization of Intracardiac Flow Patterns, Chapter 5, pages 141–170 in textbook. Pulsed Doppler Ultrasound in Clinical Pediatrics: Edited by William Berman, Jr, MD 1983, Futura Publishing Co, Inc Mt Kisco, NY Stevenson J Geoffrey, Kawabori I, Gunther Roth WG, Pulsed Doppler Echocardiographic Diagnosis of Patent Ductus Arteriosus: Sensitivity. Specificity, Limitations and Technical Features. Cath Cardiovasc Diagn 6:255, 1980.
4. Bierman FZ, Williams RG: Prospective Diagnosis of D-Transposition of the Great Arteries and Neonates by Subxiphoid Two Dimensional Echocardiography. Circulation, December 1979, Volume 60 # 7, pages 1496–1502.
5. Henry WL, Demaria A, Gramiak R, King D, Kisslo JA, Popp RL, Sahn DJ, Schiller NB, Tajik A, Teicholz LE, Weyman AE: Report of the American Society of Echocardiography Committee on Nomenclature in Standards in Two Dimensional Echocardiography. Circulation, volume 62 # 2, 1980, pages 212–217.

Index